D1480059

DISCARD

Exercise Is Medicine

EXERCISE IS MEDICINE

How Physical Activity Boosts Health and Slows Aging

Judy Foreman

OXFORD
UNIVERSITY PRESS

OXFORD
UNIVERSITY PRESS

Oxford University Press is a department of the University of Oxford. It furthers
the University's objective of excellence in research, scholarship, and education
by publishing worldwide. Oxford is a registered trade mark of Oxford University
Press in the UK and certain other countries.

Published in the United States of America by Oxford University Press
198 Madison Avenue, New York, NY 10016, United States of America.

Library of Congress Cataloging-in-Publication Data
Names: Foreman, Judy, author.
Title: Exercise is medicine : how physical activity boosts health and slows aging / Judy Foreman.
Description: New York, NY : Oxford University Press, [2020] |
Includes bibliographical references.
Identifiers: LCCN 2019009496 | ISBN 9780190685461 (hardback) |
ISBN 9780190685478 (updf) | ISBN 9780190685485 (epub)
Subjects: LCSH: Exercise therapy. | Exercise—Health aspects.
Classification: LCC RM725 .F66 2019 | DDC 615.8/2—dc23
LC record available at https://lccn.loc.gov/2019009496

9 8 7 6 5 4 3 2 1

Printed by LSC Communications, United States of America

To Mike, Robin, Owen, and Hugo, my dear ones. And to Ken, my beloved husband, with much, much love and many thanks.

CONTENTS

ACKNOWLEDGMENTS

Thanks first and foremost, to my terrific editor at Oxford University Press, Abby Gross.

Thanks also to Florence Graves, Founding Director of the recently closed Schuster Institute for Investigative Journalism at Brandeis University, not only for welcoming me as a Senior Fellow, but also for supporting this book over the years with a steady supply of fantastic research assistants. They include Yuchen He, Kimberly Milando, and most especially, Stephanie Yan. Many, many thanks to all. Thanks, also, to Lisa Button, managing editor at the Schuster Institute, for finding the perfect assistants for my project from the pool of outstanding Brandeis students. Thanks, too, to my agent, Jim Levine.

In addition, a number of scientists have gone way beyond the call of duty in responding repeatedly to my phone calls and emails to help me understand the thorniest scientific questions. They include Steve Austad, Steve Blair, Claude Bouchard, Carl Cotman, Monika Fleshner, Matt Kaeberlein, I-Min Lee, Benjamin Levine, Barbara McGovern, Martin Gibala, Steve Horvath, Jay Olshansky, Stuart Phillips, David Slovik, Bruce Spiegelman, Mark Tarnopolsky, and Henriette van Praag. Thank you, thank you, thank you.

I am also very grateful to the following scientists and physicians who helped me with specific chapters.

Chapter 1:
Steve Austad
S. Jay Olshansky
Michael Rose
Daniel Lieberman
Matt Kaeberlein
Steve Horvath
Lorenzo Galluzzi
Gary Ruvkun

Chapter 2:
Claude Bouchard
Steve Blair
Trina Hosmer
Jerome Fleg
Jeffrey Metter
Eleanor Simonsick
I-Min Lee
Claudia Kawas

Chapter 3:
Peter T. Katzmarzyk
I-Min Lee
Ken Kaplan
Benjamin Levine
C. Ronald Kahn

Chapter 4:
Katherine Beiers
T. K. Skenderian
I-Min Lee
Benjamin Levine
Arthur Leon
Jonathan Myers
Jay Handy
Timothy Church

Chapter 5:
Mark Tarnopolsky
Christopher Gillen
Martin Gibala
Mark Mattson
Marcia Haigis
Darrell Neufer
Paul McLean
Bruce Spiegelman
David Hood

Chapter 6:
Mark Tarnopolsky
Stuart Phillips
Orly Lacham-Kaplan

Chapter 7:
Lynda Bonewald
Clifford Rosen
Mark Hamrick
David Slovik

Chapter 8:
Carl Cotman
Henrietta van Praag
Mercedes Parades
Shawn Sorrells

Chapter 9:
Carl Cotman
Michael Otto
Ronald Duman
Rod Dishman
Elizabeth Droge-Young

Chapter 10:
Paul Cotter
Lita Proctor
Barbara McGovern
Heather Buschman

Chapter 11:
Monika Fleshner
Connie Rogers
Brandt Pence

Chapter 12:
Marcia Bailey
Karen Mustian
Bradley J. Behnke
Jennifer Ligibel

Chapter 13:
Mary Armanios
Masood Shammas
Steve Horvath
Matt Kaeberlein
Eli Puterman
Elissa Epel

Carol Greider
Jay Olshansky

Chapter 14:
Matt Kaeberlein
Steve Austad
Lorenzo Galluzzi
Todd Manini
C. Ronald Kahn
Irene Mazzoni
David Sinclair
Bruce Spiegelman

Chapter 15:
Benjamin Levine
Frank Hu
Claude Bouchard
I-Min Lee
Mark Tarnopolsky
Bruce Spiegelman
David Becker

Chapter 16:
Thomas Perls
Elizabeth Arias

INTRODUCTION

Aging, to most of us, especially on a bad day, is an appalling prospect, and, all too often, a grim reality. It represents a diminution of much that we have been, a penultimate phase of life, a slow, downward slide into decrepitude, disability, and dependence, a one-way street toward an all-too-literal "dead end." As a friend of mine put it, it's knowing you're on your next-to-last dog.

To a biologist, though, aging is one of the most exciting mysteries in the universe, a tale told in the chemical language of every cell and repeated in the life span of every organism. What is aging, anyway? Why aren't humans like salmon, who die immediately after laying and fertilizing their eggs? Why aren't we like mayflies, whose lives consist only of birth, reproduction, and a spectacularly fast death? For that matter, why aren't we like some clams, which can live for hundreds of years? Or like 40-year-old bats?

Why does aging even exist, and why is there *senescence*, this gradual loss of function and vigor? Why do we live so long after our reproductive years are over?

It's possible that we live a long time after reproduction because in social species like ours—as with elephants, wolves, and monkeys—it's advantageous to have postmenopausal females around to act as reservoirs of knowledge about watering holes, food supplies, and child rearing. But while this "grandmother effect" might explain long life, it doesn't explain senescence—which makes you wonder, is senescence necessary? Is it part of the evolutionary deal? Are we stuck with it?

Or could things be different? Could we have what scientists call "compression of morbidity," that is, long, healthy lives *without* senescence, then a more or less sudden demise, saving ourselves the misery of slow-motion decline, and saving the healthcare system a bundle in the process?

It turns out that while we can't get rid of senescence entirely, we can dramatically minimize it. With exercise.

Exercise is the closest thing there is to a magic bullet for preventing disease and disability, maximizing health, and prolonging life. The data are overwhelming.

For openers, there's the compelling *epidemiology*, as we'll see in Chapters 2 and 3. Exercising moderately for half an hour a day for five days a week, for instance, increases life span by 3.5 years. Even running *slowly* for just 5 to 10 minutes a day is linked to a lower risk of death from *all causes*. And, of course, it's not just running. Walking counts, swimming counts, weightlifting, dancing, gardening, jumping rope— anything that gets you moving.

Indeed, a sedentary lifestyle is now confirmed to be a stronger predictor of premature death than obesity, diabetes, high cholesterol, high blood pressure, and smoking. In other words, it's not the sheer passage of time that makes us fall apart, it's lack of exercise.

While the epidemiology gives us the big picture, it's the *molecular biology*—the tiny molecules deep inside our cells that are activated by exercise—that are now seen as the true, underlying reasons why exercise has so many beneficial effects throughout the entire body.

In contrast to the epidemiological evidence, which has been building for decades, the molecular biology is new, and forms the real questions behind this book: How *does* exercise generate so many beneficial changes in so many different tissues at the same time? How *does* exercise get fat, muscles, the brain, virtually all our organs, to "talk" to each other biochemically, like gossipy neighbors on an old-fashioned party line?

In the years that I have been working on this book, the thing that has impressed me the most is how much this chemical "cross-talk" among the organs is changed for the better with exercise. I always knew, as did almost everybody else, that exercise was good for you. What I didn't know, until I began researching this book, was exactly why exercise was so good, and how it could possibly trigger such varied beneficial effects all over the body.

Parts of the puzzle of what exercise does in different organs are still being worked out, including at the National Institutes of Health, via the awkwardly named project called the Molecular Transducers of Physical Activity in Humans.

But some parts of the story are beginning to be known. As I combed through hundreds of scientific papers, I was blown away by what exercise does for mitochondria, the power factories inside our cells.

I was dumbfounded by the powerful effects exercise has on the immune system—and the brain. The two chapters on exercise and cognition and exercise and mood became my favorite chapters in the book.

Researching this book, far from being drudgery, has been a powerful motivator. It has left me in awe—most of all about how evolution "designed" us to move, and how our very metabolisms depend on it. We clearly did not evolve to sit at computers or in front of the TV all day. We evolved to run, to plant, to harvest. And to live as vigorously as possible for as long as we possibly can.

Judy Foreman
Cambridge, MA
January 2019

HOW TO READ THIS BOOK

In figuring out the organization of this book, I decided to spin the tale mostly according to scientific logic, which I'll spell out in a minute.

But that doesn't mean you have to read it that way.

If you want to jump straight to the practical stuff, flip to Chapter 15, "The Nitty Gritty." This chapter contains many common questions about exercise and the answers I culled from my research and interviews with experts. Similarly, if you want a quick idea of what's most likely to kill you at what age, go straight to Chapter 16, "Dodging Bullets." And if you want an easy way to figure out how fit (or not) you are, see the websites in the Appendix.

In most of the chapters, I've put the big picture first and the most technical stuff—the molecular mechanisms—at the end. To me, the hard-core science is compelling, but if it's not for you, skip the tough parts. Hopefully, you'll still get the main idea.

I strongly suggest starting with Chapter 1, on the biology of aging. This chapter does get into some fairly heavy-duty science, but if you're not used to thinking in evolutionary terms, it should be a fascinating eye-opener. Until I researched this chapter, I had a pretty negative view of aging. But what I learned about the biology put a whole new spin on aging for me, and took some of the sting out of it. Because this chapter involves the basic mechanisms of aging, it's the foundation for the rest of the book.

Chapter 2 presents powerful epidemiological evidence that exercise (or, more precisely, fitness) is a powerful predictor of health and longevity. As a science writer, it was a special treat to write about something for which the data line up so beautifully. This stuff is so clear there's no need to wade in to the usual "on the one hand, on the other hand" bog.

As for Chapter 3, let me say I was horrified at what I found out. Before writing this book, I had assumed that sitting was just the low end of the physical activity curve. I didn't realize that sitting was so detrimental that it comprises a whole separate category. (Yes, I did sit for hours, weeks, years, writing this book. But in addition to exercise, I got up as often as I could for coffee and gum. And I put my printer far enough away that I had to get up to get print-outs.)

Chapter 4, on the heart, is one of the most important chapters in the book. In fact, if you only read one chapter, read this one. The biggest killer in America is heart disease, and exercise has many of its most potent benefits on the cardiovascular system. This should get you off the couch, if nothing else does.

Chapter 5, on mitochondria, kicks off the red meat of the book. I love this chapter. For one thing, I got to interview some terrific older athletes, whose feats left me both motivated and daunted. For another, I was amazed to learn how new mitochondria (the energy powerhouses inside cells) are made and how that process cranks up with exercise. If I hadn't believed in the value of exercise before, I would have been converted by this chapter.

Chapter 6, on how muscles get bigger (hypertrophy), also had some surprises for me. I hadn't realized how different the molecular processes were for building endurance and for building muscle. I still don't love pumping iron, but this chapter keeps me on track. The most exciting section of the chapter for me was discovering that muscles are hormone factories and that they "talk" chemically to bones.

Chapter 7, on bones, may startle you. Since muscles and bones are now seen as a unit, it made sense to put the chapter on bones right after muscles. I was in for some big surprises myself as I researched this chapter, too. So, spoiler alert! Exercise is still important to protect bones, but not for the reasons we used to think.

Chapters 8 and 9, on exercise and cognition, and exercise and mood, were the biggest "uppers" for me. Once again, the epidemiological data that exercise improves both cognition and mood are very strong. What surprised me was that some of the same molecular mechanisms are involved in both. Given how many people suffer from depression, and how many others face, and fear, cognitive decline with aging, I consider these chapters "must reads."

Chapter 10, on the microbiome, is fun. The science on the potential effects of exercise on the microbiome is still new and somewhat unsettled, but fascinating nonetheless.

Chapter 11, on immunity and inflammation, is one of the most important in the book. Chronic inflammation underlies many of the diseases and conditions of later life, many more than most of us would think. Exercise turns out to be a great way to keep chronic inflammation at bay.

Chapter 12 on exercise and cancer is important. Obviously, exercise can't completely protect against cancer, or cure it once you've got it. But it does lower the risk of getting it and raises the chance of living longer if you do. It's also a major tool for *coping* with cancer and potentially devastating cancer-related fatigue. (I italicized "coping.")

Chapter 13, on telomeres, focuses on one of the hottest controversies in science today and on exercise research in particular. Commercial telomere testing, a booming business online, was something I couldn't resist doing myself. You'll see how that turned out.

Chapter 14 examines exercise pills. I know, I know. The whole idea sounds crazy. But these pills are out there, with more coming along, and in many cases, the pills are based on legitimate science about how exercise affects the body. That said, I am no fan of these concoctions, as you'll see, except perhaps for people who are so sick or disabled that exercise is completely impossible.

That's it. I hope you enjoy reading this book as much as I enjoyed writing it.

CHAPTER 1
Aging

WHY *DO* WE AGE?

Aging is one of the deepest mysteries of the universe. After all, what's the point? Once you've passed your genes on to the next generation, why stick around? Why take up space and use food and other scarce resources? It's the young who need those things to live to reproductive age. So why do old animals even exist? Or old people?

Evolution has no reason to favor long life, Steven Austad, a former lion tamer and now a bio-gerontologist at the University of Alabama at Birmingham, points out. Quite the contrary, he says: "Evolution favors early, copious reproduction at the expense of later life survival."

S. Jay Olshansky, a bio-demographer at the University of Illinois, Chicago, puts it this way: "We age because Mother Nature turns her back on us once we're in the post-reproductive region of the life span. Natural selection didn't build in a program to make us fall apart later in life."

And yet here we are, a world with growing numbers of old people, even very, very old people. Was it "supposed" to be this way? Come to think of it, why is there even such a thing as menopause? Why do women live 30, 40, even 50 years past reproduction? (There's less of a question about old men—some can produce viable sperm until the day they die, though getting it to its proper destination can get iffy.)

Perhaps, as one school of thought suggests, aging exists because old animals—especially females—provide evolutionary advantages, not to the old animal herself, but to her offspring and genetic relatives. It's the so-called grandmother effect.

"If you are a human female and you are taking care of your grandchild, your act of taking care of your grandchild is a reproductive act," at least in the eyes of evolutionary biologists, says Michael Rose, a professor of ecology and evolutionary biology at the University of California, Irvine.

Actually, *grandfathers* are sometimes just as important as grandmothers because they, too, share food, and sharing is evolutionarily crucial, says Harvard University evolutionary biologist Daniel Lieberman. A hunter-gatherer mother requires enough calories to sustain not just her own body but the bodies of her children as well, Lieberman notes, which means that hunter-gatherer females who are lactating and caring for young children struggle to get enough energy. "But grandmothers and grandfathers are unencumbered—they can produce a surplus," he says. "And that energy goes toward the family. As soon as humans started sharing, there was a strong selective pressure for longevity." (Longevity, as we'll soon see, is also fostered by "nice" environments, with lots of food around.)

Among other things, older animals are handy because they know where to find long-forgotten watering holes or food supplies. Female postmenopausal killer whales (orcas) are terrific resources for their tribe—they know where scarce salmon are, and they are often the ones who lead others to food when supplies are low.

Old female elephants are great resources, too. In fact, elephant societies are famously matriarchal, with older females helping their herds survive droughts, food scarcity, poachers, and, of course, lions.

Some traditional human societies with long-lived men and women show a similar pattern, says Jared Diamond, a professor of geography at the University of California, Los Angeles, who for more than 50 years has studied New Guinea farming societies. To be sure, he says, *nomadic* hunter-gatherer societies aren't always kind to old people, who may be cast out to die or simply left behind if they can't keep up with the group's wandering. But in *sedentary* traditional societies, old folks are valuable. "In traditional societies without writing, older people are the repositories of information," Diamond says. "It's their knowledge that spells the difference between survival and death for their whole society in a time of crisis caused by rare events for which only the oldest people alive have had experience."

That's exactly what happened in 1993, when an outbreak of the hanta virus triggered a spate of deaths on the Navajo reservation in the Four Corners area of the American Southwest. The virus, originally—and unfairly—dubbed the "Navajo flu" and since renamed the Sin Nombre

(No Name) virus, is carried by deer mice. When the feces of deer mice dry up and become aerosolized, humans can unknowingly breathe the contaminated dust and come down with often-fatal pulmonary infections.

When the outbreak hit, scientists from New Mexico's health department and the federal Centers for Disease Control and Prevention flocked to the Navajo reservation to study the virus. But it was their wise decision to talk with Navajo elders that cracked the case.

The Navajo elders remembered that twice before in the 20th century, they had observed a connection between increases in rainfall, a booster crop of pinyon nuts, and a surge in the deer mouse population. In 1993, those exact conditions pertained—unusually heavy rains, lots of snowmelt, huge quantities of pinyon nuts, a surge in deer mice, and a not-new-after-all epidemic, deciphered by the oldest folks around.

Clearly, then, there are some benefits for the group as a whole to have older animals or people around. But this can't be the whole story. After all, evolution didn't "plan" for older people to hang around because evolution doesn't "plan" anything. There must be some other reasons, including genetics, why some creatures live long past reproductive age.

In the past, some evolutionary biologists thought that animals might be *programmed* by "death genes" to age and die right after reproduction. And there are species, like some fish, that *are* programmed to die right after spawning. According to this "death genes" theory, if an animal lives a long time after reproduction, it must be that, for whatever reason, death genes just didn't kick in.

But others argue against this theory. There can't be "death programs" in our genes ordering us to age and die, says Olshansky: "Death programs cannot exist as a direct product of evolution because the end result would be the systematic demise of all living things." Our internal clocks, he says, are "all about life, health and vigor, not decrepitude and death. They are present to develop and sustain life, not take it away."

Besides, if there *were* pre-programmed signals for aging and death lurking in our DNA, how would they work? They couldn't become activated *before* reproduction because no one would reproduce and the species would die out. Any genetic trait that prevents reproduction eventually would become vanishingly rare. And if such a death gene became activated *after* reproduction, natural selection would no longer be operating. And natural selection is the driver of evolution.

So, what's going on? Is aging just one big evolutionary accident?

Actually, yes. It turns out that we are not really like our cars, whose parts eventually just wear out. Our parts—our cells—can renew themselves.

Aging, in other words, is what happens when you haven't died or been killed off by predators. Yet, aging "is an accidental byproduct of surviving beyond our biological warranty period, beyond fixed genetic programs that exist for growth, development and reproduction."

Evolutionary biologist Rose puts it this way: We live a long time after reproduction "because the adverse impacts of the forces of natural selection take some time to kill us "

Natural selection, of course, is a tricky business. So is genetics. And things get really complex when it comes to trying to explain why creatures like humans age, that is, live long past reproduction, the pivot point for natural selection.

Usually, we think about genes as health-promoting ("good") or disease-causing ("bad"), with the former presumably boosting the odds of a long, healthy life, and the latter messing things up royally. But it's not that simple. There aren't just "bad" genes and "good" genes, but genes that are a bit of both. Some genes have multiple effects, that is, they are "good" and "bad" at different times. This is called "antagonistic pleiotropy," and it's one explanation of why we age.

The theory goes like this: If a gene has a beneficial effect early in life, but a detrimental effect later on, after reproduction, when natural selection is irrelevant, natural selection will favor that early beneficial gene even if the late-life effect is "catastrophic," as Austad puts it.

This means that deleterious, late-acting genes can accumulate generation after generation because they are not weeded out at reproduction. Eventually, these late-acting "bad" genes wreak havoc, causing the deterioration that we recognize as aging.

But, of course, genetics is only half the story. The other half is environment.

Ultimately, long-term survival depends not just on genes but on the interplay between genes and environment. If you are born into an environment full of hazards, your chances for long-term survival are obviously poor, no matter how good your genes. If you are born into a safer environment, your chances for longer life increase.

And this feeds into the genetics. Over generations, if you grow up in a safe environment, you can afford to postpone the age at which you reproduce. *This is key because delayed age of reproduction helps select for genes that indirectly allow for or encourage longer life.*

In other words, the hostility or friendliness of the environment "determines the time of reproduction, which determines the duration of life," Olshansky says.

This is worth pondering.

The link between environment and life span is something that has fascinated thinkers since Aristotle, thousands of years ago. Aristotle noticed that large animals like elephants live longer than little ones like mice. He guessed that some factor in the environment, maybe moisture, had something to do with it. Elephants, he figured, simply didn't dry up as fast as mice.

In truth, moisture has nothing to do with it. But large size does predict longer survival because of a safer environment: Big animals face fewer predators. Greater size means that bigger animals can go longer without food and water. Big animals also tend to live in clusters with lower population densities, which means they are less likely to catch contagious diseases. And large size also means that creatures can withstand cold and heat better.

Austad, the bio-gerontologist, discovered a dramatic illustration of this reproduction-survival principle years ago while studying opossums, which typically exhibit accelerated aging. Opossums don't live long because they live in an unsafe environment—they get picked on by owls, coyotes, wolves, feral dogs, cougars, bobcats, and, in modern times, cars. Their environment is just too hazardous for long-term survival.

For an animal in such a predicament, it makes no sense to waste resources on defenses like a good immune system, which would benefit the animal in the long run. For these animals, there *is* no long run. What *does* make sense is to reproduce as early as possible.

This made Austad wonder what would happen to opossums' chances for longer life if they did live in a safer environment with no predators around. He found an island off the coast of Georgia that contained opossums. It was perfect for his purposes—too far from the mainland for opossums to swim (and thus exchange genes with mainland opossums) and it contained few opossum predators. If the theory was right, Austad reasoned, opossums on the island should age more slowly and reproduce later than their cousins on the mainland.

That's exactly what he found.

Something similar may be going on right now with humans. All over the comparatively safe developed world, women are having children later. In the United States, the average age for the birth of a first child is now 26.3, up from 24.9 just a few years ago.

Indeed, the ability to stay fertile longer, that is, to be biologically able to delay reproduction, is one of the most striking features of America's oldest old, as data from the Long Life Family Study at Boston University show. Women whose biological clocks are ticking slowly enough that they are still capable of having a baby beyond age 33 are twice as likely to reach very old age as women who have their last baby at 29.

In other words, much of the increase in human longevity in recent times has to do with the fact that, in the developed world at least, we have made our environment safer, not that the process of aging itself has changed. Despite the horrifying headlines we read daily, we really do have fewer hostile forces—predators, diseases, food scarcity—to contend with now.

In the old days of our species, almost everybody died relatively young. Life was so hard, the environment so harsh, that nobody had a chance to age.

WHAT *IS* AGING, ANYWAY?

Aging, says Steve Austad cheerfully, is the "progressive deterioration of virtually every bodily function over time."

European researchers make it sound even gloomier: Aging is "a progressive loss of physiological integrity, leading to impaired function and increased vulnerability to death . . . the time-dependent accumulation of cellular damage."

But is this downward slide really inevitable? Does every creature on earth face the slow decline that we humans dread?

Surprisingly, the answer is no. In theory, at least, aging is not inevitable.

"Some animal species don't show aging—at all," says evolutionary biologist Rose. "There is nothing whatsoever in the basic cellular or organismal biology of animals and plants that requires aging."

The truth is that the aging process can be quite different in different critters. Lots of animals, and plants, die right after they reproduce.

But others don't age at all. In sea urchins, for instance, cells just don't degrade. Sea anemones don't age, either. For animals like these that don't age, the risk of death does not increase as time goes on, as it does with humans. It stays the same, all the way along. Take freshwater hydra—they have an equal chance of dying at age 10 or age 1,000.

And then there are the creatures, like Greenland sharks, that do age, but do so astonishingly slowly. Danish researchers recently discovered (by radiocarbon dating the lenses of sharks' eyes) that these sharks, who live in very cold water, live for more than 400 years, making them the oldest vertebrates known, second only to ocean quahogs in longevity.

What these examples show, in other words, is that we can't extrapolate from our observation of human aging to the rest of critter-kind. In reality, there is a striking variety in how—or whether—living creatures age.

And this huge variety prompts some evolutionary biologists, among them Michael Rose, to wonder if the physiological process of aging ever has to stop, or whether aging could just keep on going, more or less forever.

There's no reason to assume, says Rose, that "each and every type of physiological deterioration that has been associated with aging must continue without remit throughout late adult life." Maybe things could plateau in later life, maybe the process of aging could simply stop.

BOX 1.1 LIFE EXPECTANCY

As we think about aging, it's important to remember that this biological process, however long it lasts, is not the same thing as life expectancy, which is the average of everyone's age at death. Life expectancy has been a moving target in recent decades. For most of human history, life expectancy was drastically shorter than it is today because many, if not most, babies died in their first year of life, dragging down the average.

Worldwide, life expectancy at birth is now 68.6 years, and is projected to rise to 76.2 by 2050. In some countries, men and women at age 65 can expect to live at least 20 and 25 years more, respectively, and by 2020, people aged 65 or older are expected to outnumber children under age 5. In the United States, the population aged 65 and older is expected to double by 2050 from what it was in 2012, thanks to aging baby boomers.

Women's life expectancy at birth is generally longer than men's. That's not because they age more slowly, although that's possible, but because at any given point in time, they die at lower rates. Life expectancy at birth for US women in 2016 was 81.1 years; for men, 76.1. Surprisingly, the trend toward increasing life expectancy has been going backward in the last several years.

If aging is not absolutely inevitable, the fascinating question then becomes, can we manipulate it? Could we change the basic biological mechanisms that, as noted, deteriorate over time?

And what would it mean if we *could*? What would it mean for us as individuals if we could live both longer and more healthily? What if, instead of attacking the major diseases of aging one by one, as we do now, we pumped the big federal money into slowing the basic processes of aging themselves?

Some researchers, Olshansky among them, estimate that we could increase life expectancy by at least an additional 2.2 years, and that, more importantly, most of these extra years "would be spent in good health."

To be sure, delaying aging, and thus increasing the numbers of older people, would be economically costly in terms of Social Security and other entitlements. But these costs could be offset by raising the retirement and Medicare eligibility age. The real goal, he says, is to "compress both morbidity and mortality into a shorter period of time at the end of life."

And how exactly might we do this?

The main thesis of this book is that exercise is the closest thing we have to a magic bullet against aging. As we'll see in the chapters to come, exercise affects the deepest molecular biology of our cells, tissues, and organs—an array of effects so broad.

No pill is likely ever to match it. Why? Because, in a very real sense, the ability to exercise and the need to do it is built into our genes.

Harvard biologist Lieberman puts it this way: We humans evolved to be "especially well adapted for plentiful physical activity."

It's when we don't get the exercise that we evolved to get that things fall apart.

THE MAJOR HALLMARKS OF AGING

So what are these biological processes that underlie aging? What's going on at a biochemical, genetic, and physiological level when we age? What are the molecular "signatures"—clusters of biological markers—that could be used to predict how well, or poorly, a person is aging?

Not long ago, it wouldn't have been possible to give satisfying answers to these questions. But today, researchers have boiled down the most important changes to nine "hallmarks" of aging, as detailed in landmark papers in 2013 and 2016 by a team of European scientists led by Carlos Lopez-Otin in Spain and Guido Kroemer in France.

This gets into some heavy-duty cell biology, and we'll translate it into plain language in a minute. But for the record, the nine hallmarks are "genomic instability, telomere attrition, epigenetic alterations, loss of proteostasis, deregulated nutrient sensing, mitochondrial dysfunction, cellular senescence, stem cell exhaustion and altered intercellular communication"

Don't panic. This isn't as off-putting as it sounds. And the good news, at least in the view of some researchers, is that the beneficial effects of exercise involve all nine hallmarks of aging.

Each hallmark is a complicated web of biochemical interactions, and each of the hallmarks is intricately connected with all the others, making the process of untangling them an ongoing challenge.

But the take-home message is clear: Each hallmark has undesirable metabolic consequences. And it's our "Westernized" lifestyle—too much food and too little exercise—that accelerates this downward slide.

Among the most pronounced of the nine hallmarks are epigenetic changes, which can be measured by the so-called epigenetic clock. This is a biological metronome that "is literally an age estimate for any cell type, tissue type or organ," says Steve Horvath, a professor of human genetics and biostatistics at the University of California, Los Angeles.

Epigenetics consists of the changes to DNA that influence which genes are active but *don't alter* the DNA itself. It's a link between nature (the DNA we're born with) and nurture (what we encounter in the world around us). The key is that epigenetic changes affect which specific genes are "turned on" and when, not changes in DNA itself.

The epigenetic clock is actually one of a number of clocks that keep track of time and control what happens in the body. When should we get hungry? When should we sleep? When should we conceive babies? The most familiar of these is the one that keeps track of day and night— the circadian clock. But all these clocks are essential to life. "We could not exist without them," says Olshansky. It is these built-in genetic programs, he says, that "transform a fertilized egg into a teenager capable of reproduction."

But the epigenetic clock stands out because of its surprisingly strong relationship with chronological age. Metaphorically, it's like counting tree rings to estimate the age of a tree, says Horvath.

One of the chief epigenetic changes is a process called DNA methylation. This happens when a chemical structure called a methyl group latches on to certain stretches of DNA. Depending on where on the DNA the methyl group lands, it can control the expression of particular genes. As we age, some sites on the DNA molecule gain methyl groups, while others lose them.

Scientists know that enzymes (methyl transferases) attach methyl groups to the DNA. But what triggers DNA methylation in the first place—and how the enzymes "know" where, exactly, to attach the methyl groups—remains a mystery.

Still, the fact that the epigenetic clock works in chimpanzees, and that similar clocks can be defined for mice and dogs, suggests that these processes were "decided" by evolution hundreds of millions of years ago.

One of the most dramatic illustrations of the link between *exercise* and DNA methylation came in 2014, when researchers from Sweden's Karolinksa Institute asked a group of healthy young men and women to subject themselves to muscle biopsy tests, then ride bikes in the lab *using only one leg* four times a week for 45 minutes for three months.

Then the muscle biopsies were repeated. The scientists found that more than 5,000 sites on the genome of muscle cells had new methylation patterns, with some sites showing more methylation, and some less. The fascinating thing was that these changes showed up only in the exercised leg, not in the other leg, which served as a control. Horvath has recently shown that exercise does seem to slow the epigenetic clock, possibly by keeping weight under control.

One of the most stunning things scientists have learned from studying epigenetic clocks is that, at the molecular level, we don't all age at the same rate, as we all intuitively know from going to high school reunions.

In fact, as Horvath's research shows, not only can two people of the same chronological age be quite different in biological age, but different ethnic groups age at different speeds, too.

In a 2016 study, Horvath's team studied DNA methylation in more than 4,500 people from seven ethnic groups: two African groups, African-Americans, Caucasians, East Asians, Latinos, and indigenous people from Bolivia called the Tsimane. Latinos age more slowly at the molecular level than other ethnic groups. And the Tsimane age even more slowly than Latinos.

Men age faster than women, too. Even more fascinating—not to mention theoretically puzzling—different organs and tissues *in the same person* age at different rates. The heart can be 50 years old while the lungs are only the equivalent of 30 years old.

Breast tissue, for instance, is biologically older than many other tissues, possibly because the breast matures and differentiates faster during adolescence, pregnancy, and lactation. In obese people, the liver ages faster than other organs. In fact, the higher a person's body mass index, the higher the age of his or her liver. Infections like HIV accelerate the epigenetic clock. So does Down syndrome.

DNA methylation can actually predict all-cause mortality, regardless of chronological age. In one 2016 study, for instance, Horvath's team looked at the DNA of more than 13,000 people from the United States and Europe. The epigenetic clock was able to predict the life spans of Caucasians, Hispanics, and African-Americans "even after adjusting for traditional risk factors like age, gender, smoking, body-mass index, disease history and blood cell counts."

Other researchers, too, have also found that DNA methylation predicts all-cause mortality—independent of health status, lifestyle factors, and known genetic risks. In fact, some data suggest that there is a 35 percent increase in the risk of death for each five-year increase in DNA methylation age.

In centenarians (people over 100 years old), DNA methylation shows a youthful pattern, suggesting that these very old folks are biologically significantly younger than their chronological age.

Another hallmark of aging involves telomeres, tiny bits of DNA on the ends of chromosomes. Telomeres are like the caps on the ends of shoelaces. They keep the ends of chromosomes from being misidentified by the cell as damaged DNA, which can trigger a DNA repair process that can fuse chromosomes together, tangling up cell division. With aging, telomeres naturally get shorter, ultimately becoming unable to keep DNA in good enough shape for the cell to divide.

For about a decade, scientists have known that an enzyme called telomerase can restore missing bits of telomeres, thus allowing chromosomes to stay long and keep functioning. Although many mammals continuously make telomerase, most human cells make very little telomerase, which is why telomeres in people get shorter over time.

The question of whether exercise helps keep telomeres long (and sedentary behavior hastens their shortening) is a contentious one, as we'll see in Chapter 13. Diet does seem to play a role in telomere health, with a Mediterranean diet (fruits, veggies, olive oil, and not much red meat) possibly slowing the rate of telomere shortening.

But here's a curious thing: Telomere shortening does *not* seem to correlate with the epigenetic clock. If all the biological clocks in the body were tightly linked, one would expect the telomere clock and the epigenetic clock to be in sync. But a number of studies have shown that telomere length is not correlated with epigenetic age.

And even cells whose telomeres are well maintained by the enzyme telomerase continue to age according to the epigenetic clock. It's possible that telomeres and the epigenetic clock are independent markers of aging. But overall, these studies show that it's not possible to stop or reverse aging by reversing the telomere clock alone, says Horvath: "Rather, a comprehensive anti-aging strategy needs to find ways of slowing the epigenetic clock as well."

Another key hallmark of aging is genomic instability. This means that our DNA has become damaged over time and has lost the ability to repair itself. DNA damage is a constant—scientists estimate that the DNA in each human cell is damaged a million times a day, though in young, healthy cells, a number of processes kick in to detect and repair this damage.

Telomere shortening can be considered a specific type of genomic instability. But there are others, and they, too, are disruptive to the basic functioning of cells. One of these is a phenomenon called "jumping genes." These are rogue bits of DNA, technically called transposons, that leave their normal place on the DNA strand and insert themselves elsewhere, where they are not "supposed" to be. Transposon activity rises with age.

Loss of proteostasis, another aging hallmark, means that the normal process by which cells recycle protein goes awry. In a normal, healthy cell, proteins are routinely synthesized, folded into the right shapes, and when they become old and damaged, recycled. This recycling process is called "autophagy," or "self-eating," and it's crucial for preserving the fitness of cells from the inside. (Research on how autophagy works won a Japanese scientist the Nobel Prize in 2016.)

But if autophagy breaks down, as it does with aging, damaged proteins clump together, messing up cell function. Alzheimer's disease, which is characterized by plaques and tangles of clumped-together proteins, is an example of proteostasis failure. The good news is that exercise is a powerful stimulator of autophagy.

Another hallmark of aging involves the failure of an organism's system for detecting the availability of food in the environment. This process, called nutrient sensing, is key to survival, but with aging, it becomes deregulated.

The availability of food and the "decision" by an animal to reproduce are tightly linked. Indeed, the ability to sense nutrients evolved because animals had to find a way to tell when there was enough food around to support reproduction; if food supplies were scare, an animal had to "know" to hold off on making babies until things got better.

Delayed reproduction, as we saw with the opossums, is associated with longer life span. "When nutrients are abundant, animals, including humans, grow and reproduce—the evolutionary imperative," in Austad's words. When food is scarce, accurate nutrient sensing allows animals to spend their precious energy on maintenance and repair, not reproduction.

Discovering exactly how the nutrient sensing system works, and how it fits in with aging, is a fascinating story, and it happened in a roundabout way. Years ago on Easter Island, also known as Rapa Nui, scientists discovered an antifungal agent (now a drug) that they dubbed "rapamycin," named after the island. (Considerable research is now focused on rapamycin as an anti-aging drug, as we'll see in Chapter 14.)

Rapamycin, they discovered, acts on an enzyme that they named "mTOR," for "mammalian target of rapamycin." This enzyme is a nutrient sensor, a chemical that detects the presence of amino acids.

"When we eat food, the proteins from the food are broken down in the gut to amino acids," explains geneticist Matt Kaeberlein of the University of Washington. "When there are a lot of amino acids around, that means there are a lot of nutrients, which turns mTOR on," he says. Once turned on, mTOR sends chemical signals to other enzymes that "tell a cell it's a good time to divide or grow." In other words, more mTOR, more growth.

On the other hand, when there are no amino acids around, mTOR shuts down, telling an organism not to reproduce until food supplies are up again. Since delayed reproduction is associated with longer life span, the mTOR–aging link goes like this: Low mTOR is "good" because it is linked with slower aging, and high levels are "bad" because they are linked with accelerated aging.

There's another wrinkle here. A major reason that scientists are intrigued by mTOR is that it is also part of a pathway by which insulin and a hormone called IGF-1, or insulin-like growth factor, act. Insulin regulates cell metabolism, while IGF-1 triggers cell growth, differentiation, and tissue repair, all potentially "good" things.

But IGF-1 can also be "bad" because it turns on mTOR, potentially accelerating age-related diseases, stimulating smooth muscle growth in atherosclerosis, and even boosting cancer cell growth.

Exercise fits into all this, too. Exercise increases both IGF-1 and mTOR. In theory, this could potentially have adverse effects. But—and it's a big "but"—the exercise effect is short term and localized to specific tissues. The danger only comes if IGF-1 and mTOR are *chronically*, not temporarily, increased.

Yet another hallmark of aging involves mitochondria, little organelles inside cells often dubbed "powerhouses" because they are the factories that produce energy for everything from basic metabolism to running marathons.

Mitochondria have their own DNA, distinct from the DNA in the cell's nucleus and inherited differently (only through the mother). Like the DNA in the nucleus, mitochondrial DNA can become damaged and fail to be repaired, which becomes a significant contributor to aging. Mitochondrial dysfunction in fact is a major driver of aging and age-related diseases. The good news, as we'll see in Chapter 5, is that exercise is a powerful way to keep mitochondria from becoming dysfunctional.

Cellular senescence, another hallmark, means that cells, though still alive, can't reproduce anymore. Scientists think cells become senescent when they are damaged or when their telomeres become too short, and are in danger of becoming cancerous, and thus need to be controlled.

Senescent cells contribute to the aging process by pumping out cytokines, substances that influence how cells "talk" to each other. Among other things, cytokines promote inflammation, which in turn contributes to aging. Scientists are working on ways to get rid of senescent cells with drugs that nudge the cell to commit "suicide." In lab experiments with mice, this technique extends the life span of mice by more than 20 percent.

Stem cell exhaustion is yet another hallmark of aging. Stem cells are undifferentiated cells that give rise to many more cells. With aging, the reservoir of stem cells becomes depleted. Some researchers have been able to reactivate aging, adult stem cells with a gene called "NANOG." Others have injected cardiac stem cells from young rats into the hearts of older rats, which seems to slow cardiac aging. Rapamycin may also be able to boost stem cell function.

The final hallmark of aging is altered intercellular communication. This means that the signals, including hormones, that allow one cell to "talk" to another become dysregulated. Among other things, this tangled-up communication tends to increase inflammation.

HOW WE AGE: COMPETING THEORIES

Despite the deepening understanding of the hallmarks of aging, there seems to be no one master gene or mechanism running the whole aging process, no "hallmark" so powerful that it drives all the others. The messy truth is that aging is a mélange of interacting processes that ultimately bring down the entire biological system.

There are several theories about all this, and one of the most-studied involves caloric restriction, that is, a diet that supplies essential nutrients but is drastically reduced in calories.

In 1935, a Cornell University team observed that limiting the food intake of rodents while keeping their diets rich in vitamins and minerals allowed the males to live 75 percent longer than their better-fed controls. Follow-up research showed the effect in females, too.

Since then, other scientists have tested the idea extensively—in worms, insects, even primates. In a recent human trial, the first of its kind, caloric restriction did not show the same metabolic changes as in some animal studies, and the participants were not able to cut calories as much as researchers had wanted. Even so, caloric restriction did have a positive impact on some age-related diseases and on life-span markers such as blood pressure, cholesterol, and insulin resistance.

Overall, the bottom line is clear: Caloric restriction—limiting calories by roughly 30 percent—is a spectacularly effective way to increase the average and maximum life spans in a range of creatures, and to delay the onset of age-related diseases. It is one of the only *proven* ways to retard the aging process, though the drug rapamycin is promising as well.

But precisely *how* restricting calories slows aging is the subject of many theories. Maybe, as some researchers have proposed, it's because caloric restriction lowers body temperature. Or maybe it's that reducing energy intake triggers a "biphasic" phenomenon called hormesis. This is a process by which the body responds favorably to low levels of biological stressors that would be harmful at *high or chronic* levels.

Other researchers think caloric restriction boosts cell survival by activating a gene called SIRT (more on this in Chapter 14). Other theorists think caloric restriction promotes longevity by damping down mTOR. Caloric restriction may also preserve genome function by reducing DNA damage, specifically the damage caused by "jumping genes." Caloric restriction may also work by activating autophagy.

But other theories explain aging on the basis of "aging genes."

Back in the 1980s, scientists discovered a gene they dubbed "*age-1*" in a worm called *C. elegans*. Worms with a particular form of this gene lived longer than others. Since then, scientists using this gene have created worms that can live 10 times longer than their non-modified cousins.

In his lab at Massachusetts General Hospital in Boston, molecular biologist Gary Ruvkun has discovered that when worm insulin or a similar hormone called IGF binds to a receptor called *daf-2*, the *age-1* gene is activated.

It's a complicated pathway, but the bottom line is that low levels of insulin are a great way to extend the life span. In fact, when Ruvkun *suppresses* the insulin signaling pathway, his worms act sick and stop, or at least postpone, reproduction. And delayed reproduction—as we saw with Austad's opossums—favors longer life.

Other aging-related genes have also caught scientists' eyes.

Scientists have identified dozens of genes that, when altered, lengthen the life span in mice. Still other scientists have bred fruit flies (*Drosophilia*) for longevity by allowing only older flies to reproduce, thus creating "Methuselah" flies with dramatically extended life spans. They have even found a longevity gene dubbed *Indy*, which stands for "I'm not dead yet."

Another gene, *FoxO*, is important, too. A particular form of *FoxO* may account for the strange life of the hydra that we mentioned earlier, those jellyfish-like creatures that don't age, but do die. Among other things, this gene seems to work by preventing stem cell exhaustion.

But, of course, the real goal is to understand the genes underlying long, healthy life spans in humans, and not surprisingly, a variant of the *FoxO* gene is present in long-lived humans, too.

Other genes are at play, too, in exceptionally long-lived people. Centenarians are endowed with specific genetic profiles, Boston University researchers have found. Indeed, 90 percent of 801 centenarians in the team's New England Centenarian Study fit into one of 27 genetic profiles. These folks do what many of us wish we could do: pack sickness and disability into a very short period at the end of a very long, healthy life.

Yet another theory of aging involves the "cross-linking" of proteins, DNA, sugar, and other molecules. Cross-linking means that molecules that shouldn't stick together do, literally gumming up the works.

This is especially important when cross-links occur via sugar. In this process, called glycosylation or glycation, glucose molecules stick to proteins, forming permanent chemical bonds that prevent the proteins from functioning normally. Cross-linking is partially responsible for wrinkling of the skin and cataracts in the eye.

And when glucose attaches to collagen, it forms cross-links that make collagen less flexible. In arteries, glycosylated proteins lead to athero-sclerosis (hardening of the arteries). Glycation also contributes to the formation of beta-amyloid, a protein that clumps together in the brains of people with Alzheimer's disease.

When attached to proteins, glucose also causes "browning," what chemists call the Maillard reaction. Just as meat turns brown when it is cooked, the same chemical reaction—glucose attaching to proteins—creates a yellow or brown product in our bodies. Browning turns out to be a major part of the aging process. In diabetics, when glucose attaches to hemoglobin (a protein), it creates chemicals called AGEs (advanced glycosylation end-products), which have damaging effects. Unfortunately, we form so many AGEs over a lifetime that no single test can detect the degree of glycation in the organism as a whole.

Other scientists have theorized that aging is related to metabolic rate, hypothesizing that animals with higher metabolic rates simply wear out sooner than slower-paced creatures. Known as the rate-of-living theory, this idea has morphed into the popular notion that all animals are born with a certain number of heartbeats and when those are used up—game over.

But the facts have tarnished this theory. Parrots, for instance, have crazy-fast heart rates—600 beats a minute—yet live longer than many other animals with more leisurely heartbeats.

Another theory—the free radical theory of aging—holds that we age because of damage to DNA, cell membranes, blood vessel walls, and other body parts caused by free radicals (toxic forms of oxygen). "When iron is oxidized, we generally call the result rust," writes bio-gerontologist Austad. "When bronze is oxidized, as on ancient bronze sculpture, we call the green film patina. When we are oxidized, we call it aging."

But the free radical theory, popular several decades ago, has lost cred-ibility for lack of evidence. True, the destructive power of free radicals (called oxidative stress) is enormous. But animals, including people, are also genetically endowed with defenses *against* free radicals, specifically, genes that make antioxidants such as superoxide dismutase, glutathione, glutathione peroxidase, and catalase. In some species, at least, extended life does appear to be linked to good antioxidant defenses.

And then there's the ultimate rebuttal of the free radical theory of aging, an ugly little animal called the naked mole rat. These critters have high levels of oxidative damage and low levels of antioxidants, but still live 10 times longer than similar-sized lab rats. In fact, naked mole rats, which live underground and don't have much sex, don't seem to age at all, at least not the way most creatures do: They have the same risk of death throughout their entire lives. For reasons that still mystify scientists, naked mole rats appear to be "non-aging mammals," even though they eventually do die.

Yet another theory of aging is the idea that our cells are programmed to have only a fixed number of cell divisions, the so-called Hayflick limit. When that number—supposedly 40–60 cell divisions—is reached, the theory goes, aging (cell senescence) and death ensue. But this theory, too, has run into trouble.

Some cells, notably cancer cells, never stop dividing—they can, unfortunately, keep dividing forever. And think of those telomeres and the enzyme telomerase, which keeps restoring telomere length, thus enabling a cell to keep dividing.

But enough theory!

WHERE EXERCISE FITS IN

That's what the rest of this book is all about. But here's a quick look ahead.

As evolutionary biologists have confirmed, we evolved to run, to behave much as our hunter-gatherer ancestors did more than 600 generations ago. Exercise and physical activity are normal human behavior, from an evolutionary point of view. Sloth and gluttony are not.

Many, if not most, of the chronic diseases we now suffer from come from what Lieberman calls a "mismatch" between our genes and our environment. "We evolved to be athletes—you couldn't survive [as a hunter-gatherer] without being active. It's only since the Industrial Revolution that we could have survived without physical activity. In essence, we are Paleolithic creatures, genetically programmed to run around and eat modest amounts of food, transplanted into an environment conducive to too much sedentary behavior and too much food"

We are, quite literally, built to run—with good feet, lots of sweat glands to maintain healthy body temperature, pretty good balance in motion, and relatively long legs.

As bipedal creatures, we may not be able to run as fast as, say, lions, but our advantage is that we are capable of running at moderate speeds for very long periods of time. In fact, it's this endurance capacity that allowed our ancestors to develop "persistence hunting"—chasing an animal until it drops dead from exhaustion or overheating. Humans, says Lieberman, are actually "among the best long-distance runners in the mammalian world."

"Exercise promotes longevity," he adds. "There's no question that people who exercise more live longer and with less disability. There's nothing to debate. Removing exercise from our environment is like removing air: You get sick."

CHAPTER 2

Run for Your Life

It seems so obvious now: Physical activity is a key—some would say *the* key—to a longer, healthier life, a magic bullet, a hedge against the many ills of humankind.

We know without a doubt, for instance, that exercise lowers the risk of heart disease, some cancers, premature mortality, and even all-cause mortality. We know it lowers blood pressure and reduces dangerous blood clots. We know it helps prevent diabetes, improves brain function, and spurs muscles to make hormones that dampen chronic inflammation—and much more.

But it wasn't always so obvious.

It wasn't until the late 19th and early 20th centuries that a few scientifically minded souls began exploring what effect exercise might have on health and longevity. One of the clues came from an early study comparing the life spans of highly fit oarsmen from England's historic Oxford and Cambridge Universities to those of the rest of the population. The oarsmen lived significantly longer.

To be sure, a handful of ancient physician-philosophers—Hippocrates and Galen come to mind—had suspected that a lack of physical exercise was detrimental to health. During the Enlightenment, a perspicacious Italian physician had observed that runners (chiefly, fleet-footed messengers) were healthier than sedentary tailors and cobblers, whom he urged to exercise on holidays to counteract the harm done by many days of sedentary life.

But it wasn't until 1915 that the US Surgeon General began putting things together, documenting, among other things, that manual laborers were less likely to get degenerative heart, kidney, and blood vessel problems than less active workers. A few years later, in 1922, Minnesota researchers similarly showed that people in physically demanding jobs lived longer than those in sedentary jobs. In 1939, Philadelphia researchers, too, found that the risk of death from cardiovascular disease was higher for white-collar workers than for laborers.

At the time, though, few people were paying attention, as the world rushed to forget the horrors of World War II. Most were all too eager to embrace spiffy new labor-saving devices and to exchange physical labor for cushier, more prestigious, sedentary jobs.

But by the end of the 1940s, attitudes began to change when a Scottish physician-epidemiologist named Jeremy N. Morris published dramatic findings from his London Transport Workers Study. Morris compared the cardiovascular health of conductors on the city's double-decker buses, who climbed up and down stairs all day taking tickets, to that of the sedentary bus drivers. The conductors' heart health was significantly superior. Morris found the same pattern when he compared the fate of active postmen with that of sedentary telephone operators.

Even so, physical activity was a tough sell. Most doctors still pooh-poohed Morris's findings. But he and a handful of other British researchers stuck to their guns, eventually recruiting more than 200 pathologists to examine the hearts of people after death: The worst heart damage occurred in the most sedentary people.

Morris then dropped an even bigger bombshell when he claimed that physical activity wasn't linked just to better cardiovascular health, it was linked to a lower risk of *all-cause mortality* as well.

BOX 2.1 AN INSPIRATIONAL TALE: THE "ANTIQUE" SKIER

"I am an antique," says Trina Hosmer, 73, a passionate cross-country skier who has won 46 gold medals in age-group competitions in Masters World Championships and still runs, does yoga every day, and bikes 30–50 miles every other day—at least until serious training starts in the fall.

At that point, she cranks up her already intensive training—venturing outside of her Stowe, Vermont, home when there's enough snow to ski on, or inside on a Nordic ski exercise machine when there's not.

Hosmer and her husband, David, retired together 14 years ago from their jobs as statisticians at the University of Massachusetts in Amherst. "The writing was on the wall," she says. "It was obvious we wanted to keep skiing and we got tired of two places. So we moved full time to Stowe."

They met in 1966 at the University of Vermont, where they kept bumping into each other in math classes. He was captain of the ski team and she was soon tagging along, driving the men to competitions and bringing food. There was no women's team in those pre–Title IX days, though David often brought ski equipment for her, just in case she decided to ski.

The fateful day came one weekend at the start of a 50-kilometer race.

"I was just watching everybody warming up," she recalls. "I said to myself, 'It can't be that hard.' Three hours later, I was still going round and round at the back of the pack. I was supposed to feed the guys, but I forgot. I was hooked." She soon started training and racing with the men's team.

In 1970, she made the first US women's team for an international competition in Czechoslovakia. "I didn't know how to ski that well," she says, "but I had been a pretty good runner and I was in good shape." She made the 1972 team for the Olympics in Sapporo, Japan, too, and the team for the 1974 Nordic Skiing World Championships.

A year later, while out jogging, she went into labor with her son. Three years later, her daughter was born. Juggling kids and work for years until the kids went to college, she barely missed a day's workout. She is, of course, still at it.

In 2016, at the Masters World Cup in Finland, she not only won all three races for her age group, but her times were so good that a coach, suspecting that she was under 70, asked to see her passport to check her age.

Now that she is over 70, competition rules dictate that she has to race "in the old lady division, where the distances are cut in half," she told the Wall Street Journal.

"But that just means I can go fast the entire time."

THE FRAMINGHAM HEART STUDY

As Morris was slowly building his case for the benefits of physical activity, a handful of US researchers from the federal government—specifically, at the National Heart, Lung and Blood Institute—and Boston University embarked on what would become the grandfather of all longitudinal research, the Framingham Heart Study. It would become pivotal in establishing the exercise–longevity link.

Launched in 1948, this observational study was designed to follow thousands of people over their entire life spans to see who lived the longest and healthiest lives, and more specifically, to see what factors were linked to cardiovascular disease and deaths.

For the record, an observational, that is, correlational, study like this is different from an interventional study, in which people are randomized to get or not get a specific intervention such as a drug, diet, or exercise program. There's a built-in chicken-and-egg problem in studies that just show correlations: They can't prove cause and effect, just an association. You can't tell from correlational studies whether exercise really makes people healthier, or whether the people who exercise are healthier to begin with. After all, people who exercise also tend not to smoke, to have healthier diets, and to be more educated. And exercise, of course, is not the only thing that can help us live longer, healthier lives. Solid, nurturing relationships can, too.

At the outset, the Framingham study recruited 5,209 healthy men and women aged 30–62 from the town of Framingham, Massachusetts, and asked them to come in every two years for extensive physical exams and lifestyle interviews. The researchers kept records of participants' height, weight, diet, drinking habits, reported exercise patterns, blood tests, and even variables such as whether a person went to church regularly, had close friends, or was depressed or worried.

Over the years, the study grew. In 1971, the team enrolled 5,124 more people who were the adult children of the original participants and their spouses. In 2002, to great fanfare, the researchers added a third group, the grandchildren of the original participants.

As medical science became more sophisticated, the Framingham study did, too, adding tests to track cognitive function, genetic information, and other variables. Instead of just asking people to report on their exercise, the team also began giving participants accelerometers (devices like Fitbit) to document actual activity levels.

The payoff has been stunning. The Framingham team, which invented the term "risk factor," has now published more than 1,200 scientific papers on their findings. In the early days, emerging data from Framingham didn't show much correlation between physical activity, fitness, and cardiac risk factors, probably because most initial participants were quite sedentary.

But today, the take-home message is clear, says cardiologist Dr. Jerome Fleg, medical officer at the National Heart, Lung and Blood Institute, which runs the Framingham study. More physical activity and more fitness are both associated with reduced cardiovascular events and often with greater longevity, he says. The risks of cancer and other diseases are also reduced by regular exercise. And the main reason for greater longevity in people who exercise is that they get less cardiovascular disease.

Indeed, the Framingham team has shown not just that exercise is a powerful preventer of cardiovascular disease, but also that *lack* of exercise is a major risk factor for developing it.

As the Framingham study was getting underway, another scientist, Dr. Ralph S. Paffenbarger, also became intrigued by the link between physical activity and heart disease.

In 1951, Paffenbarger, an epidemiologist and marathon runner himself, began the California Longshoreman Study. He enrolled 6,351 longshoremen aged 35–74 whose jobs demanded that they perform a range of strenuous, moderate, and light tasks. He followed them for 22 years, until their 75th birthday, or death, whichever came first.

By 1975, his results, published in the *New England Journal of Medicine*, were indisputable: Men who did the most strenuous work had significantly fewer coronary events than those doing light or moderate work. Repeated bursts of high energy output established what Paffenbarger called a "plateau of protection" against coronary mortality. (Studies in Finnish lumberjacks and US railroad workers would come to similar conclusions.)

Paffenbarger kept at it. In the early 1960s, he began tracking a different group: nearly 17,000 male Harvard University alumni, to whom he mailed detailed questionnaires. He queried the Harvard men about their physical activities and augmented their answers with information from college records on their athletic activities during their student years. He followed up with more studies in 1972, 1988, and 1993.

To nail things down, Paffenbarger created a numerical index for various physical activities, assigning each activity a score based on how much energy it required. Sports such as bowling, baseball, golf, and light housework were categorized as needing "light" energy expenditure; more strenuous sports such as basketball, running, swimming, and tennis were assumed to require more energy expenditure. He then estimated how many calories each man expended in exercise each week.

The results were striking: The risk of a first heart attack was inversely related to how many calories a man spent per week in exercise—the more calories expended, the lower the risk. Men who expended fewer than 2,000 calories a week in exercise had a 64 percent higher risk of heart attack, a pattern Paffenbarger went on to document again and again. And there was bad news for college jocks who abandoned their athletic ways: Men who had been varsity athletes in college retained their lower risk of heart disease only if they kept exercising as alums.

Other researchers, too, began documenting strong links between exercise and health. In 1958, gerontologists embarked on the Baltimore Longitudinal Study on Aging, a massive, decades-long project. The study was not explicitly focused on exercise, but on a more basic question: What happens in normal, healthy aging? Researchers soon discovered that their original question crossed paths with research on exercise.

To be sure, even normal, healthy bodies change with age, even in exercisers, notes Dr. Jeffrey Metter, a former medical officer of the Baltimore study. As people age, they tend to exercise less overall and less vigorously. These declines in both total and high-intensity physical activity are independent predictors of all-cause mortality.

But the more important—and good—news from the Baltimore study is that many of the changes once presumed to be an *intrinsic* part of the aging process—such as hypertension, diabetes, and dementia—are the result of specific *diseases*, not an inevitable part of aging. Indeed, as other research has since confirmed, the bodies of some physically active older adults resemble those of younger people, sometimes having a "fitness age" 25 years less than their chronological age.

Like the Framingham study, the Baltimore study is ongoing and evolving, along with exercise science. So far, more than 3,000 people have participated. All pledge to show up for testing at regular intervals for the rest of their lives. To the delight of the Baltimore researchers, many people are aging so well that the team has started a project to study "exceptional aging" among people 80 or over *with no health problems*.

Many factors, of course, not just exercise, contribute to healthy aging. But exercise, the Baltimore research has found, is a cornerstone of a longer, healthier life. It's the people who exercise at moderate- to high-intensity levels who have a better chance for longer, healthier lives.

In fact, in an analysis of people aged 70–79, the Baltimore researchers have shown that, *regardless of their genetic makeup*, people who exercise are less likely to develop mobility problems than those who do not. Even people who don't start exercising until their 60s and 70s can still develop healthier hearts, including improved heart function, lower resting heart rates, larger heart mass, and stronger heart pumping action.

Study by study, the evidence for exercise, even in later life, has piled up. In fact, Honolulu researchers documented this dramatically. They followed 8,006 Japanese men for an average of 23 years and found that middle-aged men who were more physically active had a lower risk for coronary heart disease and death. That link held up much later in life, too. The Honolulu team found that older men who walked more than two miles a day had *half* the mortality of men who walked less than a mile a day.

THE REAL GOAL: FITNESS

As important as these large epidemiological studies have been for documenting a link between exercise and longevity, the more important question for scientists is whether physical *fitness* was tied to health and longevity. It's an important distinction. Physical *activity* is a behavior that can be reported and tracked. Physical *fitness* is a physiological state that must be measured in the lab, is partly determined by genetics, and can be improved by physical activity. (For a quick, noninvasive way to gauge your fitness, go to https://www.worldfitnesslevel.org/#/.)

Back in the early 1970s, preventive medicine specialist Kenneth Cooper began to explore all this, setting up the Aerobics Center Longitudinal Study, now called the Cooper Center Longitudinal Study. Cooper recruited his first patient in 1970, putting his notes on index cards and storing them in a shoebox. Today, the database for the Cooper study includes records for nearly 100,000 individuals. It's Cooper who planted the word "aerobic" in our national lexicon, and Cooper who established 10,000 steps as a daily exercise goal. Indeed, it was the work of Cooper and his colleagues that led to our current national exercise recommendations.

Cooper thought big, realizing that, to make the case for fitness, he would need data from thousands of people, so he gave questionnaires to 13,444 men and 3,972 women aged 20–87. Like Paffenbarger, he and the Dallas team tallied how many calories each person expended per week in physical activity. They concluded that most people could achieve cardiorespiratory fitness by walking briskly for 30 minutes almost every day.

By the late 1980s, one of Cooper's colleagues, Steven N. Blair, a physical activity epidemiologist who is now at the University of South Carolina, pushed fitness research even further. In one study, Blair studied 10,224 men and 3,120 women, assessing their fitness by a treadmill stress test and following them for eight years. Like Morris, Blair was interested in *all-cause mortality*—deaths not only from heart disease, but also from cancer, the second leading cause of death, and other conditions as well.

His findings electrified the medical world.

Among the least-fit men, Blair found that all-cause mortality, that is, the rate of dying from any cause, was 64 per 10,000 person-years. In the most fit men, it was 18.6, a whopping difference. For women, the all-cause mortality rate was 39.5 for the least fit, versus 8.5 for the most fit. These results held true even after statistical adjustments for age, smoking, cholesterol level, blood pressure, blood sugar level, and family history of heart disease. Maintaining or improving fitness, Blair's team concluded, is linked with lower all-cause and cardiovascular mortality *even with no change in body weight.*

But here is Blair's most important finding: Even just getting out of the least-fit category—that is, merely becoming *moderately* fit—has a huge beneficial effect on all-cause mortality.

Going from unfit to moderately fit over a 4.9-year period was linked to a 44 percent lower mortality risk. Physical activity, Blair found, not only reduces the incidence of stroke, high blood pressure, type 2 diabetes, metabolic syndrome, breast and colon cancer, excessive weight gain, injurious falls, depression, and lower cognitive function, but also can lead to better sleep and better quality of life.

BOX 2.2 AN INSPIRATIONAL TALE: THE AGELESS MARATHONER

Ed Whitlock, the legendary marathoner, was 85 in October 2016 when he set his latest distance running record: finishing the Toronto Waterfront Marathon in 3 hours, 56 minutes, 34 seconds. He is the oldest person to run 26.2 miles in under four hours.

Whitlock, who died in March 2017, has long awed doctors, one of whom noted that Whitlock is "about as close as you can get to minimal aging in a individual." Unlike many marathoners, Whitlock had no coach, didn't adhere to any special diet, didn't keep track of his mileage, didn't lift weights. The Toronto running star used to be a mining engineer. He had an astounding VO2max, the standard measure of the maximum amount of oxygen that muscles can use during exercise. His VO2max was 54, comparable to a college-age recreational athlete. Unlike many older people, especially sedentary ones, Whitlock barely lost any muscle mass since his 20s.

After his 2016 race, he told the New York Times *that he didn't feel a runner's high and did not run for health. "The real feeling of enjoyment," he said," is getting across the finish line and finding out that you've done okay."*

Even very moderate exercise is better than nothing. If you're a runner, just 5–10 minutes a day at relatively slow speeds (less than six miles per hour) is linked to a markedly reduced risk from all-cause and cardiovascular mortality. Interestingly, a 5-minute run is as good as a 15-minute walk. But even a brisk walk for 15 minutes a day reduces all-cause mortality and provides an extra three years of life expectancy. Astonishingly, just one hour of running can add seven hours to your life.

All you really have to do for better health and increased longevity is meet the US government's—and the World Health Organization's—minimum activity guidelines: 150 minutes a week of moderate exercise, or 75 minutes a week of vigorous activity. Even "weekend warriors," who pack those total minutes of exercise into one or two long runs or other vigorous activity on the weekends, lessen their risk of premature death almost as much as people who do shorter workouts all week long.

But fewer than half of American adults get even this minimal exercise. And an estimated 31 million *older* Americans don't do any exercise at all beyond the minimal movements needed for daily life.

In general, more exercise is better than less, up to a point. The biggest longevity benefits correlate with the biggest doses of exercise, with the maximum benefit occurring with exercise at three to five times the 150 minutes a week minimum. At this point, the benefits plateau, though they don't decline.

Overall, there's no excess risk of harm, even at 10 times the recommended level of exercise. But there are some caveats. Ultrasound studies done at the end of marathons have shown changes in both left and right ventricles of the heart (the former is the main pumping chamber; the latter, the chamber that supplies blood to the lungs). These changes are usually transient but could lead to problems, especially in inadequately trained middle-aged runners.

Certain biomarkers (such as troponin and brain natriuretic peptide) may be elevated, too, suggesting possible, though usually transient, heart damage in some marathon runners right after a race. Atrial fibrillation (an irregular rhythm in the top chamber of the heart) is also five times more likely in middle-aged men who are endurance athletes.

That said, a 2012 analysis of 10.9 million marathon runners showed a low overall risk of cardiac arrest and sudden death. When cardiac arrest does occur during long-distance running events, it does so rarely in half marathons (13.1 miles), but more often in full marathons (26.2 miles).

But most of us exercise much less intensely than marathoners. And for us, even when studies lump together several lifestyle variables—smoking, exercise, weight, and so on—exercise turns out to be the most important factor for health and longevity.

In a 2013 study, Blair found exactly that. He looked at smoking, body mass index, cardiorespiratory fitness, and diet in 11,240 men and women and followed them for an average of 12 years. Avoiding both smoking and low fitness would have prevented 13 percent of the deaths in this group, he found. But it was low fitness that turned out to be the more important variable, beating out smoking as a risk factor.

In other words, the case for exercise is now irrefutable. A 2008 review of 33 studies involving more than 883,000 adults showed that people who exercise have 35 percent less cardiovascular mortality and 33 percent less all-cause mortality. This translates into an extra year or two of life. A 2009 meta-analysis of studies involving 102,980 participants similarly showed that better cardiorespiratory *fitness* (as opposed to physical activity) was associated with lower all-cause mortality.

And a 2011 analysis of 80 studies involving more than 1.3 million adults nailed the case: Higher levels of physical activity were linked to lower all-cause mortality, with the biggest benefit linked to the most vigorous activity. A 2015 analysis of middle-aged and older Australians came to the same conclusion. conclusion.

BOX 2.3 AN INSPIRATIONAL TALE: THE BMX BIKING GRANDMA

Kittie Weston-Knauer, her gray hair shaved close to her scalp, is the oldest female BMX bike rider in America. She was 69 when last I checked, racing hard despite having had both knees and both hips replaced. Eyes focused straight ahead, helmet with the big chin guard locked in place, orange racing suit clinging to her limbs, Weston-Knauer looks very much the champion she is in the 2017 photograph in Bicycling *magazine.*

For 33 years, the article in Bicycling *explains, she was a high school principal in Des Moines. Now she travels all over the country to compete in bike races. She got into the sport in the late 1980s when her son Max, then 11, urged her to try. At age 40, she tried it, using Max's helmet, gloves, and bike. She was hooked. When she's not training or competing, she told* Bicycling, *she's at the gym five days a week, doing strength training and core exercises. She says her proudest moment came not during her many wins, but after a crash that paralyzed her from the shoulders down in the early 1990s, when she defied her neurosurgeons, who told her she'd never walk again. She did, and then some.*

"So I am 69, big deal," the grandmother known on the track as "Miss Kittie" told an interviewer. Racing is "fun, more fun, and even more fun."

"I'm in great shape and I want to stay that way," she added, noting that she often has to race against men and teenagers because there aren't many women racers her age.

"I do this because I'm having a blast and who would ever think that as an older woman you can have a blast out there racing with younger people."

THE 90+ STUDY

Even among the very old—people aged 90 or older—exercise pays off—big time. Way back in 1981, 14,000 residents of a retirement community in California called Leisure World filled out lengthy questionnaires about their diets, activities, vitamin intake, and medical histories, a collection of data that would turn out to be a researcher's dream.

That researcher was Claudia Kawas, a neurologist at the University of California, Irvine. Realizing what a treasure trove these data were, she set out in 2003 to follow up on those among the initial 14,000 people who were still alive, a project that became known as the 90+ Study.

To her delight, Kawas discovered that more than 1,600 were still alive and doing remarkably well in their 90s. Several factors, she found, were especially important. People who drank alcohol moderately (up to two drinks a day) lived longer than those who abstained. So did people who drank coffee (one to three cups a day). Socializing and staying intellectually engaged were also linked to longevity.

And exercise? Physical activity had a profound "dose effect" on longevity. Even as little as 15 minutes of exercise a day, she found, was linked to a significant reduction in mortality, though 45 minutes was the best.

GENETICS: THE UN-EQUALIZER

Overwhelming as the evidence for exercise is, there's a wrinkle. Exercise isn't as effective in some people as in others—the same amount of exercise benefits some of us a great deal more than others.

In 1992, Claude Bouchard, an exercise physiologist and geneticist, started the Heritage Family Study with colleagues at five institutions in the United States and Canada. The idea was to see which genes might underlie the differences in response to exercise. So far, Bouchard's project has produced more than 160 published papers, with more in the pipeline.

Bouchard began by recruiting 742 healthy, sedentary people aged 17–65, testing them on cardiovascular and other variables. His trainers put them through an exercise program for 20 weeks, then retested them. The participants included whites and blacks, men and women, and parents and children from the same families.

Some people showed a big improvement in "VO2max," a measure of aerobic capacity, that is, the body's ability to use oxygen efficiently. But others did not. The difference, which ranged from zero to 50 percent, was linked to genetics.

Moreover, even if a person shows impressive gains in VO2max, this didn't necessarily mean that the person would show equally large improvements in other measures, such as blood pressure or HDL, the "good" cholesterol. In fact, concluded Bouchard and his team, one set of genes seems to influence a person's baseline aerobic capacity, while a different set of genes influences how much that person *responds* to exercise training.

Other researchers have confirmed the role that genetics plays in responsiveness to exercise. The bottom line? Many of the differences in response to exercise are associated with genetic factors. For any given person, exercise may act on all, or just a few, of these factors.

THE TAKE-HOME MESSAGE

It's precisely because exercise acts on so many different bodily processes—blood pressure, body fat, lipid profile, insulin, inflammation, to name but a few—that it is so important.

In the next few years, researchers funded by the National Institutes of Health expect to know in much greater detail why physical activity is so beneficial. The massive $170 million, five-year project (un-poetically called Molecular Transducers of Physical Activity in Humans) aims to identify the exact biological molecules that change in response to exercise.

Those ancient philosophers who intuited how powerful exercise could be for health and longer life couldn't have known how right they were. But we do now.

"Nothing—no pill, no other lifestyle measure—has so many multifaceted consequences as exercise," says Bouchard. "Exercise will not prevent you from getting older. But it will maintain your fitness, protect your flexibility and balance, protect your respiratory fitness, normalize or improve your cardio-metabolic profile and play a big role in preventing cognitive decline."

"Exercise is unique."

CHAPTER 3
Sitting Kills

It's not just that physical activity is *good* for you. It's that a sedentary lifestyle, as a totally separate variable, is seriously *bad*. Sitting too much—all by itself—can raise the risk of disease and premature mortality, *even if you dutifully exercise*. In fact, many well-educated people *do* exercise, but they're also more likely to have desk jobs.

A large 2012 study of 240,819 healthy American adults, for instance, showed that more time spent sitting was linked to premature death from heart disease and cancer. *Even among people who exercised more than seven hours a week,* watching TV for more than seven hours a day was linked to a 50 percent greater risk of all-cause mortality and a two-fold greater risk of cardiovascular mortality.

You *may* be able to offset this somewhat with activity. But to wipe it out completely, you have to work out hard for an hour or more every day, as a 2016 study in *The Lancet* showed. That study, a meta-analysis of 13 studies involving more than 1 million people, showed, as expected, that people who sat for 8 hours a day and got almost no exercise had higher mortality rates than people who sat less and were very active. The good news was that sitting for 8 hours a day was *not* associated with higher death rates *if* people were very active—meaning 60–75 minutes of hard exercise a day.

Put bluntly, sitting kills. If you want a short, sickly life, just sit there, for 13 hours a day, like the average American. (In Western countries overall, adults spend 55–70 percent of the day—9–11 hours—just sitting.)

Before you give up in despair, though, contemplate this. Replacing just two minutes of sitting every hour with a bit of moving around helps mitigate the risks of sitting. Better yet, don't sit for more than 30 minutes at a stretch. The main idea here is that sedentary behavior is not just the absence of physical activity, but a distinct behavior with its own health risks. In fact, "sedentary physiology" is now considered a separate field of research from the long-established field of "exercise physiology."

Technically, *sedentary behavior* is defined as any waking behavior characterized by an energy expenditure less than or equal to 1.5 times the resting metabolic rate while in a sitting or reclining position. (Scientists measure activity in METs, or metabolic equivalents. One MET is the amount of energy it takes to sit still; moderate activity burns three to six METs; vigorous activity burns more than six.)

That's different from *physical inactivity*, which is defined as not reaching the recommended 150 minutes per week of moderate-intensity exercise. Physical inactivity, in fact, is believed to be "the biggest public health problem of the 21st century," says Steven N. Blair, a professor of exercise science and epidemiology/biostatistics at the University of South Carolina.

Indeed, physical inactivity causes as many deaths a year globally as smoking.

There's a caveat here: Some research studies, unfortunately, fail to differentiate between sedentary behavior and physical inactivity. And some studies simply *ask* people how much they sit. More rigorous studies track sedentary behavior objectively with accelerometers like Fitbits and smartphones that measure steps taken. Some even track activity with "magic underwear" that contains motion sensors.

BOX 3.1 AN INSPIRATIONAL TALE: THE "BUBBIE" WHO NEVER SAT DOWN

Bessie Kaplan Kemler, aka "Bubbie," my husband's grandmother, lived to be 98. My husband can't remember her ever sitting down.

A first-generation immigrant from Lithuania, Bessie was born in New York City in 1888. She stopped school after eighth grade to work as a bookkeeper, married at 21, and spent the rest of her life cooking, cleaning, and taking care of other people. She and her husband raised four sons and a daughter and might have looked forward to an easier life.

But when her daughter's husband died suddenly at 39 in a furnace explosion, Bessie, by then in her 60s, immediately took in her devastated daughter and took on the job of raising her two grandchildren: my husband, then 9, and his sister, 5.

My husband says his grandmother never sat down, though his sister says Bessie might have sat a little to watch the Lawrence Welk show. The powerhouse of the family, she did even the heaviest household chores, changing storm windows, raking leaves, and shoveling snow, on top of the endless scrubbing, vacuuming, and sweeping.

In her later years, she lived in a third-floor walk-up until three months before she died, when she moved to a nursing home. This sturdy woman, who would not have comprehended the term "sedentary behavior," died peacefully in her bed, just two years shy of her 100th birthday.

THE RISKS OF SITTING

A sedentary lifestyle not only raises the risk of getting many chronic diseases, but increases the severity of these diseases and the risk of dying from them as well.

We'll get to the details of why sitting is so harmful in a minute. The quick version is that sitting triggers a cascade of unhealthy metabolic events. It tends to increase visceral fat. Visceral fat is not an inert blob of tissue, as once thought, but an active organ that pumps out chemicals that lead to chronic systemic inflammation. This leads, among other things, to insulin resistance (a precursor of diabetes), atherosclerosis, and neurological degeneration.

It gets worse. A sedentary lifestyle is also linked to high cholesterol, metabolic syndrome, gallstones, asthma, chronic obstructive pulmonary disease, some cancers, cognitive dysfunction, dementia, osteoarthritis, low back pain, frailty, decreased functional independence, constipation, muscle weakness, chronic inflammation, depression, less healthy levels of triglycerides, HDL (high-density lipoprotein, or "good" cholesterol), and C-reactive protein (a marker for inflammation).

Perhaps most important, sitting too much raises the risk of heart disease, and the more prolonged the sitting, the bigger the risks. In fact, sitting for more than 10 hours a day increases levels of a protein called troponin, a marker for damage to cardiac cells that is normally seen in heart attacks. Sitting too much also raises the risk of blood clots.

Physical inactivity, including sitting, is so lethal—and so common—that it now accounts for an estimated 5.3 million deaths worldwide, according to a landmark 2012 study. That's 9 percent of premature mortality (death before a person's statistical life expectancy), 6 percent of coronary heart disease, 7 percent of type 2 diabetes, 10 percent of breast cancer, and 10 percent of colon cancer. If inactivity were decreased just a bit, by 10 or 25 percent, more than 1.3 million deaths could be averted worldwide.

Sitting and inadequate activity are also very expensive. According to a 2015 analysis, 11.1 percent of healthcare expenditures in the United States were associated with inadequate exercise. This could well be an underestimate since the researchers looked only at inadequate activity, not sedentary behavior per se. Worldwide, an analysis of 142 countries showed that physical inactivity cost a whopping $53 billion in 2013. This, too, may be an underestimate, because it tracked only physical inactivity, not sitting.

Even just standing—not exercising, but simply not sitting—would reduce premature deaths from all causes, a study of 16,586 Canadian adults showed. (Sadly, there's little evidence that standing desks help much.)

The case for the lethality of sitting has been building for decades. Way back in 1955, when President Dwight Eisenhower had a heart attack, his physician, Paul Dudley White, stunned fellow doctors and laypeople alike by telling Ike to get out of bed and move instead of spending the traditional six months in bed. It worked—vigorous cardiac rehab is now the order of the day.

Intrigued by Eisenhower's recovery, other doctors began documenting the dangers of bed rest. By 1965, they had shown that continuous bed rest was linked to postural hypotension (low blood pressure when standing up), tachycardia (rapid heart rate), kidney stones, loss of skeletal muscle, muscle weakness, pressure ulcers, osteoporosis, constipation, deep vein thrombosis, blood clots in the lungs, pneumonia, and difficulty with urination, among other things. Even short-term bed rest has now been linked to adverse changes in blood lipids, increased blood pressure, and impaired function of tiny blood vessels—and that's in healthy people. Bed rest for nine days has even been linked to adverse changes in the body's ability to produce mRNA (messenger RNA), which affects many biological pathways.

On the heels of the Eisenhower story, Texas researchers embarked in 1966 on what is still one of the most dramatic studies on the perils of sitting, the Dallas Bed Rest Study. The researchers, from the University of Texas Southwestern Medical Center, asked five healthy 20-year-old men to spend three weeks in total bed rest—no getting up at all, even to use the bathroom. The initial idea was to use bed rest as a model for weightlessness in space. The researchers kept track of many variables, including changes in VO2max, a measure of aerobic capacity measured in milliliters per kilogram of body weight per minute.

Thirty years later, the Texas researchers, among them Benjamin Levine, rounded up all five of the men. Levine is now director of the Institute for Exercise and Environmental Medicine at Texas Health Presbyterian, Dallas, and professor of medicine and cardiology at the University of Texas Southwestern.

The men, by then aged 50 or 51, were still remarkably healthy. Once again, they were put through numerous tests, including exercise tread-mill tests and VO2max. The astounding conclusion? *The three weeks of bed rest in 1966 caused a greater deterioration in cardiovascular and physical work capacity than 30 years of aging.* Still curious, the Texas research-ers studied the men *again* 10 years later, when they were aged 59–60. Again, the researchers concluded: *The decline after 40 years of aging was comparable to that experienced after three weeks of bed rest at the age of 20.*

"Much of what we think is an inevitable consequence of aging," says Levine, "is actually due to deconditioning."

BOX 3.2 AN INSPIRATIONAL TALE: THE SWIMMER WHO FLUNKED RETIREMENT

On June 17, 2017, Pat Gallant-Charette, a 66-year-old retired nurse and full-time caretaker of three young grandchildren, became the oldest woman to swim the English Channel.

It was just one of the open water world records for Gallant-Charette, who left Dover, England, at 4:55 a.m. and stood up on the sandy beach 18 hours later in Cap Blanc, France.

As we chat, she cheerfully rattles off her six world records as the oldest woman swimmer in marathon swimming events: the English Channel, North Channel between Northern Ireland and Scotland, Molokai Channel in Hawaii, Lake Ontario, Catalina Channel in California, and the Tsugaru Strait in Japan.

She's got one swim left in the "Oceans 7," the Holy Grail for open water swim-mers: Cook Strait, a 14-mile swim in New Zealand. After that, her next challenge is the Still Water 8, said to be the eight most challenging swims in the world.

She's still surprised at becoming a champion swimmer later in life.

"I was a spectator mom for years," says Gallant-Charette, who grew up in Maine, one of eight kids. She married at 21 and had two children. "The years went by. I got my bachelor's degree and worked as a nurse. I didn't have any dreams. I was just so busy, caught up in life."

Then, when she was 46, her adored younger brother, Robbie, died suddenly of a heart attack at age 34. Soon afterward, her 16-year-old son, Tom, announced that, to honor Robbie, he was going to do the 2.4-mile Peaks to Portland swim across Casco Bay.

"Tom, that's so sweet! I wish I could do the same," she told him.

"Ma, you can, if you try," he answered.

"That was a turning point in my life. I was filled with much self-doubt," she recalls. "I hadn't been swimming for nearly 30 years." But she started training. It took her a year to qualify. But at 47, she attempted the swim.

"I was overwhelmed, intimidated by the whole thing. I had a fear of ocean swimming. All these young athletes were ahead of me. Then something clicked. Casco Bay was beautiful, seeing the sky, the seagulls, a lobster boat going by."

She was hooked. She soon realized that she was blessed with an unusual ability to recover quickly from big races, snagging better and better times. She began having the strongest swims of her life.

Two years ago, though, she retired from nursing, eager to relax and finally do the arts and crafts she'd been putting off for years. It was a disaster.

And an epiphany.

"I did that for a week, sitting almost that whole week. I felt like I aged overnight. It was an eye-opener. Here I am, this great endurance swimmer, and I'm sitting there. After one week of arts and crafts I felt like a 100-year-old woman walking across the kitchen. You can't sit for eight hours knitting or sewing or reading. You have to get up and move."

The famous Texas bed rest study piqued interest in sedentary behavior among researchers around the world.

In the 1992 Copenhagen Male Study, Danish researchers followed 4,999 men aged 40–59 for 17 years, assessing their fitness, physical activity levels, and mortality. If a man was very fit *but also sedentary*, the team found, he was not protected against ischemic heart disease and all-cause mortality.

In 2009, American and Canadian researchers studied 17,013 Canadians aged 18–90. After 12 years of follow-up, they found a direct link between time spent sitting and death from all causes, as well as deaths from cardiovascular diseases. This link held up even after accounting for sex, smoking status, body mass index, *and physical activity level.*

A 2010 study of 53,440 American men and 69,776 American women came to the same conclusion after 14 years of follow-up. Sitting for more than six hours a day was linked to higher total mortality, *regardless of physical activity level.* A 2012 study of more than 200,000 adults similarly showed that prolonged sitting raised the risk of all-cause mortality, *independent of physical activity.*

In a whopping 2013 study, an international team pooled the results of six studies involving 595,086 adults. Again, more sitting was linked with more all-cause mortality, *even after taking physical activity into account.*

In an even larger 2014 study involving 800,000 people, sedentary folks had a 50 percent higher risk of dying prematurely. Not surprisingly, the risk of being sedentary is just as true—if not more so—for women and for blacks.

Finally, in 2015, a huge University of Toronto review and meta-analysis of 47 studies found that greater sedentary time was linked to an increased risk of all-cause mortality, cardiovascular disease mortality, cancer mortality, cardiovascular disease incidence, cancer incidence, and type 2 diabetes incidence, *regardless of physical activity.*

The take-home lesson is unmistakable: Unless you work out really hard for an hour or more a day, you can still be at risk of bad health outcomes and increased risk of death if you sit for the rest of your waking hours.

WHY SITTING IS SO DANGEROUS

To be honest, it's not fully clear exactly *why* sedentary behavior is so unhealthy, partly because, while researchers have been studying exercise physiology for decades, they have only recently begun probing the effects of sitting still.

But there are already some clues. For starters, think evolution.

Obviously, we did not evolve to sit in cars, at desks, or to hunt and gather in supermarkets. We evolved walking around on two feet and chasing bison over cliffs.

Yet we still have the genes of our active ancestors. Which means that today, with our sedentary lifestyles, we expend much less energy every day than they did. Even the few remaining hunter-gatherers today expend at least 600 calories a day more than the average sedentary American.

The most visible consequence is the rise of obesity, defined as having a BMI, or body mass index, of 30 or more. Currently, 35 percent of adult men and 40.4 of adult women are obese. Kids are fat these days, too—among children aged 2–19, 17.0 percent are obese and 5.8 percent are extremely obese.

Sitting makes us fat because it lowers the amount of food that is converted into energy. This excess body fat then raises the risk of heart disease, diabetes, arthritis, and some cancers in multiple ways.

So let's look at some of those pathways.

Scientists have long known that obesity is the main driver of diabetes, especially type 2 diabetes, the most common form in adults. Diabetes now afflicts more than 100 million Americans.

The key actor here is fat. Fat tissue, especially the deep belly fat called visceral fat, doesn't just sit there. It is metabolically active, pumping out chemicals called adipokines that trigger inflammation and suppress insulin pathways. The result is that the body becomes less responsive to insulin, a condition called insulin resistance or insulin insensitivity, which can lead to diabetes. Put bluntly, visceral fat triggers insulin resistance and, ultimately, diabetes.

It's worth pausing for a moment on insulin. Insulin, which is made in the pancreas, is one of the most crucial hormones in the body. Its basic job is to take sugar out of the blood and escort it into muscle and other cells where it is needed. But insulin also does something else: It shuts *off* the ability of the liver to make glucose when glucose is not needed in the circulation, notes C. Ronald Kahn, a senior investigator at Boston's Joslin Diabetes Center.

The system works like this: To get glucose (sugar) out of the blood and into each cell, it has to be conveyed across the cell's membrane. This is done by proteins called glucose transporters.

But not all glucose transporters are alike. Some, like those on liver and pancreas cells, are passive; they simply let glucose flow in freely. Others, like those on fat and muscle cells, only let glucose into a cell if insulin binds to nearby insulin receptors. This binding then signals the glucose transporter to release its glucose into the cell.

If a person fails to make enough insulin or if insulin receptors become insensitive to insulin, blood sugar rises. Things get particularly nasty when insulin resistance occurs in muscle, fat, and liver cells. This happens when fatty acids and triglycerides, which are triggered by excess visceral fat, are high.

Here's the cool part.

Exercise makes muscles more sensitive to insulin, which in turn reverses insulin resistance and lowers blood sugar levels. The really interesting thing is that exercise allows glucose to enter muscle cells even when there's no insulin around, a major way in which exercise combats high blood sugar and diabetes. It's almost as if exercise were insulin.

By contrast, sitting around and not exercising pushes the system the other way, triggering the loss of insulin sensitivity in skeletal muscles and the body as a whole. Indeed, physical inactivity is one of the most important proximal behavioral causes of insulin resistance.

An Australian study illustrates the point. In that study, 67 men and 106 women without diabetes wore accelerometers (activity monitors) on their trunks and shoulders during all their waking hours for seven consecutive days. They were also tested for blood sugar levels. The results? The more time they spent sitting, the more their blood sugar levels rose. In a Finnish experiment with 10 pairs of identical male twins in which one twin exercised regularly and the other did not, researchers found significantly better glucose metabolism in the active twins.

It's a shockingly sensitive system. Even in studies of superbly trained men with excellent insulin sensitivity, that sensitivity drops after as few as 38 hours without exercise to the levels of sedentary people. In fact, even just one day of sitting—in young, healthy, fit men and women—can lead to insulin dysregulation unless caloric intake is reduced to match reduced physical activity.

Sitting is even bad for thin folks—sitting after a meal leads to a spike in blood sugar. Getting up after a meal can cut such spikes in half. Indeed, standing up and walking around just a little can double energy expenditure within minutes.

In many other ways, too, sitting and moving around activate quite different metabolic pathways. Sitting leads to negative changes in artery function and structure, for instance, while physical activity remodels blood vessels in a healthy direction.

Not surprisingly, sitting has some of its worst effects on muscles, just as, inversely, exercise exerts some of its best effects via muscles. Prolonged sitting, for instance, can make muscles so weak that you get a painful curvature of the back. Sarcopenia, or muscle wasting, is another major risk of sedentary behavior. (So is winding up in a nursing home if your leg muscles get so weak that you can't get on and off the toilet seat by yourself.)

BOX 3.3 THE TRAGIC TOLL OF TOO MUCH TV

Among the biggest contributors to sitting too much are those ubiquitous screens—for TV, video games, and computer work.

In 2008, Australian researchers reported on a study of 2,031 men and 2,033 women, all of whom met the recommended guidelines for physical activity, spending at least 2.5 hours a week in moderate to intense exercise. But many also spent a lot of time watching TV. Result? There was a linear association between TV watching and increasing waist circumference, systolic blood pressure, blood sugar levels, and other variables.

Indeed, a strong association between too much TV and all-cause mortality has since been shown over and over. Too much TV has also been linked with some cancers.

Interestingly, sitting around watching TV may be worse than sitting at work, perhaps because people eat and smoke more while watching TV than while working. In one Harvard study, each two-hour increase in TV watching was associated with a 23 percent increase in obesity and a 14 percent increase in diabetes, while each two-hour increase in sitting at work was associated with only a 5 percent increase in obesity and a 7 percent increase in diabetes.

In Hawaii, researchers tracked 61,395 middle-aged men and 73,201 middle-aged women of different ethnicities for an average of 13.7 years. For women of all ethnic groups (except Japanese), time spent sitting in front of the TV was linked to overall and cardiovascular mortality, while sitting at work was not. For men, this link did not hold up, possibly because men and women behave or snack differently while watching TV.

Sitting too much also means that you miss out on some of the most important benefits from using your muscles. Just as visceral fat is now known to be a metabolically active organ, muscles, too, are now seen as busy chemical factories, pumping out hormones called myokines that have powerful anti-inflammatory effects. (See Chapter 6.) Altered myokine function, in fact, is a major link between sedentary behavior and chronic diseases.

The list of woes goes on. Sedentary behavior is linked to a failure of mitochondria, the tiny energy factories inside cells. (See Chapter 5.)

It may also affect telomeres, which are powerful markers of health and longevity. (See Chapter 13.) Telomeres are tiny regions of DNA that sit on the ends of chromosomes, like the caps on the ends of shoelaces. Their job is to keep DNA from unraveling during cell division. As we age, it's normal for telomeres to get shorter and shorter.

But sedentary behavior may have an adverse effect on telomeres. In a recent Swedish study, researchers recruited a group of sedentary, overweight men and women, all aged 68, and took blood samples. They then told half the group to start a modified exercise program and to sit less. The other half was told to try to lose weight and generally be healthy. Six months later, both groups went back for blood tests.

The group that had begun exercising and had reduced sedentary time showed remarkably longer telomeres than six months earlier. Telomeres in the control group got shorter. But here's the fascinating part. It didn't seem to be exercise per se that held the magic. It was sitting less. Within the exercise group, people who simply stood up more often appeared to show the most beneficial effect on telomeres.

A 2015 University of Mississippi study involving 6,405 people compared telomere length and "screen time." For every hour increase in sedentary screen time, there was a 7 percent increase in the likelihood of having the lowest telomere lengths. Sedentary behavior was also linked to shorter telomeres in other studies.

There are, of course, many other mechanisms by which sedentary behavior accelerates the deterioration of our bodies. But for now, it's time to move on.

In the chapters to come, we will focus on more positive things—the many and varied ways that exercise changes our organs, tissues, cells, genes, and molecules in a healthy direction, offsetting at least some of the downward slide of aging.

So hang in there. The best is yet to come.

CHAPTER 4

The Heart of the Matter

SUPERSTARS

Katherine Beiers was 85 when I spoke with her not long ago from her home in Santa Cruz, California. She cheerfully admitted that she looks her age.

But she sure doesn't act it. Beiers has run 41 marathons since her first at age 51 in 2003. She's run the last 10 in a row, including a horrifying finish that didn't count in 2013 when the bombs went off at the Boston Marathon.

"My son was running it, too, two and a half hours ahead of me," she recalled. "I could see the finish line, I almost got there. But the runners were coming toward me. I realized something big had happened, there were sirens, helicopters, and runners crying and upset."

Like many runners from that marathon, Beiers immediately went back the next year, and the next, and the next. In 2017, at 84, she was the oldest runner in the event, finishing in 6:04:07, a time she remembers precisely and that the Boston Athletic Association, which organizes the race, confirms. There were six guys over 80 in that race, too, but they were all 83 or younger.

It takes grit to run a marathon at any age, but especially as one gets older. Then again, no one would ever accuse Beiers of lacking grit.

She was 29 and living in France with her husband, an Air Force physician, when he was killed in a plane crash. Suddenly a widow with three kids under age four—the youngest was just nine days old—she gathered up the kids and moved back to live with her sister in Los Angeles.

After a few years, she hungered for a small town in which to raise her kids, and drove around California looking for the perfect place. She found it—Santa Cruz. A former children's librarian in Brooklyn, New York, she began working on a Master's in Library Science, soon landing a job as a librarian at the University of California, Santa Cruz.

The Santa Cruz campus was "so beautiful, a national park," she told me. In her mid-40s, she started going out for a run on her lunch hour. "It took me three months to run a mile without stopping," she laughed. "I never thought I'd do two miles. But five other runners took me under their wing. I knew so quickly that this was what I was looking for. I had energy in the afternoon. I felt good about myself. I had something other than work and kids."

She went on to become second in command at the library, mayor of Santa Cruz, and, of course, a marathoner. These days she walks up the hills, but still runs five or six miles four days a week, except in pre-marathon season, when she cranks it up to a couple of 20-mile runs a week. "I can run 10 miles and play bridge that night with people a lot younger," she says. I could almost hear her grin over the phone.

In 2017, after running Boston, she flew to Paris the next night, met a friend, and hopped on a train to Spain, where she spent the next 36 days walking the Camino de Santiago, 15 miles a day for 500 miles. She was the oldest person. No problem.

"I was in really good shape."

Beiers, of course, is not the only older athlete to be not just inspirational, but proof that the human body is capable of a lot more than we typically expect. True, Beiers and other geriatric superstars are statistical outliers, the extreme end of the fitness curve. But the sheer fact that such highly fit older people exist shows that decrepitude isn't nearly as inevitable as we often assume.

Harriette Thompson, for instance, a runner from North Carolina who has cancer and didn't even take up running until her 70s, finished the 2015 San Diego Rock 'n' Roll marathon in an unofficial time of 7:24:36. She was 92, the oldest woman to run competitively for 26 miles 385 yards. Two years later, at 94, Thompson became the oldest woman to finish a half-marathon.

Cincinnati marathoner Mike Fremont has also battled cancer. In fact, when he was 70, he thought he had just three months to live. But he changed his diet, hung on, and in 2017, at age 95, was still going strong. In fact, he holds the world record for his age group in both the half and full marathons.

And of course, there's Boston's Johnny Kelley, a legendary figure for years. There's now a statue downtown entitled "Young at Heart," depicting Kelley as a 27-year-old winning his first Boston Marathon and at 84, crossing the finish line for the last time. In all, he ran 61 Boston Marathons, and at age 65, quipped to the *New York Times*, "For me, the race these days is to try to beat the girls to the finish and to wave to all my old friends along the course." He died at age 97.

BOX 4.1 SHOULD FITNESS BE A VITAL SIGN?

Cardiorespiratory fitness is defined as the ability of various organs in the body—including the lungs, heart, blood vessels, and muscles—to take oxygen from the outside world and get it to the mitochondria, especially in muscle cells, to perform physical work. Cardiorespiratory fitness is the most powerful predictor of survival.

Fitness can be, and usually is, measured as VO2max, as gauged by walking or running on a treadmill. VO2max is the maximum amount of oxygen the heart and lungs can efficiently supply the muscles. In general, VO2max declines 8–10 percent per decade, with women's decline slower than men's; the decline accelerates after age 70.

But exercise helps offset this decline. In distance runners aged 60–80, for instance, VO2max is 30–40 percent higher than in non-exercisers the same age. Other studies agree. But genetics counts, too, accounting for as much as 47 percent of a person's VO2max response to exercise.

Fitness can also be expressed in METs, or metabolic equivalents. One MET is the oxygen cost of sitting quietly; 10 METs involves expending 10 times the energy needed at rest.

The gold standard test to measure fitness is running on a treadmill, but this is a fairly expensive method. Medical staff must be present to monitor vital signs and must be ready to intervene if the patient has a heart attack. A cheaper method is to calculate fitness from non-exercise algorithms. A doctor can estimate fitness, for instance, by timing how long it takes a person to walk 400 meters, or, better yet, a longer distance like a mile or two.

But here's the catch. Many physicians do virtually nothing to test patients' fitness, a fact that infuriates exercise scientists, among them Jonathan Myers, an exercise physiologist and health research scientist at the Veterans Affairs Palo Alto Health Care System. Many doctors, he says, were quick to embrace statin drugs to lower cholesterol, a pharmacological fix. But many fail to prescribe exercise, despite overwhelming evidence that even small increases in fitness are linked to 10–30 percent less risk of cardiovascular problems.

Some professional groups have tried to change this. The American College of Sports Medicine has a vigorous campaign called "Exercise is Medicine."

And in 2016, the American Heart Association made a big splash when it announced that fitness should be considered a "vital sign," like body temperature, heart rate, respiration rate, and blood pressure. And, to be fair, that idea is taking hold in some places, including the Kaiser Permanente health system in California. But overall, fitness is still the only major risk factor not routinely assessed at medical checkups.

A little push at the annual physical wouldn't hurt, given that only half of Americans over 18 meet the government's minimum guidelines for exercise, a dismal fact that has economic, as well as health, implications. Inadequate exercise is linked to 11.1 percent of all healthcare expenditures.

FITNESS SAVES LIVES

Surprising as it may seem, older runners are actually the fastest-growing segment in the running world and, not surprisingly, they are a pretty fit bunch. And it's not just runners who are surpassing expectations, but Masters swimmers, hardy cyclists, champion rowers, on and on.

How can so many older athletes like Beiers defy the odds so strikingly? It's not rocket science: They work out, hearts pumping, legs churning, often for the sheer joy of it, day after day, decade after decade. To be sure, many older people have exercise limitations because of musculoskeletal injuries, not cardiovascular problems.

Still, of all the beneficial things that exercise, especially aerobic exercise, can do for the body—and we have seen many in previous chapters—the most important is its effects on the cardiovascular system. That's because cardiorespiratory fitness is the biggest single contributor to a lower all-cause risk of death.

You can think of this the other way around, too. *Poor* cardiorespiratory fitness is a more important risk factor than hypertension, obesity, smoking, high cholesterol, or diabetes in raising the risk of death. Put starkly, among both healthy people *and* those who already have coronary artery disease, the least fit have more than four times the risk of dying from any cause than the most fit. And, of course, there's a vicious cycle at work here, too. People who are healthy to begin with are precisely those who *can* exercise and thereby keep protecting their health, while the less healthy can't.

Researchers are careful, as we'll see in a minute, to separate two things. One is *physical activity*, which is usually measured by people's self-reports of how much exercise they do or, in more recent years, objective studies by accelerometer devices such as Fitbits. The other is *cardiorespiratory fitness*, which is measured by specific, medical tests. Fitness is a better predictor of all-cause mortality. But fitness and physical activity usually go together, and both count. Both are strongly, and independently, linked to decreased heart disease.

The reason is obvious, says I-Min Lee, an exercise epidemiologist at the Harvard T. H. Chan School of Public Health. Heart disease is the leading cause of death in the United States, killing more than 600,000 adults a year, with stroke killing an additional 140,000. Exercise, she says, is powerful precisely because "it can prevent the largest killer."

Other epidemiologists and cardiologists agree, among them Arthur Leon, a professor in the school of kinesiology at the University of Minnesota. "The biggest reason exercise boosts longevity is because of its beneficial effects on the heart," he says, adding that epidemiological studies for 50 years have consistently shown an inverse association between coronary heart disease and regular physical activity or cardiorespiratory fitness.

That's because exercise has a favorable effect on virtually all risk factors of cardiovascular disease. In other words, exercise affects all those things that doctors test to see how our hearts are doing. That includes blood pressure, heart rate, glucose and insulin, lipids such as high- and low-density lipoprotein and triglycerides, and inflammatory markers such as C-reactive protein.

Exercise increases cardiac output and leads to faster recovery from physical work. It protects the lining of blood vessels. It makes blood vessels and the heart bigger and stronger. It prevents the accumulation of proteins that have become stuck together because of excess sugar in the blood. It slows inflammation that leads to atherosclerosis.

To be sure, as we hit our 40s and 50s, "things go south—our hearts and arteries start to shrink and stiffen, which makes hearts less able to pump blood to the muscles," says Benjamin Levine, director of the Institute for Exercise and Environmental Medicine at the University of Texas Southwestern Medical Center.

Once you hit 65, even a year of vigorous training can't fully reverse the *structural* damage from cardiac stiffening, though exercise can make the heart *function* better. "Structure is hard to change," says Levine, who himself has been training regularly for 40 years.

On the other hand, *lifelong* training at the level of competitive Masters athletes—people who have trained for at least 25 years six or seven days a week with at least 30 minutes a day of vigorous activity—completely prevents cardiac stiffening, Levine says. "That level of training keeps the heart and large blood vessels youthful."

Most of us, of course, don't do that level of exercise, or even aspire to. But even modest amounts of exercise (four or five exercise sessions a week throughout life) can prevent some cardiac stiffening. And high-intensity interval training (see Box 4.4) *can* actually "reverse decades of sedentary aging," Levine says

Indeed, after more than five decades of research, the data on the cardio-protective effects of fitness are now so vast, and so compelling, that we need only hit a few highlights here.

To wit:

In 1989, as we noted in Chapter 2, exercise epidemiologist Steven Blair, now at the University of South Carolina, reported on his research involving 10,224 men and 3,120 women. After eight years of follow-up, Blair found that higher levels of physical fitness, as gauged by treadmill tests, clearly delayed all-cause mortality. But the most stunning finding? That just getting out of the least-fit category was key. Since that pivotal study, Blair and his colleagues have kept at it, documenting over and over the powerful link between fitness and lower risk of mortality.

Exercise physiologist Myers has, too. Among more than 6,000 men who were undergoing treadmill testing to detect potential heart problems, Myers found that the best predictor of an increased risk of death (aside from age) was performance on the treadmill test. In fact, he found, every 1-MET increase in treadmill performance was associated with a 12 percent increase in survival. In another study, this one in men aged 65–90, Myers showed that exercise capacity was an independent predictor of all-cause mortality, even in later life.

This pattern has been shown by now in thousands of men and women, with the protective effect of fitness holding up regardless of age, ethnicity, weight, smoking status, alcohol intake, and many other health conditions.

The large meta-analyses clinch the case. In one meta-analysis of 33 studies involving more than 100,000 people, researchers showed that each increment of fitness was linked to a 13 percent lower risk of all-cause mortality and a 15 percent lower risk of cardiovascular disease. Another huge analysis of a 160 randomized controlled trials similarly showed that exercise dramatically raised fitness and other biomarkers of health.

Have you ever wondered where that widely touted goal of getting 10,000 steps a day came from?

It wasn't science, says Harvard T. H. Chan School of Public Health epidemiologist I-Min Lee, who does 13,000 steps a day herself. "It came out of thin air," she says. "The Japanese character for 10,000 looks like a man walking, that's where the number came from."

In reality, getting just 7,000–8,000 steps a day is enough to meet the government guidelines of 150 minutes of exercise per week. "You can even begin to see benefits at half of that, 3,500 steps a day," Lee says.

PHYSICAL ACTIVITY COUNTS, TOO

As with *fitness*, the link between *physical activity* and longevity is also beyond debate, buttressed by hundreds of studies, many involving thousands of people followed for many years. Taken together, the studies show that more aerobic exercise is better than less, and more *vigorous* exercise is better than less vigorous; in other words, there's a clear "dose-response" effect.

Again, a few highlights.

In 1989, a study of more than 3,000 American railroad workers followed for 20 years showed that those who did the most leisure-time physical activity had the lowest risk of death from coronary disease and all other causes. In 1996, Finnish researchers followed more than 1,000 men for up to 10 years and found that those who expended fewer than 800 calories a week exercising had almost three times the risk of all-cause mortality as men who expended at least 2,100 calories a week in exercise.

In 2008, German researchers did a meta-analysis of 33 studies involving 883,372 people. Regular physical activity was linked to a 33 percent reduction in all-cause mortality and a 35 percent reduction in cardiovascular mortality. That amounts to a year or two of additional life. In 2009, a different German meta-analysis of 38 studies also showed a dose-response effect.

In 2017, a huge study of 130,843 people in 17 countries (poor countries as well as rich) found that people who were physically active at work or play had a 28 percent lower risk of death and a 20 percent lower risk of heart attack or stroke. The more exercise a person did, the lower the risk of death.

Finally, the icing on the cake.

Harvard epidemiologist Lee asked 16,741 older women to wear a high-tech accelerometer (fancier than a Fitbit) for at least 10 hours a day for at least four out of seven days. (The device, ActiGraph GT3X+, is worn on the hip and is sensitive enough to pick up movement in all directions.) The results were astounding. As expected, the women who did more physical activity a day had lower mortality rates than those who did less.

But what was dazzling was the size of this effect. Self-report studies, in which people simply try to recall how much exercise they've done, generally show a 20–30 percent reduction in mortality risk with moderate to vigorous exercise. This accelerometer study showed a whopping 60–70 percent mortality risk reduction. Interestingly, light physical activity like slow walking did not reduce mortality rates, a finding that fits with some other research.

BOX 4.3 CUT MORTALITY RISK BY 31 PERCENT

The best way to increase cardiorespiratory fitness is aerobic exercise that involves major muscle groups—in other words, things like running, jogging, cycling, swimming, and dancing in a continuous, rhythmic fashion.

Ideally, exercise should be of moderate to vigorous intensity and should be done at least five times a week for 30–60 minutes each time. But it can also be spread over multiple sessions of 10 minutes or more a day. The government's guidelines call for 150 minutes a week of moderate to vigorous exercise, or 75 minutes a week of intense activity, or some combination that expends as much energy as either regimen alone.

The good news is that even as few as 5–10 minutes of running a day at a 10-minutes-per-mile pace, or 15 minutes a day of moderate-intensity exercise, yield significant cardiac and longevity benefits. The government's minimum guidelines are enough to lower mortality risk by 31 percent. Doubling or tripling the minimum lowers mortality risk by 37 percent. The maximum benefit comes at three to five times the minimum. After that, adding more exercise has diminishing returns, though there's no harm at even 10 times this amount.

FOR HEART DISEASE, TOO?

It's not just healthy people who can extend their life span with exercise. People with cardiovascular disease can, too, though extreme exercise, like hard workouts every day, may pose a risk.

A 2004 British meta-analysis of 48 studies involving 8,940 people with coronary heart disease, for instance, found that exercise-based cardiac rehabilitation was linked to lower all-cause and cardiac mortality.

In 2008, Montreal Heart Institute researchers studied more than 14,000 people with suspected or proven heart disease and found that after almost 15 years of follow-up, people who said they exercised the most had the lowest rates of all-cause and cardiovascular mortality. In 2016, an international research team reviewing 66 studies involving 14,486 participants also found that cardiac rehabilitation reduced heart disease deaths.

And in 2017, a large international team studying 15,486 people with stable coronary heart disease in 39 countries similarly found that more physical activity was linked with lower mortality, a finding echoed by still other researchers.

Exercise may actually be *better* for people with clogged arteries than surgically implanted stents, although stents have recently been shown not to be very effective anyway. In a German study of 101 men with blocked arteries, those randomized to 12 months of exercising for 20 minutes a day had fewer hospitalizations and repeat stent procedures than those only given stents. The cost was less, too.

As for *heart failure*, there's a strong beneficial effect of healthy behaviors, including exercise, for this, too. Heart failure happens when the heart isn't pumping enough to supply oxygenated blood to the rest of the body. The result is fatigue, shortness of breath, and an inability to do normal activities like climbing stairs. People with heart failure may also have a low ejection fraction—the volume of blood that the heart can spurt out with each beat.

It's clear that being physically fit lowers the risk of getting heart failure in the first place, partly by improving VO2max and endothelial function and lowering levels of stress hormones.

In a large study of heart failure risk, Swedish researchers followed roughly 34,000 men and 31,000 women aged 45–83 for 13 years. Being physically active for more than 150 minutes per week, along with not smoking, having normal weight, and eating a modified Mediterranean diet, dramatically reduced the risk of heart failure. Even taken one by one, each of these healthy behaviors significantly reduced heart failure risk.

A team of American and British researchers, who followed more than 4,000 men and women for 21.5 years, came to similar conclusions. So did researchers studying 18,346 Finnish men and 19,729 Finnish

In recent years, many, though not all, studies have shown that HIIT (high-intensity interval training) may lead to greater beneficial changes in cardiorespiratory fitness than moderate-intensity continuous training.

In 2012, Danish researchers studied more than 5,000 healthy women and men aged 21–90 and found that it was the intensity of cycling, not the duration, that had the most benefits for reducing all-cause and coronary heart disease mortality.

The American Heart Association says that both HIIT and longer, more moderate regimens can be effective in increasing cardiorespiratory fitness in healthy people and people with cardiovascular disease.

Some cardiologists are conservative about recommending HIIT for people with preexisting cardiovascular disease lest it trigger adverse events. But a number of studies show that even in people with coronary artery disease, congestive heart failure, metabolic syndrome, and obesity, HIIT can improve cardiorespiratory fitness at least as well as, and often better than, continuous, moderate-intensity training.

The big advantage of HIIT training is that it boosts fitness significantly, despite a much lower time commitment than longer, more moderate workouts. HIIT training may also burn more calories than traditional workouts, especially in the two-hour post-exercise recovery period.

(For more on high-intensity interval training, see Chapter 5.)

women. Researchers studying 84,537 women as part of the Women's Health Initiative agreed.

HOW EXERCISE WORKS

Exercise produces its cardiovascular effects through a variety of mechanisms. In fact, exercise affects so many bodily systems that affect the heart that we can only focus on the main ones here: autonomic tone, platelets and blood clotting, heart rate variability, endothelial function, blood pressure, heart and artery size, inflammation, atherosclerosis, lipids and cholesterol, obesity, glycation, and diabetes.

Granted, this sounds daunting. But this is the heart of the book (pun intended), so let's start with my favorite inspirational tale, about diabetes. Diabetes, as has long been documented, significantly raises the risk of heart disease. Fortunately, diabetes is also one of the diseases most amenable to prevention and treatment by exercise.

Jay Handy is 55 now, handsome and oozing energy. He bounded into a popular Harvard Square restaurant in Cambridge, Massachusetts, recently to meet me, giving me a strong, enthusiastic hug. We hadn't spoken in years since I interviewed him for my weekly health column for The Boston Globe *in 2004.*

Handy was in town for a reunion with his Harvard Business School buddies and I seized the opportunity to connect with him again. As I set up my laptop, Handy started patting his arms. "I have to give myself insulin," he said, chatting all the while. He had an insulin pump attached to his left arm, but he had to move it to different places on his body every three days, so it took a moment for him to remember where it was. He glanced at his blood sugar monitor (the size of a cell phone), then hit a button on a device that told the pump to inject insulin.

It had been 13 years since I first interviewed Handy for my column, which began like this:

"For ordinary mortals, just finishing an Ironman Triathlon is almost unimaginable. You swim 2.4 miles, dodging hundreds of other adrenaline-crazed swimmers, then hop on your bike to pedal for 112 miles, then don running shoes and run, jog or limp your way through an entire 26.2-mile marathon. If you actually want to win, you do this in roughly nine hours."

Jay Handy, at that time 41, not only did all this, he did it with type 1 diabetes, which he had had since age 13. During the race, he had to check his blood sugar every hour, then eat carbohydrates or inject insulin, depending on whether his sugar was too high or too low. He had rigged his bike so that he could prick his finger, dab a drop of blood onto a test strip, and put the strip into a monitoring device taped to his handlebars—all with one hand. Handy finished that marathon, as he put it, "dead last, but still alive."

Back then, Handy was only the third person with diabetes ever to race an Ironman. He has now done four Ironmans, and told me that 3,500 other people with diabetes have now done the race.

Today, Handy works out every day, runs marathons with his wife, still works in finance, and started a biotech company dedicated to curing diabetes with gene therapy. He also meets one-on-one with young diabetic athletes, coaching them on how to manage their diabetes and still compete.

"That's the best," he says, grinning," helping kids learn that they can thrive with diabetes, and that exercise holds the key."

DIABETES

"Why is diabetes so bad?" Timothy Church, an adjunct professor at the Pennington Biomedical Research Center in Baton Rouge, Louisiana, asks rhetorically. "It's a pretty fundamental concept. When you have a stroke, it's in your brain. When you have a heart attack, it's in your heart. When you have cancer, it's in one organ. When you have diabetes, it's in your whole body. Diabetes is basically a failure of the body to control blood sugar."

Cells need sugar, of course. "But high levels of sugar in the *blood* are toxic to every cell, every system in the body," Church says. "If you have diabetes and don't control your blood sugar, you are poisoning every system in the body."

Diabetes, of course, is a serious enough problem in its own right, but it packs an extra punch because of its effects on the cardiovascular system. At least 68 percent of older people with diabetes die from some form of heart disease, and 16 percent die of stroke. Adults with diabetes are two to four times more likely to die from heart disease than adults without diabetes.

"Being diabetic is so bad that in the clinic, we consider someone with diabetes to have the same risk as someone who has already had a heart attack," says Harvard epidemiologist I-Min Lee.

Among other things, people with diabetes do not make as much nitric oxide, the beneficial blood vessel dilator, as people without diabetes. People with diabetes are also subject to increased oxidative stress that can damage the cardiovascular system. And diabetes raises the risk of potentially fatal blood clots.

All of this is exacerbated with age and lack of exercise.

As we age, we face an increased risk of insulin resistance, the precursor to diabetes. In fact, insulin resistance itself is a predictor of cardiovascular disease, though exercise mitigates this risk.

Insulin is the hormone, made in the pancreas, whose job is to take sugar out of the blood and escort it into muscles and other cells where it is needed. Insulin also does something else: It shuts *off* the ability of the liver to make glucose when it's not needed in the circulation.

(For the record, there are two main types of diabetes. Type 1, juvenile diabetes, is a failure of the pancreas to make insulin because the immune system mistakenly attacks insulin-producing cells in the pancreas. In type 2, which is manageable with exercise, weight loss, and medication, the problem is insulin resistance.)

If a person fails to make enough insulin or becomes *insensitive* to its effects, blood sugar levels rise. In that sense, diabetes is a disease of muscles, the largest consumers of blood sugar in the body. When muscles are "happy and chewing up blood sugar all day long, it's great," says

Church. "When muscles are not happy, they ignore insulin and sugar stays in the blood. That's 'insulin resistance.'" And when muscles can't draw sugar from the blood, and blood sugar gets too high, nerves and blood vessels become damaged.

Both aerobic and resistance training can increase glucose uptake in muscle cells, thereby reducing insulin resistance. (By contrast, *not* exercising pushes the system other way, triggering loss of insulin sensitivity. Being both diabetic *and* unfit is truly dangerous—these folks have twice the mortality risk of people who, though still diabetic, are physically fit.)

Exercise helps by making muscles more sensitive to insulin. Exercise can even allow glucose to enter muscle cells when there's no insulin around, notes C. Ronald Kahn, chief academic officer at Boston's Joslin Diabetes Center. Among other things, exercise helps sugar get into muscles by increasing levels of a carrier protein called GLUT-4. Exercise also increases production of a protein called AMPK, which helps break down fats that can interfere with glucose transport molecules.

Not surprisingly, highly fit people have been consistently shown to have better blood sugar control than less fit people. In an Australian study, for instance, 67 men and 106 women without diabetes were asked to wear specialized accelerometers (activity monitors) for seven consecutive days. They were tested for blood sugar levels. The more time they spent sitting, the more their blood sugar levels rose.

It's a shockingly sensitive system. Some data suggest that even in superbly trained men with excellent insulin sensitivity, that sensitivity drops to the levels of sedentary people after as few as 38 hours without exercise. In fact, just one day of sitting—and this is in young, healthy, fit people—can lead to insulin dysregulation unless caloric intake is reduced to match reduced physical activity.

And ponder this: Sitting around after a meal triggers a spike in blood sugar. But getting up after a meal can cut such spikes in half. In other words, it pays to get up and wash the dishes or walk the dog.

OBESITY

There's no way to say this nicely. The United States is a fat, fat, fat country, with 70.7 percent of Americans now officially obese or overweight, according to government statistics. Obesity is defined as a body mass index (BMI) of 30 or more. Overweight is defined as a BMI between

25 and 30. And we're not alone in our excess: Obesity is now the fifth leading risk factor for mortality worldwide.

The exact physiological causes of obesity are complex and interwoven, as are the ways that obesity affects the cardiovascular system, says Church.

But the basic culprit is a no-brainer: too much food and too little exercise = energy imbalance. (For the record, you can lose weight by reducing the former, or increasing the latter, but the math is against you if you try to do it all by exercise. A 160-pound person walking at a 20-minute per mile pace burns just 255 calories in an hour—the calories in one small muffin!)

In biochemical terms, excess body fat is a metabolic disaster. People think of fat as an inert blob of tissue, but the opposite is true. Fat is metabolically active, a genuine endocrine organ that constantly pumps out molecules called cytokines and adipokines. Adipokines shut off normal glucose metabolism, with the result that glucose does not get into cells and stays in the blood, forcing blood sugar up.

"Obesity not only increases CHD [coronary heart disease] directly," write exercise epidemiologists Kokkinos and Myers, "but also enhances it indirectly through its adverse effects on several established risk factors, including insulin resistance and hypertension." Both visceral fat and lack of exercise can trigger insulin resistance.

Indeed, obesity, especially excess abdominal fat, is a major hallmark of metabolic syndrome, a cluster of problems including hypertension, poor lipid profiles, and insulin resistance. About 27 percent of Americans now have "metabolic syndrome," which raises the risk of coronary artery disease. Exercise improves all of the components of the syndrome.

It's not just that exercise combats obesity by burning off excess calories. Vigorous exercise suppresses the hunger hormone, ghrelin, and increases the appetite-suppressing hormone, peptide YY.

GLYCATION

Sugar (glucose) binds to many proteins throughout the body, with often terrible effects. When proteins or fats are exposed to sugar in the blood, the sugar bonds to these molecules, creating so-called advanced glycation end-products, or AGEs. Exercise can reduce AGEs. AGEs affect almost every cell in the body, playing a major role in aging and in direct damage to blood vessels from diabetes. This process, called glycation, "pretty much damages everything it touches," notes Pennington scientist Church.

When sugar binds to collagen, for instance, it leads to "cross-links" between molecules, which results in stiffening of connective tissue and blood vessel walls. When LDL (low-density lipoprotein) particles become glycated, they stick around too long, which is dangerous. And when HDL (high-density lipoprotein), the "good" cholesterol, becomes glycated, it *shortens* the half-life of HDL, making it less protective against atherosclerosis.

Sugar molecules can also attach to hemoglobin. High levels of glycosylated hemoglobin, a hallmark of diabetes, are directly linked to cardiovascular disease, as well as to damage to the retina and nerve pain. Glycosylated hemoglobin is measured with a test called A1C. Hemoglobin is the protein in red blood cells that carries oxygen. Typically, red blood cells live for three months, which is why A1C tests can reflect blood sugar levels over the preceding three months. Each *increase* of 1 percent in A1C is linked to a 28 percent increase in mortality risk, while each percentage point *drop* in A1C is linked to a 35 percent reduction in damage to small blood vessels.

AUTONOMIC TONE

The autonomic nervous system regulates involuntary functions such as heart rate and smooth muscle tone in the intestines. It has two parts, the sympathetic nervous system, which generally revs things up—speeding up heart rate, constricting blood vessels, and increasing blood pressure—and the parasympathetic system, which calms things down, slowing heart rate and relaxing sphincter muscles. Good autonomic tone is a healthy balance between the two.

But chronic imbalance—especially over-arousal of the sympathetic system, which keeps the body in a constant, revved-up "fight-or-flight" state—is a powerful risk factor for adverse cardiovascular events. Exercise helps reverse this. With exercise, the heart contracts more forcefully, increasing blood flow through the arteries, which nudges the system toward a lower resting heart rate, lower blood pressure, and greater heart rate variability. Improved autonomic tone reduces the risk of sudden death with exercise.

PLATELETS AND BLOOD CLOTTING

When a blood vessel is cut or injured, it triggers the activation of tiny platelets, which change from their normal, round conformation to a spiny shape. This allows them to stick to each other and to blood vessel walls.

Platelets then hook up with other proteins to form fibrin strands that form a net. This net catches more platelets along with blood-clotting factors that produce a molecule called thrombin, which helps attach the clot firmly to the vessel wall. Once the blood vessel heals, this process is reversed.

Obviously, blood clotting is a life-saving mechanism. Otherwise we'd bleed to death. But it has a dark side as well. Heart attacks can be triggered when a blood clot breaks off an artery wall and travels to the heart, blocking coronary blood flow. Platelet activation also triggers inflammatory molecules that contribute to atherosclerosis. Although acute exercise sparks an *increase* in platelets and clotting factors, this acute response goes back to normal within hours; regular exercise helps prevent over-activation of platelets.

HEART RATE VARIABILITY

Heart rate variability is controlled by the constant flow of hormones from both the sympathetic and parasympathetic nervous systems. Having high variability in heart rate is a good thing. It means that the heart is able to slow down more quickly after exercise. Overall, people who exercise regularly have higher heart rate variability, fewer adverse cardiac events, and lower all-cause mortality. In contrast, low heart rate variability is powerful trigger of life-threatening arrhythmias.

ENDOTHELIAL FUNCTION: BLOOD VESSEL LININGS

Although it sounds frightening, one of the major things that exercise does is create "shear stress" inside blood vessels. It's the perpendicular force of increased blood flow against vessel walls that causes this stress on the walls, which in turn temporarily increases the risk of cardiac events during exercise, especially in sedentary people.

In the long run, though, there's a beneficial response: the release of nitric oxide (NO), which dilates blood vessels. (If you have trouble remembering the importance of nitric oxide, think Viagra: It's nitric oxide that makes Viagra work, by dilating blood vessels in the penis, allowing more blood in, creating stiffening.)

The improved ability of blood vessels to dilate allows blood vessels to be more elastic, that is, to expand and contract with blood pressure and blood flow. This in turn allows blood to get more readily to skeletal muscles and to the heart. Nitric oxide also makes platelets less sticky, thus less likely to clump together in clots.

"Exercise doesn't physically change the endothelial lining of blood vessels," exercise physiologist Myers says, "but it allows blood vessels to react to stress in a more healthy way." This benefit holds up even in people who already have coronary artery disease.

BLOOD PRESSURE

More than 70 percent of older people have age-related stiffening of the larger arteries, which leads to hypertension, or high blood pressure. Hypertension is a powerful risk factor for stroke, heart failure, coronary problems, and kidney disease. In fact, hypertension is a leading risk factor for death, accounting for almost 13 percent of total deaths in the world.

The risk of death doubles with every 20-millimeter mercury increase above 115 in systolic (the top number) blood pressure, and with every 10-millimeter increase above 75 in diastolic (the bottom number). (In 2017, the American College of Cardiology and the American Heart Association announced a new definition of hypertension—130/80—instead of 140/90, putting nearly half of US adults into the high blood pressure category.)

The good news is that regular aerobic exercise, in older as well as younger people, decreases the stiffness in blood vessels and triggers nitric oxide, which leads to better blood flow and lower blood pressure. Even low-intensity exercise such as walking can reduce blood pressure somewhat. Large prospective studies have shown that fitness is strongly linked to less hypertension, regardless of body weight.

One way exercise accomplishes this is by lowering levels of catecholamines—stress hormones such as adrenaline and noradrenaline. These hormones increase the contractility of the heart, increase cardiac output, and increase the stroke volume (the amount of blood pumped with each heartbeat). These stress hormones go up during exercise, then drop down afterward. Resistance training also reduces systolic and diastolic blood pressure, but not as dramatically as aerobic exercise.

BIGGER, STRONGER HEARTS AND ARTERIES

Exercise increases the flow of blood to the heart by making coronary arteries bigger. It also increases the number of tiny blood vessels (capillaries). In rats, for instance, exercise increases the number of capillaries for each heart muscle from one to three.

Like blood vessels, hearts get bigger with exercise. In trained athletes, the wall of the left ventricle, the main pumping chamber, gets thicker, though this benefit disappears if the athlete stops training. (The enlargement in athletes' hearts is different from, and healthier than, thick heart walls in people with heart disease.) In fact, athletes' enlarged hearts do not lead to long-term cardiac disease—quite the contrary. Older athletes who have trained intensively all their lives have hearts and blood vessels as big and wide open as healthy 30-year-olds.

INFLAMMATION

One of the most important things that exercise does is reduce inflammation all over the body, including in the cardiovascular system. (See Chapter 11.)

Doctors measure inflammation with a marker called CRP (C-reactive protein), which goes up with inflammation. Elevated CRP and inflamed arteries are associated with a higher risk of heart attack, stroke, and death in both healthy people and those with cardiovascular disease. In fact, people with the highest CRP have three times the risk of death as people with the lowest.

Exercise can lower CRP significantly, often by as much as 20–30 percent. In one study, people in the most-fit group had 80 percent lower levels of CRP than people in the least-fit group. This pattern held true regardless of weight and other cardiovascular risk factors.

An acute bout of strenuous exercise temporarily increases CRP, probably due to joint and muscle inflammation, but regular, sustained exercise suppresses it. Exercise also reduces body weight, insulin resistance, and LDL, all of which, if too high, can trigger higher CRP.

In a study of runners training for a marathon, nine months of training yielded a decrease of 31 percent in CRP. Other research shows that people who exercised five or more times a week had 37 percent lower CRP levels than those who exercised once a week or less. In a study of data collected from nearly 14,000 people on a government database, the most active people had CRP levels almost 50 percent lower than sedentary people. Even in people undergoing cardiac rehabilitation, three months of exercise lowers CRP.

ATHEROSCLEROSIS

Atherosclerosis, the buildup of plaque in artery walls, is now seen as a disease of inflammation, also called a "response to injury" process.

The idea is that some factor, often a pathogen or LDL, migrates to the inside of artery walls (the endothelium). As LDL builds up, free radicals (toxic forms of oxygen) land on it. This "oxidized" LDL "looks" like foreign tissue to the immune system, which then attacks it. In this inflammatory reaction, white blood cells called macrophages try to destroy the oxidized LDL by engulfing it, a process that creates so-called foam cells.

The foam cells then become filled with fat and form atherosclerotic plaques, which obstruct blood flow. Plaques lead to clogged arteries to the heart, as well as to clogged arteries in the neck, arms and legs, and kidneys.

Exercise works in part by reducing oxidation of LDL by free radicals. It also decreases triglycerides, a fatty molecule that contributes to plaque. In animals, exercise can actually reverse atherosclerosis. In people, with the exception of a few studies, including research by preventive medicine guru Dean Ornish, it's proved harder to show this effect.

Blocked blood vessels can also cause peripheral artery disease (PAD), which causes pain in the legs during walking. Exercise increases the amount of walking a person can do before calf pain from poor blood flow sets in.

The two best-known types of fats (lipids) in the blood are little pack-ages made of fat on the inside and proteins on the outside—the lipo-proteins. They come in two flavors, LDL, the "bad" cholesterol, and HDL, the "good" cholesterol. (The body makes its own cholesterol, which is needed to produce hormones and vitamin D, and we also get cholesterol from the diet.)

LDL is considered "bad" because it deposits cholesterol on the walls of arteries, where, as we just saw, it can be oxidized. The higher the level of LDL, the greater the chance of heart disease.

In a randomized controlled trial of 217 men and women, Japanese researchers asked half the group to exercise and improve their diets, while the other half did not. After almost a year and a half, the exercise-diet group had better cardiorespiratory fitness and beneficial changes in LDL.

By contrast, HDL is "good" because it takes cholesterol *away* from arteries into the liver, where it is metabolized and excreted or used for digestion. The net effect is a reduction of cholesterol in blood vessel walls. HDL levels above 60 milligrams per deciliter are linked to reduced risk of heart disease.

Here's the important part: Regardless of age, race, or sex, exercise is linked to beneficial effects on blood lipids, in part by boosting HDL, although how big a benefit you get depends partly on genetics.

In one meta-analysis involving more than 1,400 people, aerobic training yielded significant increases in HDL and total cholesterol, regardless of whether people lost weight or not, though the question of whether just raising HDL alone has a causal effect on cardiovascular health is controversial.

In a different meta-analysis, Japanese researchers found that every 10-minute increase in exercise time yielded a measurable increase in HDL; interestingly, in this study, it was the duration of exercise, more than its intensity or frequency, that made the difference. Other researchers have come to similar conclusions.

IS INTENSE EXERCISE EVER BAD FOR THE HEART?

Yes, but only in rare cases. (Sex can count as intense exercise, too, by the way. In a study of 4,557 cases of cardiac arrest, only 34 incidents occurred during or within one hour of sex.)

The incidence of a major cardiovascular problem, including sudden cardiac death during aerobic exercise, is very rare in healthy people, and even in endurance athletes like Olympic marathoners or Tour de France cyclists.

And for most of us, the dutiful joggers of the world? Not to worry. In a study of Rhode Island joggers, the estimated risk is one death during jogging for every 7,620 male joggers per year, or, put differently, one death per 396,000 man-hours of jogging. In a 12-year study of 21,48 male physicians, the risk of sudden death after vigorous activity was also low—one death for every 1.42 million episodes of exercise. For light exercise, the risk was truly miniscule, one death per 23 million person-hours.

Not surprisingly, the risk is higher in people with heart disease, but it's still low: During outpatient cardiac exercise programs, for instance, it's one death in 60,000 participant-hours. (Overall, of course, cardiac rehabilitation *lowers* the risk of mortality by 25 percent.)

To be sure, there has to be *some* level at which harm occurs. Researchers don't yet know where that line is, but they do known that the danger zone is way beyond what most people do. (They also know that the risks vary by sport. In triathlons, which include swimming, biking, and running, most sudden deaths and cardiac arrests occur during swimming, while most trauma-related deaths occur during biking.)

In a 2015 study that followed nearly 38,000 healthy, fit people for an average of 11.5 years, researchers could find no upper limit to the mortality benefit of intense exercise. On the other hand, a different 2015 study involving 1.1 million healthy women followed for nine years found that while *moderately* active women did have fewer coronary events, women who did *daily strenuous* activity had a higher risk of coronary heart disease.

That doesn't totally surprise cardiologists like Missouri's James O'Keefe, who put it this way to *The New Yorker* in 2014: "Darwin was wrong about one thing. It's not survival of the fittest but survival of the moderately fit."

Still, the net result of exercise, by and large, is a good thing. The fitter you are, the less likely you are to die of anything, including a heart attack. As Benjamin Levine, the Texas exercise researcher, writes, "Although it would be foolish to argue that extraordinary endurance training can never be harmful, it is equally inappropriate to frighten individuals who wish to undertake competitive endurance training."

It's true that about one-third of marathon runners experience dilation of two chambers of their hearts, as well as increases in cardiac enzymes and patches of damaged, fibrous tissue in heart muscle, changes that could be an underlying cause of arrhythmias and even sudden death. But many such changes go back to normal without causing problems.

In young people who die during intense exercise, the chief worry is undiagnosed, inherited cardiac abnormalities. With older people, there's concern about atherosclerosis, though there's little evidence that intense exercise accelerates risk, except in people with advanced atherosclerosis who undertake high-intensity training. Atrial fibrillation (a fast, irregular heartbeat in the two upper chambers of the heart) is also a potential concern for older athletes.

But here's the take-home message: In terms of sudden death during exercise, it's being sedentary, then abruptly exercising like crazy, that's the problem. Overall, regular exercisers have less than half the risk of sudden death during exercise as sedentary folks who suddenly exercise.

To be sure, it's not a great idea to exercise if you're in a rage. A 2016 study of 12,461 people found that the combination of hard exercise and emotional upset or anger can raise the risk of heart attack.

But all that means is this: Calm down, then exercise. Regularly.

CHAPTER 5

The Energy-Converting Machine

THE TRACK STAR AND THE MUSCLE TWITCH

Olga Kotelko, a Canadian track and field superstar with more than 30 world records and 750 gold medals to her credit, didn't even start training until she was 77. One of 11 children born to Ukrainian parents who immigrated and ran a farm in Saskatchewan, Kotelko played baseball as a kid, but wasn't a serious athlete. She married young, but the marriage broke up while she was pregnant with her second daughter, after her husband took a knife to her throat.

As a single mom, she earned a college degree at night and taught in a one-room school. When she retired from teaching, she took up slow-pitch softball for a while, but gave up her spot on the team to a 55-year-old.

That's when she got serious, taking up track and field. She kept at it, decade after decade, racking up medals into her 90s, pooh-poohing her osteoporosis and a cancerous tumor (of unknown origin) in her right lung. In 2010, she carried the torch in the Vancouver Olympics, and was still competing a month before her death from a brain hemorrhage in 2014. She was 95.

But what is even more astounding to scientists who study aging and exercise is the strength of Kotelko's mitochondria, the tiny organelles inside cells that pump out energy. Normally, after age 65, people have at least some defective mitochondria.

Not Kotelko. Researchers at McGill University in Montreal took a biopsy of Kotelko's muscle tissue and examined roughly 400 muscle fibers. They couldn't find a single defect—testimony, quite likely, to the power of exercise to beef up and protect our mitochondria.

And to think it all starts with a muscle twitch.

The second you move a muscle—whether starting your morning run, hoisting your toddler onto your hip, or just scratching your head—that one contractile motion starts a remarkable cascade of chemical signals that, ultimately, make you stronger and healthier.

To be sure, this "muscle-centric" view of the world may seem a bit startling. It appears to relegate the stuff we've always regarded as primary—like the heart and lungs—to second-class status, mere "service functions" whose main role is to supply contracting muscles with the necessary fuel and oxygen.

But in truth, it *is* contracting muscles—and their voracious metabolic needs—that actually drive the show.

So, that muscle twitch. Right from the get-go, there's a fork in the road. If you're lifting weights—resistance training—your body goes down one fork, which ends with your muscles getting visibly larger and stronger. (That's the focus of the next chapter, Chapter 6.)

If you take the other fork—endurance exercise like running, walking, or swimming—your body goes down the other trail, which ends up with something invisible to the naked eye but no less important: a dramatic blossoming of mitochondria, the "powerhouses," or energy machines, inside cells that allow you to turn food and oxygen into the energy needed not just for big movements like walking around, but for every cellular function in the body, from breathing to thinking to digesting food to making babies.

Of course, as with everything else in the body, it's a bit more complicated than that. It's not even clear yet exactly how a muscle cell "decides" whether to go the mitochondria (energy) route or the bulking up (hypertrophy) route.

"Everyone in the world is trying to understand that, to understand how endurance exercise leads to mitochondrial biogenesis while exercise with fewer, more intense muscle contractions against resistance leads to hypertrophy," says Dr. Mark Tarnopolsky, a mitochondrial disease specialist at McMaster University.

What *is* clear is that there is some chemical "cross-talk" between the molecular pathways that lead to bigger muscles and those that lead to more mitochondria. Running, for instance, is mostly an endurance activity, but running uphill brings a bit of resistance into the equation.

Similarly, lifting weights is mostly a process of muscle enlargement, or hypertrophy, but if you lift weights fast, that adds an endurance component to the training.

"For most people," says Christopher Gillen, a biology professor at Kenyon College, "there's probably an overlap between resistance and endurance training—their exercise is neither pure resistance nor pure endurance."

You don't have to be a physiologist to see the different methods at work. Just look at bodybuilders and marathoners. The bodybuilders have obvious, bulging muscles. By comparison, the marathoners, though equally or even more fit, look skinny, even cadaveric. But if you could peek inside their muscle cells, you'd be astounded. All those training miles create cells teeming with healthy mitochondria.

We'll get to the specifics of how mitochondria multiply (a process called mitochondrial biogenesis) in a minute. But first, a basic question: Where do mitochondria come from in the first place?

A TINY LIFE FORM GETS EATEN

A freakish thing happened one day, roughly 1.5 billion years ago in the galaxy we call home.

A tiny life form got eaten. Unceremoniously, so far as we know, nothing too violent. Just one little life form quietly swallowed up by a bigger, fancier cell. It's believed that this portentous meal happened only once in all of evolution. The rest is history—the history of us, even of life itself.

That tiny life form, a bacterium, was a primitive little thing. It was a genuine cell, but it didn't have much inside it except a small circle of DNA. Originally the DNA consisted of 1,300 genes, but almost all were "lost," sliding into the cell's nucleus over evolution, leaving a handful of only 13 genes (depending on what counts as a gene) coiled tightly in a circle. But the bacterium that got eaten on that fateful day had a special trick. It could use oxygen—which had been in the atmosphere for about 3 billion years—to make energy from food.

Once this bacterium was swallowed by the bigger cell, it became the organelle (or tiny organ) that we call a mitochondrion, a kind of immigrant guest-worker earning its keep in its new country. It was a happy arrangement—the engulfed bacterial cell was able to rely on the protective environment of its new host, and the bigger, host cell got to use oxygen, by this time abundant in the environment, to make energy.

For more than 100 years, scientists had suspected the ancient origins of this foreign DNA inside our cells. But it was evolutionary biologist Lynn Margulis who fleshed out the story in stunning detail, earning her the National Medal of Science. Her hypothesis is known as the endosymbiotic theory. Other scientists have since fine-tuned the theory.

Among other intriguing things about mitochondria, the mitochondrial genetic material is inherited in all offspring, male and female, only from the mother's egg cells. (Egg cells are crammed full of mitochondria.) That's why, when evolutionary biologists trace human origins back to "Mitochondrial Eve," who is believed to have lived about 200,000 years ago, the genes they track all follow the female line. (There are mitochondria in sperm, too. In fact, that's what gives sperm the energy to swim toward their encounter with an egg, but the sperm mitochondria don't get into the egg at the time of fertilization.)

Mitochondria get passed on when a cell divides—some of the mitochondria wind up in one daughter cell and some in the other, whereupon the mitochondria immediately start making copies of themselves to boost their numbers in their new cellular homes.

But, like all immigrants, mitochondria cling to bits of their own history and maintain a degree of independence inside their host cells. They keep their own biological rhythms, dividing when they "feel" like it, usually when a signal from the host cell raises the alarm that oxygen levels are low. In other words, mitochondrial division is independent of the host cell's cell division cycle. Mitochondria reproduce in their own ways, too: Sometimes they fuse with one another to make one bigger organelle; sometimes they divide in two by fission.

It's a busy life—mitochondria are almost constantly dividing, fusing, and changing shape. They are at their busiest in cells, like muscle cells, that need a lot of energy. In fact, as we'll soon see, it's precisely when a muscle cell contracts that mitochondria "know" they'd better rev up their activity and replicate themselves to produce more energy.

Mitochondria, which are found in differing amounts in different types of cells (liver cells have thousands; red cells, none), are best known for making energy, and we'll get to how they do that in a moment.

But mitochondria also do other important things for the cells they live in, including passing chemical messages around, helping control the cell's life cycle, and, when they sense through molecular signals that the time is right, telling the cell to commit suicide, a process known as apoptosis. They also secrete proteins—including a handful dubbed "SHLP" (pronounced "schlep")—that seem to protect against diabetes and help kill cancer cells.

Like people, mitochondria can get sick. In fact, abnormal, dysfunctional, or damaged mitochondria are a cause of a number of serious illnesses, including cancer and Alzheimer's and Parkinson's diseases.

Not surprisingly, mitochondrial diseases are most severe when the damaged mitochondria are in muscle, brain, or peripheral nerve cells because these cells need more energy than other types of cells. In fact, one of the chief hallmarks of aging—sarcopenia, or muscle loss—is due in part to deleterious mutations in mitochondrial DNA.

Sick mitochondria, as we saw in Chapter 1, are a major hallmark of aging. "In fact, the thinking now is that the demise of mitochondria is responsible for our demise," says mitochondria expert Darrell Neufer, who directs obesity and diabetes research at East Carolina University.

As we age, mitochondria change their normal shapes, becoming rounder; their numbers also decline. Luckily, as Olga Kotelko's example shows, exercise can dramatically offset this decline.

For most of us, mutations in mitochondrial genes eventually pile up with age. And because mitochondrial function is so tightly involved in important chemical signaling pathways in cells, when mitochondria begin to fall apart, life span itself can be affected. In fact, there's talk that doctors may soon begin testing the mitochondrial content of our cells (the so-called bioenergetic health index) to see how healthy, and how old, we actually are.

The good news is that when mitochondria do get sick or damaged— or even when a cell just senses that there are too many mitochondria around—cells have developed an efficient way to get rid of them: garbage disposal, or more elegantly, quality control. The process by which damaged or malfunctioning mitochondria are eaten up is called mitophagy, part of the general process of autophagy. It's the *failure* of this mitochondrial garbage disposal process that is a major hallmark of aging.

THE LITTLE ENGINE THAT COULD

Before we get to the cool stuff—how exercise leads to *massive* increases in mitochondria—let's have a brief tour through the basics. Granted, this is a little technical, but stay with me. It's awe-inspiring to realize that all this energy-producing magic in our human cells came about through evolution.

So, for starters: A muscle cell has three routes—metabolic pathways—to convert the food we eat into the chemicals, that is, the energy, we need to move around.

At any given moment, there's always a small amount of ATP (adenosine triphosphate, the energy molecule) sitting around in the fluid of the cell. There's not a lot of it, just enough to power "a second or two of exercise," notes biologist Gillen. (By contrast, during a 2-hour run, muscles may potentially consume as much as 132 *pounds* of ATP!)

Within seconds of a nerve telling a muscle to contract, the muscle cell uses a goodly chunk of this stored ATP. That means the cell must act quickly to re-synthesize its ATP stores. The first thing the cell tries is a process called the phosphagen system. It's anaerobic; that is, it does not involve oxygen.

At virtually the same time, the second system, glycolysis, kicks in. This involves the breakdown of glucose for fuel. Like the phosphagen system, it is anaerobic. The production of ATP by glycolysis takes place *outside* the mitochondria in the gel-like stuff (cytoplasm) of the cell. This gives us enough energy for 30 seconds to two minutes of exercise—not a lot, but enough to get us started. It also produces lactic acid, which can make muscles sore.

Them comes the big gun, the third, and most powerful, energy-producing system—the aerobic system, which *does* use oxygen and takes place *inside* the mitochondria.

This three-part system is remarkably adaptive. Let's say you're walking slowly to your car. That's aerobic, but it's so mild you don't need to breathe hard and your heart doesn't need to speed up very much. In fact, you could probably keep this low-level aerobic exercise up almost forever.

Then suddenly, you decide to sprint to your car. For this, you need a big uptick in energy to get you through this "rest-to-work" transition. Your heart rate goes up. You breathe harder. Your blood starts transporting this freshly inhaled oxygen to the mitochondria.

But this takes time.

"There's a disconnect between what the aerobic system can supply at this point and what the actual demand is," explains Martin Gibala, a professor of kinesiology at McMaster University. Energy has to come from somewhere, and in a hurry. So the phosphagen and glycolysis systems come to the rescue, anaerobically, to temporarily fill the energy gap.

Finally, as the heart and lungs get *lots* more oxygen to the mitochondria, the aerobic energy system cranks up for real. The need for more energy drives the system, or, as Neufer, the East Carolina University mitochondria expert, puts it, "As soon as demand goes up, the mitochondrial wheel turns faster."

It's a beautiful thing, when you think about it, this intricate energy-conversion system. Without such an elegant system, we could not survive, much less run marathons. And at the heart of it are these tiny organelles, the mitochondria.

Every mitochondrion in the body is built the same. It has a fatty, skin-like outer membrane, a bit of space, then, deeper inside, a fatty inner membrane that is curled up like rotini pasta. The many folds of the inner membrane provide lots of surface area for the machinery of energy production to work.

Embedded in each stretch of the inner membrane are five "protein complexes." Each of these protein blobs, awkwardly shaped like a Nestle's "Chunky," straddles the membrane in such a way that one part of each "Chunky" sticks out on one side of the membrane and the other part sticks out on the opposite side.

Lined up in single file, the five protein complexes comprise the electron transport chain. It's a biological assembly line Henry Ford himself would have been proud of. (As mystery buffs may know, it doesn't take much to bring this entire assembly line to a grinding halt—a single dose of cyanide will do the trick.)

In this assembly line, electrons (negatively charged particles) are passed hand to hand, like the baton in a relay race, from one Chunky complex to the next. As this happens, protons (positively charged particles) slip into the space between the two mitochondrial membranes. The protons then flow *back* across the inner membrane, driving an enzyme called ATP synthase to make ATP. This process is so efficient that the chemical energy from one molecule of glucose is turned into 32 molecules of ATP. But it's a delicate dance, keeping the electron chain humming along. Things can go wrong at any step along the way.

BOX 5.2 FROM CANDY BARS TO ENERGY

In slightly more detail, here's how it actually works.

Start with, say, a candy bar, although all three major types of food—carbohydrates, fats, and proteins—can be used for energy.

The sugar in the candy bar is first taken apart in a 10-step process—that's the glycolysis system we mentioned earlier. The result is a substance called pyruvate. Like a player on a chess board, pyruvate has two possible moves once it's formed. It can head to a mitochondrion to propel the process of aerobic metabolism. Or it can go on a different pathway and be converted to lactate; this happens when the demand for oxygen is greater than the supply. (The terms "lactate" and "lactic acid" are used interchangeably, even though they do not exactly describe the same molecule.)

For now, let's assume the pyruvate is headed for the mitochondria. It is first transported into the mitochondrion, then chemically transformed into a substance called acetyl CoA, which kicks off the famous Krebs cycle, also known as the citric acid cycle or the TCA cycle.

Compounds produced by the Krebs cycle are then transported to the electron transport chain, which works by passing electrons along from one complex to the next. Oxygen is needed to react with the electrons as they move through the chain. The process is called oxidative phosphorylation.

If there is not enough oxygen around—which happens if you're exercising so hard that your body can't supply oxygen fast enough to meet the demand for energy—it needs to rely more on anaerobic sources. This point is reflected in the so-called anaerobic or lactate threshold, the point at which lactate levels start to rise exponentially in the blood.

At this point, the other pathway for pyruvate kicks in. Instead of pyruvate going into the Krebs cycle, the cell uses the pyruvate to produce lactate. It's kind of a rescue mission. When there's not enough oxygen to make ATP the normal way, the cell uses its pyruvate anaerobically. You can't fail to notice this development when you're exercising at your max—you're gasping for air, everything hurts, and your "perceived exertion" is extreme, as Gillen notes. Despite its bad reputation among athletes, lactic acid is actually a fuel.

Acute endurance exercise is fueled primarily from the oxidation of fats and carbohydrates. With lower-intensity exercise, the body uses mostly free fatty acids. As the intensity of exercise goes up, the body relies increasingly on intramuscular glycogen, the predominant fuel for exercising at more than 65 percent of VO2max.

The other important thing that happens during normal, aerobic energy production is that free radicals, toxic forms of oxygen, are produced. Chronically elevated levels of free radicals are bad—they lead to a number of neurological disorders, as well as DNA damage and other problems. But if free radicals are stimulated in a pulsed fashion—as happens with exercise—this leads to production of natural anti-oxidants, which is good.

One implication is that, because pulsed production of free radicals is good, anti-oxidant supplements are not a good idea because they offset many of the benefits of exercise!

EXERCISE MASS-PRODUCES NEW MITOCHONDRIA

I'm up on the starting block, staring at the Harvard University pool. The stands go quiet. It's the annual US Masters Regional swim meet. I've been training hard for months. Glory—and the chance to go to Nationals—all depend on how fast I can swim 1,000 yards, a bit more than half a mile.

"Swimmers, take your mark!"

The gun goes off. I fly off the block, dolphin kick like mad underwater, surface, right arm starting the stroke as it breaks the water.

I churn through the water, settling into my pace. I'm breathing hard but rhythmically, not gasping, flipping my turns at the wall. It seems to take forever, then, suddenly, the race is over.

I did it! I'm not even too tired! How did this happen?

A tiny, but important, molecule I had not even heard of at the time—PGC-1 alpha—made me a champ.

PGC-1 alpha was discovered about 20 years ago by Bruce Spiegelman, a professor of cancer biology at Harvard Medical School. It is the coordinator of a cascade of chemical reactions inside muscles that runs the process called mitochondrial biogenesis, the creation of new mitochondria.

It's this creation of new mitochondria, which is induced by endurance training, that allowed me to swim so hard and long without serious fatigue.

"Flies that can't make PGC-1 alpha can't fly because flight is so energy demanding," notes Spiegelman, a runner who presumably has loads of PGC-1 alpha himself, not just from running, but from weightlifting and kickboxing, too.

To be sure, none of this was obvious until the mid-1960s, when John Holloszy, a physiology professor at Washington University in St. Louis, began wondering exactly what was going on inside the muscle cells of rats running their little hearts out on tiny treadmills. Before then, scientists had a general idea that endurance exercise was good for you for many reasons, including getting more blood to tissues and strengthening the cardiovascular system.

But what Holloszy saw under his microscope was astounding.

As he wrote in a breakthrough paper in 1967, Holloszy found that, compared to rats who lolled around all day, rats who ran strenuously on treadmills had lots more mitochondria in their muscle cells. Because of all these mitochondria, the running rats were able to produce more energy, that is, more ATP. Interestingly, as Holloszy discovered, this explosion of new mitochondria only happens if the rats run long, hard, and regularly, not if they just do mild exercise.

Holloszy kept at it. In 1984, he showed that as a consequence of greater numbers of mitochondria induced by endurance exercise, muscles in trained animals are better able to use blood glucose and glycogen (a stored form of glucose) and to rely on fat for energy when they need to.

Since Holloszy's groundbreaking work, other scientists have taken up the challenge of piecing together the exact molecular steps between endurance exercise and the creation of new mitochondria. Among these molecular sleuths is muscle physiologist David Hood of York University in Toronto.

What happens, explains Hood, is this: A signal from a nerve causes a muscle cell to "depolarize," that is, to change voltage across its membrane. This depolarization then causes the muscle cell to release a flood of calcium from its hiding place in a structure called the sarcoplasmic reticulum. In turn, this flood of calcium causes the muscle to contract. (High-intensity exercise in particular boosts this process.)

All of this happens very fast. Literally within milliseconds of being released, calcium is sucked back into the sarcoplasmic reticulum. This happens again and again, with each flood of calcium triggering the mitochondria to start working harder. The very first muscle contraction triggers all the steps that eventually lead to the creation of more mitochondria. (A grisly little tidbit: If calcium didn't flow in and out of the sarcoplasmic reticulum but stayed in the fluid of the cell, the cell would be in a hyper-contracted state all the time—exactly what happens with rigor mortis when a person dies.)

But here's the thing: New mitochondria are only created in muscles that you use—if you pedal a bike with just one leg, the muscles in your other leg won't get new mitochondria. This makes sense, notes Hood, given that "mitochondrial adaptations produced by exercise are initiated by stimuli within the contracting muscle."

What's really cool is how a muscle cell figures out when it's time to crank its mitochondria up a notch. What happens is that, as muscles contract, mitochondria wake up and go on high alert, "sensing" (chemically) that they need to work harder. They do this by "noticing" a change in levels of one cellular chemical relative to another.

This change in the chemical balance is an alarm bell. It tells the cell that there is "an energy crisis, a threat to homeostasis. Cells don't like to lose energy—it's a metabolic stress," says McMaster University mitochondrial disease specialist Tarnopolsky. The change in chemical balance then triggers an important chemical called AMPK.[1,2]

---

1. AMPK is 5' adenosine monophosphate-activated protein kinase.
2. AMPK is normally triggered by exercise, but it can also be triggered by a drug called AICAR. Interestingly, AMPK from muscles also seems to explain why even the skin of endurance exercisers looks healthier and younger.

AMPK (along with another chemical called p38MPK) kicks off mitochondrial biogenesis by revving up yet more molecules, most importantly, the one that made me a champ in the pool: PGC-1, the central player in orchestrating the body's adaptation to exercise.[3] PGC-1 alpha is a kind of genetic galvanizer: It tells genes—both genes in the cell's nucleus and those in mitochondrial DNA—to start making those Chunky protein complexes for the electron transport chain. It's an awesome process, managing moment-to-moment coordination of the two separate genomes, nuclear and mitochondrial.

Both genomes have to be involved because each protein complex in the electron transport chain is a hybrid, made up of proteins from genes in the cell's nucleus and proteins made from the genes of mitochondrial DNA. It's no mean trick for a cell—making proteins from two different genomes at the same time. A mistake at any step in the process can lead to a defective electron transport chain and thus the failure to make sufficient energy.

Yet we do it every day.

Once the newly synthesized proteins are formed into protein complexes, the complexes are plunked gently into their proper places in the inner mitochondrial membrane, ready to start churning energy through the electron transport chain. (Exercise is the major way to stimulate new mitochondria, but in the lab, scientists can use electrical stimulation of muscle cells to do the same thing. Exposure to cold temperatures also stimulates PGC-1 alpha, but sitting naked in a freezer might be less attractive, even to non-exercisers, than going for a walk or a run.)

PGC-1 alpha is such an important player in all this that when scientists artificially ramp up PGC-1 genes in mice, the animals become ultra-endurance champions. Compared to normal mice, they have vastly more mitochondria and can run twice as far before needing to rest.

In fact, PGC-1 alpha can be induced by a single bout of exercise. In general, however, it takes six to eight weeks of hard exercise to generate 30–100 percent more mitochondria. Interestingly, there's some evidence that having a nice massage right after exercise may speed up this process.

The evidence for the benefits of abundant mitochondria is overwhelming.

---

3. PGC-1 alpha is peroxisome proliferator-activated receptor gamma coactivator 1-alpha. There are actually at least two forms of PGC-1, alpha and beta, and the beta form may be even more responsive to exercise.

Muscles with a lot of mitochondria are much slower to fatigue. Contrarily, mitochondrial density is much lower in sedentary people, one reason their muscles fatigue easily.

Indeed, muscle cells loaded with mitochondria can offset many of the effects of aging and muscle disuse. Adopting or resuming an active lifestyle can improve mitochondrial function enough to significantly improve endurance and boost muscle mass.

The implication is obvious: Healthy, abundant mitochondria are a must for health and longevity. So now, the question becomes, what's the best way to get more of them?

HIGH-INTENSITY INTERVAL TRAINING (HIIT)

You can tell at a glance that Mark Tarnopolsky, the physician and mito-chondria expert at McMaster University, and his fellow McMaster researcher, kinesiologist Martin Gibala, practice what they preach.

Tarnopolsky is 54, though he looks years younger. Slender, with the taut, coiled energy of a greyhound, he leans back in the chair in his office and ponders a personal question.

"How much do I run? Well, let's see. I exercise seven days a week. On three days a week, I run for an hour or 70 minutes—before and to work. On two other days, I bike for 75–80 minutes. On Saturdays and Sundays, I do two hours of running or cross-country skiing or three hours of biking. Then, every day, I do 200 push-ups and 200 sit-ups. I've done this for 35 years."

His VO2max, the gold standard of fitness, is a phenomenal 70. "When I was young," he adds, a tad ruefully, "it was over 80, at its highest, 87."

A short walk across campus, Martin Gibala, 48, seems barely able to contain his abundant energy. He jumps up and effortlessly demon-strates the deep squats he tells his 83-year-old mother to do every day to stay fit enough to avoid a nursing home. His eyes sparkle when he leaps up again and again to draw diagrams on his white board, illustrating how mitochondria produce energy.

Gibala and Tarnopolsky are among the world leaders in the study of how endurance exercise boosts mitochondrial metabolism and in the hot new specialty of high-intensity interval training—workouts in which you alternate very short but extremely hard, all-out effort with low-intensity exercise or rest.

The goal of interval training is to get the benefits—including increased mitochondria—that you would get from, say, 45 minutes of moderate intensity effort in as few as 10 minutes, and maybe from as little as one minute of exercise.

(Beyond mitochondria creation, if your goal is burning up calories, interval workouts help with that, too. Although you do burn more calories in a 50-minute moderate workout than in a 10-minute interval workout, take heart: You actually burn lots of calories in the recovery period after the interval session, too.)

To say high-intensity interval training is revolutionizing exercise science is an understatement. The main reason people give for not exercising is lack of time—high-intensity interval workouts solve that problem. So long as interval workouts are intense enough, the shorter, harder workouts can be just as effective, and perhaps even more so, than longer, less intense workouts.

Even running just 5–10 minutes a day at relatively slow speeds is linked to markedly reduced risks for death from all causes and cardiovascular disease. (See Chapter 4 on high-intensity workouts for people who already have heart disease.)

In 2012, when Gibala and colleagues wrote a review article on high-intensity interval training for the *Journal of Physiology*, a prominent scientific publication, the field—and the lay press—went wild. As word spread, Gibala's paper became the most accessed paper in the journal in 2015. Since then, Gibala's string of impressive findings have been featured prominently in major newspapers and TV outlets across the country, prompting exercise enthusiasts—including me—to take up the challenge.

Recently, Gibala has been pushing the envelope, trying to see how low he can go, that is, how short an intense workout can be while still keeping the benefits. It's no accident that his 2017 book is titled *The One-Minute Workout*.

Before we delve deeper, we need a quick definition of HIIT, high-intensity interval training, and a variant called SIT, for sprint interval training. In general, HIIT is defined as "near maximal" efforts performed at an intensity that is about 85–95 percent of maximal heart rate; SIT involves efforts performed at "all-out" or supramaximal heart rates. The key is that exercise be intense enough that the body perceives it as stressful, so you get the really big benefits.

In lay terms, moderate intensity means things like walking fast, doing water aerobics, biking on level ground, and playing doubles tennis; vigorous activity means jogging or running, swimming laps fast, cycling fast or uphill.

Protocols vary, but the most famous is the Wingate test, developed in the 1970s in Israel. It calls for a 30-second all-out effort, followed by four minutes of recovery. This pattern is repeated four to six times during one workout session. This amounts to three to four minutes of hard exercise per session with three sessions a week for two to six weeks.

Don't skip the rest period, by the way, not that you'd really be tempted to.

"The recovery period is important," says Gibala. "If you allow recovery, the subsequent effort can be done at a higher work load. If you just train as a single block of exercise, the adaptations are not as good as if you give breaks, go hard, then take another break. You get more mitochondrial biogenesis if you do intervals than if you work out at a moderate rate continuously. Brief bursts of intense exercise are remarkably effective."

So, I gave HIIT a try. It was exciting, but tough. Okay, full disclosure: It was miserable. For what it's worth, Tarnopolsky agrees.

He prefers longer, more moderate-paced endurance workouts: "You couldn't pay me enough to do Wingate sprints four times a week in the gym and give up running. For me, it's running and biking. I see the city, the country, the environment, whereas sitting on a bike in a gym is just yuk." Some research affirms Tarnopolsky's view, finding that, outside of a gym, it's tough to make HIIT feasible.

But Gibala loves his daily high-intensity 30-minute interval workouts. And he's also backed up by research, including studies suggesting that some people actually do find HIIT *more* enjoyable than continuous moderate running.

Recently, exercise physiologists have developed modifications of HIIT that can be easier to tolerate. The easiest to remember—and least miserable—is the "10-20-30" routine. You run, bike, swim, row gently (at about 30 percent effort) for 30 seconds, increase your pace to moderate (about 60 percent effort) for 20 seconds, then go as hard as you can (90–100 percent effort) for 10 seconds. Rest, walk slowly or barely at all, for two minutes, then repeat. Do this pattern four or five times. It takes only 12–15 minutes.

A French centenarian cyclist, Robert Marchand, recently was tested in a lab at the University of Evry-Vald'Essonne by exercise scientist Veronique Billat.

At 101, Marchand had set the one-hour record for riders aged 100 or older, a feat that attracted not just cycling enthusiasts, but Billat as well. She invited him to her lab and began tweaking his rather leisurely workout program. She tested his VO2max, which in most people begins to decline at 50, even with exercise. His scores were impressive, to say the least.

Then Billat got him to do about 80 percent of his weekly workouts at an easy pace, and 20 percent at a very difficult intensity. He had to increase his pedaling speed to between 70 and 90 revolutions per minute, way more than his usual 60. The result? By two years later, at 103, his VO2max had increased 13 percent, the aerobic equivalent of a healthy 50-year-old. He went on to record an even faster time at his next event, at age 103.

The impressive thing, in terms of fitness benefits, is that this alternation between higher-intensity and lower-intensity activity even works with simple walking, and even in people who are unhealthy to begin with.

In 2013, Danish researchers reported on a study of people with type 2 diabetes. They randomized the people into three groups. One group, the controls, did no walking exercise. The second and third groups both walked five times a week for 60 minutes, expending roughly the same amount of energy. The second group walked continuously—at a moderate rate—for the whole 60 minutes while the third group, the interval walkers, alternated three-minute repetitions of walking at low and high intensities.

The VO2max scores in the interval group improved significantly over the four-month study; scores for the control group and the steady walkers *did not improve.* Only the interval walkers lost body mass and visceral fat. And this is just walking, not cranking like mad on an exercise bike.

As we'll see in the following chapters, good things happen all over your body when you do HIIT and exercise hard.

But since our interest in this chapter is mitochondria, here's the take-home lesson: HIIT is wonderful for increasing production of new mitochondria. The metabolic signals for mitochondrial biogenesis depend less on how *long* you work out than on how *hard*. For mitochondrial biogenesis, it's *intensity* that counts most, not duration.

The evidence for this has been pouring out of research labs, particularly Gibala's and Tarnopolsky's labs. They've shown that sprint interval training doubles endurance capacity; that sprint interval training and traditional exercise are comparable in their ability to boost muscle oxidative capacity, even though the sprint protocol takes much less time; that HIIT doubles levels of PGC-1 alpha. That even just one *minute* of all-out intermittent exercise three times per week delivers significant increases in the oxidative capacity of muscle cells.

In a particularly clever experiment, Gibala and MacInnis asked volunteers to train on exercise bikes with one leg performing HIIT and the other, traditional, less-intense cycling. The HIIT leg muscles wound up with significantly more mitochondria.

I could go on, but I won't. The message is abundantly clear: Healthy, abundant mitochondria are a key to longer, healthier life. And while all endurance exercise can boost mitochondria, for the biggest gains in the shortest amount of time, HIIT can't be beat.

CHAPTER 6

Bigger, Better, Stronger

THE OTHER ROAD TAKEN

Remember that fork in the road at the beginning of the last chapter, the point at which a muscle had to "choose" between producing more energy or becoming stronger and more buff?

Well, we're back at that same fork again, only this time, we're going down the other path. In the last chapter, we focused on how endurance exercise forces muscles to build more mitochondria, the tiny organelles inside cells that burn food to produce the energy that moves us around.

This time, we're focusing on how muscle cells get bigger, a process called hypertrophy, which is triggered most often by resistance exercise. (It can be triggered by genetic mutations, too, such as the rare one that made a five-month-old baby so strong he could do the iron cross, a gymnastics maneuver that involves suspending oneself by the arms between two rings. Stay tuned—we'll come back to him.)

In the last few years, scientists have been teasing apart the differences between the mitochondrial biogenesis and hypertrophy pathways, and the differences are astounding. At the basic levels—genetic, molecular, and cellular—the pathways for hypertrophy are surprisingly distinct from those that make more mitochondria. From a practical standpoint, it's abundantly clear that resistance training is better than endurance training for maintaining gains in strength and muscle mass.

Right up front, a major point: Resistance training (colloquially known as weightlifting) doesn't make muscle cells increase in *number*. That would be *hyperplasia*, which is a hallmark of cancer, not *hypertrophy*. But it does make each muscle cell that is exercised—and only those that are exercised—grow in size and strength. (Sadly, and just as with endurance exercise, the process is reversible. If you stop resistance exercise, your muscles shrink back again, but, contrary to popular opinion, they do *not* turn into fat cells.)

Strong muscles are not just a vanity issue or an obsession for bodybuilders. Healthy muscles are important for everybody, and increasingly so, the older we get. As we age, muscles normally get weaker and smaller, a problem called sarcopenia. It's serious. If you don't have the muscle strength to get out of bed or off the toilet seat by yourself, you raise the risk of falling, becoming disabled, and, all too often, heading for a nursing home.

Beyond those basics, skeletal muscle mass is also an important "sink" for glucose, that is, for holding glucose and helping maintain lower and steadier blood sugar levels. Without sufficient muscle mass, you can develop insulin resistance, a precursor to diabetes. Skeletal muscles are also important for maintaining body temperature—that's why we shiver when we're cold. In extreme conditions like starvation, muscle tissue can even break down into substances that you can use for fuel.

In recent years, scientists have discovered that muscles are also endocrine organs—little hormone factories. They crank out chemicals called myokines that travel through the bloodstream to distant parts of the body to boost the immune system, make bones grow, and help repair damaged tissues, among many other things. Myokines also act on nearby muscle cells and even on the very muscle cell that produced them in various beneficial ways.

All of this means that resistance exercise, which for years has played second fiddle to endurance in exercise guidelines, is hugely important. After all, as we'll see in a minute, resistance exercise can do some of the same things, like combatting depression, that endurance exercise can. It can even have effects, at least according to one study, that you might never have imagined—like potentially making kidney dialysis more effective if you lift weights during the procedure.

The main mission of the roughly 650 skeletal muscles in our bodies is to convert the chemical energy from food into motion and work. Unlike the smooth muscles in organs like the bladder and blood vessels, and cardiac muscles in the heart, skeletal muscles are under voluntary control—we can "tell" them to make us smile or frown, lift weights, or run from predators.

To do this, they have only two choices: contract or relax. They work in pairs—when one of the pair contracts, the other extends. When your biceps muscle (the flexor) contracts and pulls your lower arm up toward your shoulder, its opposite partner, your triceps (the extensor), relaxes. To get your arm straightened out again, your biceps has to relax and your triceps must contract.

BOX 6.1 RATCHETING UP

A skeletal muscle is composed of individual, cylindrical muscle cells called muscle fibers. Picture a nice, long chunk of rigatoni, the hollow, tube-shaped pasta. That's a muscle fiber. It's surrounded by a membrane called the sarcolemma. Inside the riga-toni, packed tightly lengthwise like long hair in a ponytail, are the myofibrils, which contain the actual contractile proteins.

Each myofibril is divided into sections (called sarcomeres) that are marked by thin, dark, protein-containing lines. The sarcomeres of adjacent myofibrils line up next to each other. Each sarcomere is made up of thin and thick filaments. The thick filaments consist of bundles of the protein myosin. The thin filaments are composed of the other important protein, actin.

When a muscle contracts, the thick and thin filaments slide over each other. The "head" of a myosin molecule latches onto the adjacent actin molecule, hangs on for dear life, and pulls. It's like a rower in a shell: The rower reaches forward, "latches" onto water in the "catch," which acts like an anchor, then pulls hard against this pivot point.

In the muscle, this ratcheting process shortens the sarcomere and thus contracts the myofibril. This makes the muscle fiber shorten; when enough fibers shorten, the whole muscle shortens, which pulls on tendons connected to bones, creating movement.

Muscle contraction is a highly organized event. It starts with an initial stimulation, triggered by an impulse sent from a motor nerve (neuron) straight to muscle fibers. When the nerve signal gets to the muscle, calcium ions are released into the cell fluid, which triggers the muscle contraction. Together, the motor neuron and the muscle fibers it innervates are called the motor unit. The bad news is that with age, the number of motor units declines. But here's the good: You can slow this decline. Resistance exercise triggers the nervous system to "reorganize" itself to recruit more motor units and improve the synchronicity of motor units at the cellular level.

In a 2010 study at McGill University, for instance, scientists showed that *runners* in their 60s had roughly the same number of motor units as active 25-year-olds; *sedentary* 60-year-olds, however, had fewer motor units. In a 2016 follow-up study of 80-year-olds, world-class octogen-arian athletes had far more motor units than sedentary people the same age. (For the morbidly curious, or medically minded, drugs like curare can block the functioning of the motor unit, causing paralysis. The poison botulinum is even worse. It can be fatal because it blocks the functioning of motor units in muscles necessary for breathing.)

And in a 2018 study of avid male and female cyclists aged 55–59, researchers found that, even though cycling is an endurance rather than a resistance exercise, the thigh muscles of these cyclists retained their size, muscle fiber composition, and other markers. In fact, the people who logged the most miles every month had the healthiest muscles.

BOX 6.2 THE AMAZING RBG

Supreme Court Justice Ruth Bader Ginsburg was 84 not long ago when a book by her long-time trainer, Bryant Johnson, took the fitness world, and many of her admirers, by storm.

In his book, The RBG Workout: How She Stays Strong—And You Can, Too! *Johnson notes that Ginsburg came to him in 1999 at the urging of her late husband, after her battle with colon cancer. At the time, she herself said, "I looked like an Auschwitz survivor."*

So she hit the gym.

After nearly 20 years under Johnson's tutelage, Ginsburg can do 20 pushups in one session. (I can't!) She hits the Supreme Court workout room twice a week at 7 p.m. sharp, dressed in sweatpants or leggings and her "Super Diva!" shirt. Then she works out, hard, for an hour. First, there's five minutes on the elliptical or jogging on the treadmill, a few stretches, then strength-training, with presses, curls, pull-downs, row, squats, pushups, planks, and kicks.

In early 2017, a writer for Politico, Ben Schreckinger, attempted to do the workout Johnson puts Ginsburg through. He noted dryly that Ginsburg had told him, "I hope he makes it through." He barely made it through the one-legged squats. (I tried, too, and I could only do a few.) Then came pushups. Ginsburg does real pushups, not from her knees. Schreckinger grunted his way through the pushups.

Ginsburg does not.

HYPERTROPHY: HOW MUSCLES GET BIGGER AND STRONGER

So, how do we get these muscles to get bigger? You pick up, say, a 10-pound barbell, or maybe the 20-pound one, or the 50, for a biceps curl. You bring it slowly up toward your shoulder. You lower it, then repeat.

You keep going until you really can't lift the thing, until absolute muscle fatigue sets in. It doesn't matter whether you lift light weights lots of times or heavy weights a few times, so long as you get to fatigue.

Congrats! You've just torn your muscles!

And that's a good thing, because it's the process of creating microscopic tears in muscles, followed by a cascade of inflammatory chemicals that rush in to repair these tears, that causes muscles to grow in bulk. Much of the growth of muscle tissue happens after the workout and during sleep.

It's these tiny tears and the resulting inflammation, not the buildup of lactic acid, as used to be thought, that cause muscle soreness a day or two after a workout. The worst soreness, by the way, comes from "eccentric" exercise, that is, exercise that involves lengthening a muscle, like running downhill, although weightlifting involves some eccentric movement, too.

(By the way, you might think that taking anti-inflammatory medications like ibuprofen could offset this essential muscle repair and rebuilding process and wipe out all your hard work. Luckily, that's not true.)

To build muscle, two things have to happen. You need to eat protein (especially whey protein), especially right after and up to 24 hours after resistance exercise. The point is to achieve "positive protein balance," meaning you are making new proteins faster than you are breaking them down. And you have to activate tiny cells called satellite cells, which fuse with muscle fibers to help make them bigger. It takes what exercise physiologists call "progressive overload," that is, increasing resistance, to activate this highly synchronized process.

Let's talk first about satellite cells, adult muscle stem cells that have the capacity to renew themselves and fuse with muscle fibers.

Satellite cells have fascinated muscle physiologists ever since 1961, when a Rockefeller Institute scientist named Alexander Mauro discovered them in the muscles of frogs' legs; that same year, independently, Sir Bernard Katz, a German-born British biophysicist, discovered the same thing.

As Mauro observed in his groundbreaking paper, when a muscle is in a resting state, satellite cells nestle so close to the muscle fiber that Mauro described it as a form of "intimacy."

Think of it this way, suggests Stuart Phillips, director of the Centre for Nutrition, Exercise and Health Research at McMaster University: The muscle fiber is like a skyscraper with a scaffold around it. When the muscle is resting, nothing much happens—satellite cells just sit quietly underneath the scaffolding. But when the muscle "is twisted and stretched and torn by exercise," Phillips says, the satellite cells swing into action. (For perspective, the satellite cells are the size of people working on the scaffold around the skyscraper.)

Back in the mid-1980s, scientists discovered that they could kick-start satellite cell activation by putting little chunks of crushed muscle into a lab dish filled with satellite cells. The crushed, traumatized muscle pumped out chemical signals that nudged the satellite cells to swing into action. Since then, a number of chemical signals have been shown to activate satellite cells.

Chemically, the message from damaged muscle is simple, says Phillips: "We need help here." Satellite cells then fuse with the muscle, adding their material to the fiber.

The interesting thing is that what a satellite cell adds to a muscle is its nucleus, its most important possession. "The nucleus is like the brain," says Phillips. When a satellite cell donates its nucleus to the muscle, "it's like adding another brain to the muscle cell, another control center."

The reason this is so important is that it's the nucleus that contains DNA, the template for RNA, which controls the manufacture of proteins, including those all-important contractile proteins, myosin and actin. Unlike other cells, in fact, muscle cells have multiple nuclei, a fact that allows them to make lots of protein. By donating their nuclei to muscle cells, satellite cells essentially give muscle cells extra capacity to make myosin and actin. Some scientists think that satellite cells may also donate mitochondria to muscle cells, which might give muscles a new boost of energy.

The good news is that the pool of satellite cells in humans can increase in as few as four days after a single bout of exercise. (Of course, if you stop training, the pool decreases again rapidly.) As we age, this reservoir of satellite cells decreases, but resistance exercise can offset this decline.

BOX 6.3 RED, REDDER, WHITE

It wasn't until the 1960s that curious researchers, using surgical samples of muscle tissue, identified different types of muscle fibers in mammals. The three major types are muscles that contract at three different speeds—slow, medium, or fast—and in three different colors: really red, red, and white.

The reddest fibers, like those in the flight muscles of ducks, are "slow twitch" because they contract slowly, can contract for long periods of time, and are resistant to fatigue. They are red because they contain a lot of a protein called myoglobin and a lot of mitochondria. They also store a lot of fat and use it as fuel, which is why duck breast meat is so greasy. These slow-twitch muscles are also called type 1. They have a rich blood supply and are great for endurance—think of those flying ducks flapping their wings for long distances. The second type, a kind of slow-twitch muscle, called type 2A, is reddish, but not as red as type 1.

The third type is type 2B. These muscles are white—like the breast meat of turkeys. These white muscles twitch fast and fatigue fast. They respond powerfully and quickly in big spurts of power, but they don't have many mitochondria, have a smaller blood supply, and lack color because they have less myoglobin. That's why they're not good for endurance.

Most people have more or less equal numbers of fast- and slow-twitch muscles, although long-distance runners tend to have more slow-twitch muscles—for endurance—while sprinters have more fast-twitch muscles for immediate, short-lived power. A person's ratio of white to red twitch muscles has a strong genetic component; identical twins are born with identical fast-to-slow muscle ratios. Critters that need to jump fast, like rabbits and frogs, are loaded with white fibers. Interestingly, muscles can switch types to some extent. If you're training for an endurance event, your muscles can be "reprogrammed" to create more mitochondria and a better blood supply.

THE MOLECULAR CASCADE: HOW IT BUILDS MUSCLE

As the satellite cells are busy fusing and donating their nuclei to muscle cells, other things also start happening when a muscle contracts against resistance. In fact, at least two separate chemical signaling pathways inside muscle cells begin humming along. *Both pathways have the same "goal": to increase a protein called mTOR*, which, down the line a few steps, leads to production of the muscle proteins, myosin and actin.

As we noted in Chapter 1 on aging, biologists who study aging and cancer consider mTOR a "bad" actor in that, among other things, it can trigger cancer. That's why the drug rapamycin is such a hot area of research—the drug inhibits mTOR and thus may suppress cancer, as well as some of the processes of aging.

For muscle hypertrophy, however, mTOR is a "good" thing because it powers new muscle protein production. In other words, when mTOR is *selectively* activated, that is, *only in muscle tissue*, not all over the body, it is highly beneficial.

So, what are those two pathways to muscle protein synthesis?

One involves a protein that many athletes have heard of and even buy on the Internet: IGF-1, or insulin-like growth factor-1, which increases with resistance exercise.

IGF-1 is actually one of the later steps in the chemical chain reaction that leads to muscle hypertrophy. What starts this chain reaction is the molecule called PGC-1 alpha that we met in Chapter 5. (In that chapter, we focused on its role in triggering formation of new mitochondria after *endurance* exercise.)

But it turns out that while the *main* version of PGC-1 alpha drives creation of new mitochondria, a *different* version of this protein, called PGC-1 alpha 4, drives muscle growth (hypertrophy), after *resistance* exercise.

"It's pretty amazing that two proteins made by a single gene regulate the effects of both types of exercise," says Bruce Spiegelman, who discovered the molecules. Spiegelman is a professor of cell biology at Harvard Medical School. The two different versions occur because the mRNA (messenger RNA) that encodes the proteins can be "spliced," or put together, in slightly different ways in the cell.

In the muscle-building cascade, PGC-1 alpha 4 increases levels of IGF-1 and at the same time *suppresses* a protein called myostatin, whose job is to inhibit muscle cell growth. Resistance training decreases myostatin, adding to muscle growth. It's a kind of push–pull system that leads, in Spiegelman's words, to "robust skeletal muscle hypertrophy."

The triggering of IGF-1 then leads, through yet more chemical steps, to activation of the big gun for muscle protein synthesis, mTOR.

Now, that second pathway. At the same time that the IGF-1 pathway is buzzing along, the other pathway to mTOR gears up, as if evolution "wanted" to be sure of redundant ways to get enough mTOR.

In this second pathway, resistance training triggers an enzyme called FAK (focal adhesion kinase) that senses how much resistance the muscle is working against and, through a different series of steps, eventually activates mTOR. This activation leads to the synthesis of new myosin and actin, which are then added to the myofibrils, bulking them up.

Though the signaling cascades can work fast, muscle growth is actually a somewhat slow process—it can take several weeks or even months to get visibly larger muscles. It also takes adequate rest between exercise bouts to get maximum muscle growth. (If you get discouraged at insufficient muscle growth, take heart. It may not be your fault: There are significant *genetic* differences, and some sex differences, in how muscles respond to training.)

In order for mTOR to make the new myosin and actin proteins that will be added to muscle cells, the body needs a hefty supply of protein from the diet to supply the necessary amino acids. For the record, there are 20 amino acids (some researchers now count 22), of which 11 are "essential." This means you have to eat them—your body can't make them on its own.

Of these 11, the most important for muscle building is leucine, an extremely potent stimulator of mTOR. In fact, leucine and resistance exercise are not just additive, but synergistic, for the formation of new protein, meaning that consuming leucine, which is found in whey, is crucial. (Whey is what's left over from milk in cheese production.)

In other words, milk is a better protein source than soy because it contains whey, which raises amino acid levels in the blood faster than other proteins. Consumption of leucine is important for older people with sarcopenia (muscle wasting), especially if they are inactive.

But eating sufficient protein of other kinds is important, too. On a practical level, this means that if you're young-ish, you should consume 20 grams of protein after resistance exercise, and if you're older, 40 grams.

While some athletes believe it's necessary to consume protein right away, within 20–30 minutes of a workout, scientists say that's not necessary. Protein synthesis lasts for about 24 hours after exercise, so what is important is to consume adequate protein during this period.

If you eat more protein than you need to make more muscle, it doesn't do any good metabolically. (Contrary to popular belief, it probably doesn't do much harm, either. There's no evidence of a link between protein intake and kidney disease or between protein and bone loss, so long as you consume adequate calcium and vitamin D.)

Getting bigger and stronger, though, is not the only thing that muscles do. As we'll see in the next section, muscles also do something that scientists have only begun to appreciate in the last decade or so.

MUSCLES AS HORMONE FACTORIES

It may sound crazy, but muscles make hormones. In other words, muscles are actually secretory (endocrine) organs.

Scientists began suspecting the existence of muscle-derived hormones in the early 1960s. Since then, they've been discovering myokines at what Swiss researchers Svenia Schnyder and Christoph Handschin call "a breath-taking pace."

Much of the credit for unraveling the secrets of muscles as hormone producers goes to Danish researcher Bente Klarlund Pedersen, who has shown that contracting muscles pump out hundreds of hormones and hormone-like substances that can travel back and act on the contracting muscle itself (a kind of self-stimulating feedback loop), travel a short distance to act on neighboring muscles, or travel through the blood to distant organs.

In 2003, Pedersen came up with a name for the collection of chemicals secreted by muscles: "myokines." These chemical messengers are quite the communicators—they "cross-talk" (chemically) to other organs, including the liver, adipose tissue, the pancreas, the immune system, bone, and brain. This elaborate network of communication—a veritable gossip fest—helps explain why exercise has so many effects on so many parts of the body.

One myokine, IL-6 (interleukin-6), is an inflammatory substance that promotes fever. It's activated when muscles contract and not when muscles are just resting. When muscles contract, IL-6 is released in huge quantities into the bloodstream.

But IL-6 is a Jekyll and Hyde actor. When it's acting as a pro-inflammatory, "bad" cytokine, it can lead to chronic, low-grade inflammation and insulin resistance. When stimulated by exercise, however, it seems to be a "good" actor by triggering production of *anti-inflammatory* cytokines such as IL-1ra and IL-10. (We'll talk more about exercise, inflammation, and the immune system in Chapter 11.)

Contracting muscles also produce IL-8, which promotes blood vessel growth; IL-15, which shrinks adipose tissue; and BDNF (brain-derived neurotrophic factor), which helps activate satellite cells. Interestingly, exercise also acts directly on the brain, which pumps out its own BDNF, as we'll see in Chapters 8 and 9.

The effects go on. With exercise, muscles release VEGF (vascular endothelial growth factor), which lands on receptors on capillaries and stimulates blood vessel growth, as we saw in Chapter 4.

Muscles also release myokines, including FGF-2 (fibroblast growth factor), that stimulate bone growth, as we'll see in Chapter 7. In fact, a particularly important myokine called irisin not only stimulates bones, but also helps turn white fat into brown, the fat that produces heat. And a myokine called cathepsin B, which is triggered by running, can act on the brain, helping to improve memory.

And then there's that intriguing protein called myostatin, which is also made in muscle cells. Its job—and this sounds counterintuitive—is to damp *down* muscle growth. In animals that lack the gene for myostatin (such as Belgian Blue and Piedmontese cattle), the animals wind up with muscles that grow to enormous size.

In the lab, scientists have created "mighty mice" by eliminating the myostatin gene. Precisely why we humans would have a way of slowing muscle growth might seem a puzzle, except that, in evolutionary terms, if we grew too big for the available food supply, we might not survive.

All of this brings us back to little Liam Hoekstra, the five-month-old baby we mentioned earlier, with muscles so powerful that he could do the iron cross. (In the extremely difficult iron cross, a gymnast hangs with legs straight down, a bit like Christ on the cross, with both arms spread out, hands clutching the rings and attempting to keep the rings still.)

It turns out that the not-so-little baby, born in 2005, has a rare condition called myostatin-related muscle hypertrophy. In other words, Liam was born unable to make myostatin. Because this natural muscle growth suppressant was missing, Liam's body developed extra-big muscles. As one of his amazed doctors put it, "He was able to grab both of my hands and nearly do an iron cross. This is not something that happens for most men, and here is this kid with this kind of power."

Not surprisingly, the idea of blocking myostatin is not lost on some competitive athletes, who reportedly seek myostatin-inhibiting drugs to boost their muscle mass.

SARCOPENIA

Sarcopenia, which means loss of muscle mass, is an all-too-common feature of aging, though it's really caused by disuse, not the sheer passage of time per se. Muscle weakness and loss of muscle mass is a set-up for many of the sad events of later life—falls, broken hips, disability, loss of independence, and, in many cases, the need for a nursing home. It's a depressing downward slide—people over 50 lose on average one pound of muscle every year.

But that's what happens *without* strength training, also called resistance exercise or weightlifting. *With* strength training, older people can significantly offset sarcopenia. Indeed, strength training has been shown to increase not just muscle *mass,* but muscle *power* as well. (Power is strength multiplied by speed—how fast you perform a strength challenge.)

In fact, older adults who do strength training can achieve gains in both power and strength similar to those of younger people. But you do have to do specific resistance workouts—running won't do it.

If you need further motivation, consider this: Australian research shows that people who lifted small weights while undergoing kidney dialysis not only got stronger muscles but got improved kidney function as well.

And that's just the beginning. In addition to boosting muscle mass, resistance exercise can be an effective antidepressant in older people. It can improve both blood sugar control and depression in diabetics, too.

It can offset mitochondrial depletion. It can reduce lymphedema (swelling following lymph node surgery) in breast cancer patients. It can help ward off increases in belly fat. It can boost cognitive function in older people. It can reduce the risk of all-cause mortality in cancer survivors.

And perhaps most important, strength training can improve older people's ability to get out of a chair or off the toilet, climb stairs, bathe, prepare meals, and generally take care of themselves.

In other words, to live an independent life, think of the judge. If Ruth Bader Ginsburg, a two-time cancer survivor, can do her workout at age 84, maybe you can, too.

CHAPTER 7

Boning Up

THE BAD NEWS

In 2016, when *New York Times* science writer Gina Kolata wrote that, contrary to medical dogma and widespread belief, walking and modest strength training do not actually strengthen bones much, outraged readers swamped her inbox.

But she was right. As Kolata pointed out, it *is* true that sitting too much, prolonged bed rest, or traveling as an astronaut in weightless space does weaken bones. But the reverse of this, that exercise in adulthood, even weight-bearing exercise, can significantly build bone, alas, is not true.

Exercise in later life can *slow* the rate of bone loss, but it can't really rebuild bone. That's true for both women and men, but is most pronounced in women after menopause, when levels of the hormone estrogen decline sharply. Though babies are born with 270 bones, the immature bones fuse as kids grow. By the time we're in our early 20s, we're down to 206 bones.

And then things get worse.

"When hormones decrease with aging, you can exercise all you want, but you will still lose bone mass," says the aptly named Lynda Bonewald, a cell biologist who heads the Indiana Center for Musculoskeletal Health at Indiana University. "Almost every study says that exercise is beneficial," she adds. "But does it block bone loss? No. Does it block the effects of aging? No, though it can delay those effects."

Exercise does have a small effect on the spongy material inside bone called the trabecula and can slightly thicken the tough outer shell called cortical bone. But these effects are too modest to make bone significantly stronger or to prevent osteoporosis, says Clifford Rosen, a senior scientist at the Maine Medical Center Research Institute and an expert on bone biology.

Unfortunately, Rosen adds, even high-intensity exercise, weightlifting, or running "just don't seem to have much of an impact on bone density," though exercise can help protect against further bone loss.

Why did so many of us ever think exercise *could* restore lost bone? "It was magical thinking," Rosen says. "Exercise was supposed to be good for everything, therefore it was good for bone. Everybody in the field wanted to believe that."

As an intervention in adults, endurance and resistance exercise can produce some improvements in bone, but the effect is "pretty minimal," agrees cell biologist Mark Hamrick at the Medical College of Georgia, who studies the molecular communication between muscles and bones. In studies for the past 50 years, he says, the evidence for exercise having a significant impact on bone is not as strong as the evidence for bone-building medications.

Depressing, isn't it? But not totally.

That's because the bigger problem for older people is not so much osteoporosis—weak bones—per se as falls and resulting fractures. And exercise *can* help prevent falls by increasing muscle strength (see Chapter 6) and by improving balance with specific exercises, including Tai chi.

Osteoporosis only comes into the picture when it makes bones so fragile that even a minor fall results in a broken bone and when it affects vertebral bones in the spine. In fact, many older people *without osteoporosis* fall and get fractures because of weak muscles, poor balance, poor physical functioning, and general frailty.

So let's talk fractures.

Fractures may sound benign, but they are deadly serious, not just because of the immediate pain and immobility, but because they can lead to lasting disability, loss of independent living, and even death. Hip fractures are particularly common and deadly in women, but men get them, too.

Every year, more than 300,000 older Americans are hospitalized for a hip fracture, 95 percent of which are caused by falling, usually falling sideways. Overall, a 50-year-old American white woman has a 15–20 percent lifetime risk of a hip fracture.

It may not be obvious why a seemingly "simple" thing like a broken bone can be so deadly, but a major cause of death is being immobile for a long period of time while the hip heals. Immobility can lead to fatal blood clots, pneumonia, infections, and a worsening of conditions such as chronic obstructive pulmonary disease (COPD).

For both men and women, there's a five- to eight-fold increased risk of dying in the first three *months* after a hip fracture. In the first *year* after a fracture, one in every four patients age 50 or older dies. This means that for people living independently before a hip fracture, only half ever walk independently again; 20 percent move to a long-term care facility and never return home.

But it's not all bleak. The good news is that higher levels of physical activity are linked to a lower risk of fractures in both older women and older men.

In a study of 61,200 postmenopausal women, for instance, researchers found that the risk of a hip fracture was *lowered* by 6 percent for each *increase* of one hour per week of walking. Walking for at least four hours a week was linked to a 41 percent lower risk of hip fracture. Studies in men have come to similar conclusions.

BOX 7.1 FALLS

Given that falls are the leading cause of injury and injury-related death for older Americans, here are some common-sense tips from the Centers for Disease Control and Prevention and the National Institute on Aging.

Practice balancing on one leg while holding on to a chair. Consider learning Tai chi. If you start to fall, try not to fall sideways—fall forward or onto your rear end. Get your vision and hearing checked regularly. If you can't see or hear an obstacle, the chances of falling increase.

Some medications, including blood pressure pills, heart drugs, diuretics, muscle relaxers, tranquilizers, and opioid pain relievers, can make you dizzy and more prone to falls. Get enough sleep—fatigue increases the risk of falls, as does alcohol.

Get up slowly from sitting or lying—getting up quickly temporarily lowers blood pressure and raises the risk of falls. Use a cane or walker if need be, and be careful on wet or icy surfaces. Wear non-skid shoes. Use a rubber bath mat in the shower. Don't climb on chairs to reach high objects.

Install handrails on stairways and make sure there's good lighting, especially in hallways and stairways. Don't leave objects, including scatter rugs and electrical cords, in areas where you walk. Get a mobile phone so you don't have to run to answer a call. Consider hiring a monitoring company that can respond to an emergency call 24/7.

And try not to trip over the dog!

You might think that bone is like a chunk of cement—hard, inert stuff that is just there for skeletal support. And bone *is* hard, especially the smooth outer surface called cortical bone.

But the inside stuff, the trabecular bone, is more porous, spongy, and slightly flexible, which allows bones to bend a bit under stress, a feature that helps protect against fractures. The bone matrix is living tissue that also contains inorganic material such as hydroxyapatite, made of calcium and phosphate. It's this mineral material that gives bone its rigidity and strength.

While we mostly think of bone only in terms of its skeletal support, it actually has a number of other important functions. It acts as a storage site for minerals, even heavy metals like lead. And the bone marrow, deep inside the bones, makes the cells of our blood and immune system.

Just as important, bone, like muscle and fat tissue, is now known to be a highly active hormone-secreting organ. For instance, bone makes a molecule called FGF-2 (fibroblast growth factor), which triggers cell proliferation all over the body. It also produces osteocalcin, a hormone that helps regulate glucose metabolism. Bone also makes IGF-1 (insulin growth factor), which stimulates hormones that tell other tissues to grow.

In addition, bones are highly sensitive regulators of calcium, a process that is governed by the parathyroid gland in the neck. Calcium sensors in the parathyroid gland keep track of calcium levels in the blood. If calcium drops too low, the parathyroid gland secretes a hormone called parathyroid hormone (PTH), which tells bones to give up some calcium and send it into the bloodstream. It's as if the body "knows" that, in a pinch, it can sacrifice bone to the more important process of keeping blood calcium levels healthy.

BOX 7.2 CARTWHEELS AND HANDSPRINGS

Decades ago, as a high school cheerleader, and proud of my swirly blue skirt and blue sweater with the big "P" on the front, I routinely did what I can barely imagine doing now.

I would jump down into a squat, then pump my arms, push hard with my legs and leap up high, arching my back so that my saddle-shoe–clad feet would tap the back of my head, forming a brief but near-perfect circle. Then I'd unfold and bounce down to the ground, then up again, chanting P-E-L-H-A-M for the local, albeit mediocre, football team.

My favorite mode of locomotion in those days, when decency allowed, was cart-wheeling down the block. At home, my goal was to do as many one-handed hand-springs across the backyard as space allowed. Secretly, I wanted to become a serious gymnast. But in those pre-1972, pre–Title IX days, my high school, like most others, didn't have the coaching or the harnesses and other equipment a girl like me needed to learn forward flips, back flips, and other tricks without landing on her head.

So Olympic glory was not in the cards. But there was a huge benefit to all that adolescent jumping and tumbling: strong bones, bones that to this day have served me well, with nary a trace—so far—of osteoporosis, the bone-thinning disease so common in later life, or its precursor, osteopenia.

As my teenage experience shows, the bone-building process is at its strongest in childhood and adolescence. And the bones that end up the strongest are those that get stressed the most through physical activity.

"You can see it in tennis players," says David Slovik, an endocrinologist and osteoporosis specialist at Massachusetts General Hospital in Boston. "If a tennis player is right-handed, the bone density in that arm is greater than in the other arm. Invariably, bone density is higher in the area that is stressed a lot. It's the body's adaption to mechanical loading. The reverse is true, too. If a person has a stroke and is immobile on one side, bones in the weaker side are less dense than in the healthy side."

The reason that bones end up unequally strong is that bones are always changing—constantly being formed and torn apart. It's a process called remodeling, in which specific cells called *osteoclasts* break down existing bone, while other cells called *osteoblasts* create new bone tissue. Once-ignored cells called *osteocytes* turn out to run the whole show, and we'll get to how muscle-building exercise plays into this in a moment.

While it takes about two *weeks* to break down bone, it can take three *months* to build up bone. And that's in a healthy, young person. A young skeleton, for instance, can be completely remodeled. But with aging, remodeling slows down, with some bones not being remodeled for decades. In fact, it can take 10 years to remodel a complete adult skeleton. Even as early as our 30s and 40s, remodeling begins to tip more toward destruction than formation, meaning that we begin losing more bone than we build.

This remodeling process is controlled significantly by hormones, chiefly estrogen. In men, testosterone helps build bone, but men need estrogen, too, which they make, thanks to an enzyme that converts testosterone to estrogen. In women, when estrogen levels crash at menopause, bone loss starts rapidly. (Estrogen replacement therapy protects against some bone loss, but cannot build new bone.)

"Once you hit menopause, the osteoblasts, the bone builders, don't have as much of an effect. There's both an increase in bone breakdown and a decrease in formation," says Slovik. That leads to a net loss of bone—the amount of bone restored by remodeling never equals what was there in the first place.

Estrogen is a key player in this because it can keep osteocytes, the master controllers of the remodeling process, alive for decades.

Here's how it works.

Osteocytes are sensors of mechanical "loading"; that is, they can detect how much stress is put on bone by movements like walking or jumping. Even the simple act of contracting a muscle changes the fluid pressure around the osteocytes, allowing them to detect mechanical loading.

Once osteocytes sense a change in mechanical load, they pump out chemical signals that both boost *osteoblasts*, the bone builders, and *turn off* genes that block bone formation. In other words, by directly boosting the bone builders and simultaneously *blocking the blockers* of bone formation, osteocytes use a two-pronged approach to promote bone formation.

The bad news? With age, the ability of muscles to generate force declines, and the ability of bone to respond to mechanical loading decreases.

BOX 7.3 OSTEOPOROSIS

Osteoporosis, which affects roughly 10 million Americans, is one of the most-dreaded complications of aging. It causes one in two women and one in four men to break a bone in their lifetime.

Thanks to more aggressive screening, more and more people, especially older women, are being diagnosed with osteopenia, a precursor of osteoporosis. This has forced many women to decide whether to take medications like Fosamax (a so-called bisphosphonate) or skip the meds and hope for the best.

This question is agonizing. Some studies have shown an increased risk of two rare but serious side effects from bisphosphonates: osteonecrosis (bone disease) of the jaw, and an unusual type of thigh fracture. These studies have scared women to the point that fewer are being screened, which could lead to more people getting fractures in the future.

"People are too afraid of bisphosphonates," says Slovik of Mass General. "People say they don't want medication, they just want exercise. But exercise is not enough. It's important, but it doesn't have as big an effect as we would like."

The actual risk of jaw necrosis from Fosamax is small, he adds, and the risk is highest in cancer patients who take bisphosphonates in high doses and for long periods of time.

Fosamax (alendronate) is not the only medication for osteoporosis and osteopenia. Binosto is also an alendronate. Other bisphosphonates include risendronate (Actonel, Atelvia), ibandronate (Boniva), zolendronic acid (Reclast, Zometa), and denosumab (Prolia, Xgeva). All have been linked to osteonecrosis of the jaw and the atypical thigh fractures.

Bisphosphonates work by lowering the activity of osteoclasts and thus slowing the breakdown of bone. The problem is that bone breakdown is part of the cyclical remodeling process that involves bone building as well as breakdown. This means, weird as it sounds, that drugs that boost bone breakdown too much or for too long can actually slow bone rebuilding.

Another drug, called Forteo (teriparatide), can actually build bone by boosting the activity of osteoblasts. But it, too, has raised fears. In rats given extremely high doses, Forteo was linked to an increased risk of bone cancer. So far, there is no evidence of an increased cancer risk in people taking Forteo. A newer bone-building drug, Tymlose (abaloparatide), was approved in 2017. (Both Forteo and Tymlose are synthetic versions of the parathyroid hormone [PTH].)

Finally, scientists are working on a new approach: drugs called senolytics that target "senescent" cells, aging cells that give off toxic chemicals. The hope is that these drugs can help protect bones.

HOW MUSCLE AND BONE "TALK" TO EACH OTHER

"Bone and muscle are a unit. It's tremendously logical that muscle would talk to bone," says Bruce Spiegelman, a professor of cell biology at Harvard Medical School. In fact, muscle strength is now seen as a good predictor of bone strength.

The chemical "cross-talk" between muscle and bone actually goes both ways. Osteocytes, those masters of the remodeling process, produce chemical signals that directly support muscle mass, and muscles make substances that keep osteocytes alive and functional.

Bones make osteocalcin, a hormone that normally declines with age. But researchers have shown that old mice injected with osteocalcin can run just as fast as younger mice, presumably because osteocalcin boosts muscle function, including the ability of muscle to use glucose and fatty acids for fuel.

But most of the research focuses on communication the other way, from muscles to bone.

One of the first clues was the observation that if a bone fracture was covered by flaps of muscle, it healed faster than bone that was not in close physical contact with muscle. This was a strong clue that chemicals secreted by muscle, including IGF-1 and FGF-2, could influence bone. Even in the test tube, these chemicals stimulate bone growth.

But it's not just IGF-1 and FGF-2 that help bones grow. Perhaps even more important is the hormone irisin, which we talked about in the previous chapter, on muscle growth.

Irisin, discovered about a decade ago by Spiegelman, is a myokine, that is, a hormone made in muscles in response to exercise. The beneficial pathway goes like this: Exercise raises irisin production in muscles, and irisin, in turn, boosts bone mass.

In a 2015 study, for instance, researchers from Italy, Norway, and the United States injected irisin into young mice and found significant increases in cortical bone mass. They subsequently found that irisin can actually *restore* lost bone, as well improve muscle atrophy. Irisin seems to work both by boosting osteoblasts and by decreasing the activity of osteoclasts.

Now dubbed "the exercise hormone," irisin has achieved star status among athletes and in the popular press, not just because of its effects on bone, but because it can also convert calorie-storing white fat into brown fat and may even slow formation of fat tissue.

WHAT EXERCISE CAN AND CAN'T DO FOR BONES

"If you run a young pig on a treadmill, the bones get bigger," says Mark Hamrick, the muscle and bone researcher from Georgia. "But not an old pig." And what's true for pigs, alas, is true for humans as well.

On the bright side, even though exercise can't *build* bone in later life, we can use exercise, especially high-impact, weight-bearing exercise, to help *preserve* the bone we've got left.

It's abundantly clear that exercise in youth builds strong bones, and that this benefit sticks around for quite a while. Compared to sedentary folks, for instance, people who were elite athletes in their youth have greater bone mass and bone strength later on, even if they've stopped training.

Jumping in particular—think cheerleaders—has been shown to boost bone density in young people. In one study involving premenopausal women, jumping 20 times with a 30-second rest between jumps and doing this twice daily can boost bone density to some degree. A different study of premenopausal women involving both jumping and weightlifting also showed some increased bone density.

But what, if anything, these data mean for older women is unclear.

A 2009 Spanish review of the research suggested that while high-impact exercise can enhance bone mass, this is not true in postmenopausal women, precisely the group most prone to osteoporosis and fractures.

On the other hand, British researchers found that both young and older women who performed brief bursts of high-intensity, weight-bearing exercise had stronger bones than those who didn't. But this study showed a simple association, not causality.

Randomized, controlled studies have been largely discouraging. A 2006 randomized study found that moderate-intensity aerobic (not resistance) training did nothing for bone mineral density. A 2017 randomized study of resistance and aerobic training also found no effect on bone mineral density, though this study was in breast cancer survivors who were taking estrogen-blocking medication.

In other words, exercise can't build bone in older people, but it can help *preserve* bone, as a 2017 systematic review and meta-analysis of 11 randomized trials involving more than 1,000 postmenopausal women showed.

A different 2017 systematic review of 10 randomized studies also showed that high-impact exercise preserved bone density in both peri- and postmenopausal women. Interestingly, this study looked not just at exercise, but at standing on a vibrating platform, which also helped preserve bone.

Granted, it may seem like cheating to exercise purists, but other research also suggests that standing on vibrating platforms may boost bone density. In a 2013 Taiwanese study of postmenopausal women, six months of standing on a vibrating platform for five minutes three times a week yielded about a 2 percent increase in lumbar spine bone density.

As for me, I am one of those exercise purists. True, I can't do all those flips and cartwheels and jumps of my youth, but I can still jog, swim, lift weights, and crank through 50 minutes several times a week on an elliptical machine.

It may take longer—and take more motivation—but for me, at least, genuine exercise is a lot more fun.

CHAPTER 8
Exercise and Cognition

A WHIRLWIND TOUR OF THE BRAIN

If we could gaze into the brain—a three-pound chunk of grayish, highly folded tissue—we'd be just as amazed as we are when we look up at night and ponder the stars. Indeed, it's often said that there are 100 billion neurons (nerve cells) in the brain, roughly the number of stars in the Milky Way.

Actually, that's not quite right. In 2009, scientists used fancy counting techniques and concluded that the human brain is made up of "only" 86 billion neurons and about the same number of glial cells, important non-nerve cells that act like glue holding the neurons together. As for the stars, the Milky Way wins hands down, with an estimated 200–400 billion stars.

The brain, arguably the most fascinating thing in our universe, is responsible for cognition, perception, emotion, decision-making, and consciousness. It's so complex that scientists are still trying to figure out how the firing of each individual neuron fits in with the big things the brain does, like feeling fear at the sight of a snake, or solving a math problem. The brain circuits involved in these complex processes have to pass electrical signals along intricate chains involving hundreds, even thousands, of individual neurons.

THE BIG PICTURE: EXERCISE AND BRAIN FUNCTION

It's not news that the brain begins to decline as we age, starting, sad to say, in midlife, and sometimes earlier.

Cognitive tasks that demand fluidity, such as reasoning, as well as tasks that can't be solved on the basis of personal experience, decline. It takes longer to process information. The volume of gray matter shrinks. The hippocampus (the memory center) gets smaller, too. It can be harder to concentrate. Blood flow to the brain decreases. Hence all the not-so-funny jokes about CRS, or "can't remember shit."

On the other hand, knowledge-based or so-called crystallized abilities such as verbal knowledge and comprehension stay fairly strong throughout life. Compared to young people doing the same task, brain scans show that older people often have to "recruit" extra brain regions to get the same job done. But the good news is that this recruiting works, allowing healthy older brains to function reasonably well. (There's a name for this recruiting phenomenon: HAROLD, which stands for hemispheric asymmetry reduction in older adults.)

But the even better news, and the focus of this chapter, is that older people who are aerobically fit don't have to recruit extra brain regions the way unfit older people do.

In fact, there is overwhelming evidence that regular exercise, especially the aerobic kind, can slow cognitive decline. Exercise helps keep the brain healthy well into later life, helping maintain brain function and brain volume in specific regions. To improve cognitive function, one way is to exercise at moderate intensity for 45–60 minutes per session on as many days a week as possible.

Aerobic exercise seems to have its biggest benefits in protecting executive function, the very function most sensitive to aging.

Exercise also protects brain function by controlling inflammation. (We'll talk about exercise and inflammation in Chapter 11.)

This is not to say that other factors, like healthy eating (particularly the Mediterranean diet, with all its fruits, veggies, fish, olive oil, and red wine), formal education, and staying socially connected and intellectually challenged have no value. Quite the contrary.

Indeed, a landmark 1995 study from the John D. and Catherine T. MacArthur Foundation tracked 1,192 people aged 70–79, looking for factors associated with successful cognitive aging. It concluded that four factors are key: education, a personality characteristic called self-efficacy, strong respiratory function, and strenuous physical activity.

Carl Cotman, part of the MacArthur team and founding director of the Institute for Memory Impairments and Neurological Diseases (MIND) at the University of California, Irvine, recalls thinking about those findings while "wandering around one day, dreaming away, as professors will do, wondering why physical activity would improve cognitive stability and offset age-related decline." It's a question that propels him to this day.

Since the MacArthur study, Cotman and others have found that, of all the factors, exercise is the most powerful way to protect the brain. The inverse is also true, notes Cotman. *Lack* of exercise—that is, physical *inactivity*—is "the number one modifiable risk factor for Alzheimer's disease."

This is compelling in part because many people assume that brain training games—now a multi-million-dollar industry—would be the most effective.

Not so. In a 2010 six-week study dubbed Brain Test Britain, for instance, researchers from Cambridge University put 11,430 television (BBC) viewers through brain training several times a week on cognitive tests designed to improve reasoning, memory, planning, visual-spatial skills, and attention.

The participants did get better on those specific tests. But "no evidence was found for transfer effects to untrained tasks, even when those tasks were cognitively closely related," the researchers found. Other research has found much the same thing.

In other words, if you really want to protect your brain as you age, "put on your shorts and go exercise," as Richard A. Friedman, a psychiatrist at Weill Cornell Medical College, put it in a *New York Times* piece about the British study.

To be sure, there are, and probably always will be, exercise deniers. There's that famous quote rightly or wrongly attributed to Mark Twain: "I take my only exercise as pallbearer at the funerals of my friends who exercise regularly." Or the quote attributed, rightly or wrongly, to Henry Ford: "Exercise is bunk. If you are healthy, you don't need it, and if you are sick, you shouldn't take it."

Worth a laugh, but wrong, as we'll show in this chapter.

We'll focus first on the brains of healthy people—on the many big, observational studies that compare folks who exercise with those who don't. Such studies are important even though, by definition, they can show only correlation, not causation.

Then we'll look at interventional studies, which can get closer to finding causation. In these studies, scientists randomly get some people but not others to exercise and then track what happens in their brains. After that, we'll see what effect exercise has on the risks of serious brain diseases such as Alzheimer's dementia, mild cognitive impairment, and schizophrenia.

And last, but most exciting to me, we'll get to the mechanisms—the specific molecules triggered by exercise that may be capable of literally changing the brain by causing new neurons to grow or making old neurons more potent, especially in the hippocampus. (As we'll see, one new controversial study has challenged that idea that new neurons can grow in the adult human hippocampus, but another new study confirms that they do.)

But first, a little inspiration to get us going: Remember Olga Kotelko, the nonagenarian track star we mentioned in Chapter 5? As we noted there, Kotelko, with all her exercise, had phenomenally healthy and plentiful mitochondria.

Well, it turns out that her 90-plus-year-old brain was unusually healthy, too. In brain scans done at the University of Illinois, the white matter in Kotelko's brain looked different from that of other 90-plus-year-olds studied: Her hippocampus was bigger than that of typical nonagenarians.

That's probably no fluke. The link between exercise and at least modest and "sometimes substantial" better brain function later in life has been shown again and again in observational studies. Overall, people who habitually do a lot of physical activity are "significantly protected" against later cognitive decline, and even those who exercise at only a "low to moderate" level get some protection.

Since the late 1970s, researchers have been piecing together exactly what exercise does for the brain, with the early studies focusing on a relatively simple phenomenon—reaction time. Older people who were athletic were found to have significantly faster reaction times than non-athletic older people. The implication was novel, and clear: Lack of fitness, not age per se, may be the bigger culprit in reduced mental processing.

In the 1980s, other researchers began probing the exercise effect. One team collected data on 2,747 youngish folks (aged 18–30), including tests of their cardiac fitness on treadmills. In the study, called Cardia, the scientists then followed up 25 years later, testing the same people, now middle-aged, on verbal memory, executive function, and psychomotor speed. The results were strikingly linear—the higher a person's level of fitness 25 years earlier, as measured by the treadmill tests, the better his or her brain was functioning in midlife.

To be sure, not all researchers think that the fitness–brain link is absolutely linear. But the trend strongly suggests it is. A different study that also used treadmill fitness tests, for instance, started tracking people in their 40s. Of the 1,100 people studied, those who were sedentary in midlife had greater brain shrinkage 20 years later.

In yet another large prospective study, epidemiologists from University College London followed more than 10,000 civil servants aged 35–55 until they were 46–68 years old. Low levels of physical activity were closely linked to worse cognitive functioning later in life.

An even longer study, this one by researchers from Iceland and the US National Institute on Aging, found that exercise in midlife was associated with better cognitive function 26 years later.

Even over shorter periods, exercisers do better cognitively as time goes on. In one such study, researchers followed people for just six years. Even in that relatively short period of time, the people who were the fittest at baseline had better cognitive function six years later.

The trend seems to continue almost endlessly. Even in old age, keeping up a moderate level of exercise seems to postpone cognitive decline, according to a study of healthy older men in Finland, Italy, and the Netherlands. An American study of more than 18,000 older women aged 70–81 found the same thing. The American study also showed that the positive effects of exercise on the brain vary dramatically with the duration and intensity of the exercise.

Varying the kind of exercise you do may be important, too. A University of Pennsylvania study that followed more than 5,000 healthy people for 10 years found that the more *different* types of exercise a person did, the better the cognitive function 10 years later.

Even just walking at a reasonably brisk pace helps.

In a University of Pittsburgh study of 299 people whose average age was 78, researchers led by psychologist Kirk Erickson documented a linear effect of exercise on cognition. Walking 72 blocks a week was the magic number—enough exercise to protect the brain. More than that didn't provide extra protection. In other studies, the same Pittsburgh researchers also showed that higher aerobic fitness is associated with greater hippocampal volume, better memory, and more gray matter volume in the prefrontal cortex.

"What's really striking," Erickson told an audience at the annual Society for Neuroscience meeting in 2016, "is what's happening in the hippocampus."

Thanks to evolving brain scanning technology, the evidence for the link between exercise and brain volume is becoming even stronger. Not only have researchers recently been able to show that fit older people have less age-related atrophy in the prefrontal and temporal cortices than unfit older people, they are finding that fit older people also have better neural connections—"connectivity"—between the prefrontal cortex and other parts of the brain.

Even when researchers simply ask people to *recall* how much they exercise (a less reliable measure of fitness than treadmill testing), the link between exercise and brain health shows up. In a study of nearly 6,000 women aged 65 or older (dubbed "Women Who Walk"), researchers tested cognitive functioning at baseline, then again six to eight years later. Once again, the results were linear: The more active a woman was, the less likely she was to have cognitive decline as she aged.

In another recall study, people in their 60s, 70s, and 80s were asked to remember how much they had exercised in their youth (youth being defined as ages 15–25). Even long ago, youthful exercise—as opposed to *current* exercise habits—boosted "cognitive reserve" and delayed later-life deficits.

While most observational studies look at exercise and brain function, some do the opposite—they focus on *inactivity* or sedentary behavior and its potential links to brain function. Again, the basic pattern holds. In a large study of more than 17,000 people aged 50 or older in 11 European countries, researchers showed that over a 2.5-year period, physical *inactivity* was associated with a decline in cognitive function.

The same thing happens in sluggish rats. Left to their own devices, rats normally love nothing better than scampering along on running wheels. Like humans, they don't do well when not allowed to run. In one study, rats were divided into two groups. One group had running wheels in their cages, the other did not. After three months, the brains of sedentary rats, but not the runners, showed significant detrimental changes.

Finally, as every writer knows, a good story needs a punch line, a "kicker." Here's mine: A 2016 British study looked at 162 pairs of healthy twins whose average age was 55. When the study began in 1999, all the women were tested in the gym on a machine that measured leg power—kicking. They were also all given a battery of cognitive tests.

Ten years later, they were put through the memory tests again. The women whose legs were stronger at the outset had fewer age-related changes in their brains 10 years later. When researchers looked at a subset of twins in which one sister was a better kicker at the outset, it was that better kicker, the stronger one, who had better brain function later.

Now, *that*'s a kicker!

BOX 8.1 WHAT'S WHERE

The brain is organized into sections. The largest chunk is the cerebrum, which is divided into two hemispheres, left and right, connected by a bundle of nerve fibers called the corpus callosum. The left hemisphere controls the muscles on the right side of the body, and the right hemisphere, the muscles on the left. The left brain also controls speech and language, while the right brain is believed more essential for creative things like artistic ability, though in fact, we all use both most of the time.

The outermost layer of the cerebrum is the cerebral cortex ("cortex" means a surrounding layer, like the bark of a tree). The cortex is where complex thinking takes place. Underneath the cerebrum is the brainstem, which connects to the spinal cord, relays information between the brain and the rest of the body, and helps control the heart, breathing, and consciousness. Behind that lies the cerebellum, which helps with motor control, coordination, and balance.

The brain also comes in two colors: white and gray. White matter refers to axons, projections of nerve cells that are coated in a whitish covering called myelin; gray matter is everything else, including the actual cell bodies of neurons and glial cells, the "glue" that holds neurons together.

The cortex consists of four separate, interconnected lobes. The frontal lobe (behind the forehead) is where thinking, planning, and decision-making (or "executive function") occur. The parietal (behind the top of the skull) processes sensory information, including taste, touch, and temperature. The occipital lobe (at the back of the skull) handles visual information. And the temporal lobe (behind the temples) processes sound, language, and, just as important, contains the hippocampus (the memory center) and the amygdala (the emotion- and fear-processing center).

Although most neurons in the brain are created before we're born, there are two areas where new neurons have been shown to grow in rodents: the hippocampus and the olfactory bulb. In humans, the growth of new neurons in the olfactory bulb stops shortly after birth. The extent and duration of new neuronal growth in the human hippocampus is still a matter of debate. While one recent study suggests that new neurons are formed in the human hippocampus only until adolescence, another recent study confirms neurogenesis until old age. This latter finding is consistent with earlier, landmark research.

When scientists actually compare brain function in people who are randomized to an exercise program with those who are not, the case for a positive effect of exercise on the brain gets even stronger.

To be sure, not all interventional studies show a clear-cut effect. One 1991 study found no differences in cognitive function in older people who were assigned to aerobic exercise, those who did yoga, and those who did no exercise. But, as the authors note, the people in this study were functioning at a very high level to begin with.

A 2015 study also found no clear effect of exercise, but for the opposite reason. The researchers from the LIFE study randomized 1,635 older people at eight US medical centers to a walking, resistance, and flexibility training group or a health education group for two years. There was no difference in cognitive outcomes at the end of the study. But, as the researchers suggest, this may be because the level of physical activity was set too low to make a difference or because the participants themselves were physically unable to do much activity.

By and large, though, interventional studies for decades have shown positive results.

Back in the 1980s, researchers asked some people aged 55–70 to participate in an aerobic exercise program for four months, asked others to do strength and flexibility exercise, and had a third group do no supervised exercise program at all.

At the end of the study, the aerobic exercisers did significantly better on cognitive tests than either of the other two groups. Similarly, in a 1999 study of 124 previously sedentary people aged 60–75, those randomly assigned to aerobic exercise for six months improved substantially on executive function tests compared to people who just participated in stretching and toning.

In a 2006 study of 59 healthy people aged 60–70, half were assigned to aerobic exercise for six months, and half to a toning and stretching group. Significant increases in brain volume, in both white and gray matter, were found for the aerobic group, but not the stretching group. Other studies also show that aerobic exercise can slow the rate of hippocampal loss by an impressive one to two years.

In terms of executive function (planning, problem-solving, and other high-level brain activity), a 2008 study assigned 57 people aged 65–79 to either aerobic exercise or strength-and-flexibility training for

10 months. Only the aerobic exercise group improved on the Stroop Word-Color test, which tests executive brain functioning.

In a 2010 study of 24 men and women aged 65–78, researchers assigned some to an aerobic exercise program and the others, again, to a stretching program, three times a week for 12 weeks. This team studied several outcomes, including cognitive function before and after the intervention. Only the aerobic group improved in executive brain function.

In a 2015 randomized trial, a University of Kansas research team compared sedentary people aged 65 or older to those getting aerobic training for 26 weeks. Cardiovascular fitness is a good predictor of better cognitive function.

Some researchers have even used a particularly tricky cognitive test in which people undergoing brain scans are asked to focus on a single, central object while ignoring irrelevant, distracting objects. Using this method, researchers from Illinois and Pennsylvania tracked brain function with functional magnetic resonance imaging (fMRI) in older people randomly assigned to an aerobic exercise group or a non-aerobic stretching and toning group for six months. The aerobic group was better able to ignore the misleading information.

An even more powerful way to examine the relationship between exercise and cognition in later life is a meta-analysis, in which researchers pool data from numerous studies to get a larger sample.

In a 2003 meta-analysis of 18 interventional studies of exercise and cognitive function in older people, researchers Stanley Colcombe and Arthur Kramer at the University of Illinois, Urbana, asked a straightforward question: Does aerobic fitness have a "robust and beneficial influence" on cognition? The answer was "an unequivocal yes." And the biggest benefits were for executive processing, the very function most affected by aging.

In a 2008 systematic review, researchers writing for the Cochrane Database of Systematic Reviews examined 11 randomized clinical trials of aerobic training and cognitive function. Eight of the 11 studies confirmed that aerobic exercise was linked to improvements in cognitive capacity. Since then, other meta-analyses and systematic reviews have come to similar conclusions.

While aerobic exercise has been more extensively studied for its potential benefits to the brain, studies on resistance exercise—weight training—are beginning to catch up.

In one study, 62 older people were divided into three groups: One group did no exercise, one did moderately difficult resistance training, and one, high-intensity resistance training. After six months, both moderate- and high-intensity resistance exercise had beneficial effects on cognitive functioning, a finding supported by other studies.

BOX 8.2 CHEMICAL MESSENGERS

Unlike stars in the Milky Way (at least as far as we know), our 86 billion neurons "talk" to each other using chemical signals, with each neuron getting input from thousands of others.

The communication works like this. An electrical signal passes down an axon— a long, skinny branch of the nerve cell—until it reaches its end point at the synapse, a tiny structure that allows signals to pass between two nerve cells. At the synapse, a neurotransmitter (chemical messenger) takes the message across the fibrous synapse to waiting dendrites, the receiving branches of the next cell.

The neurotransmitter slides into a receptor on the receiving cell, much as a key fits into a lock. As soon as the neurotransmitter lands, ion channels in the receiving cell's membrane open up, which converts the signal back into electrical form. When the electrical charge in the receiving cell reaches a certain threshold, that cell then sends an outgoing signal along its axon to the next neuron. In our always-busy brains, this process repeats over and over.

The two most important neurotransmitters in the brain are glutamate, an excitatory (stimulatory) messenger, and GABA (gamma-aminobutyric acid), an inhibitory messenger that does the opposite, calming things down. (Some general anesthetics work by reducing the effects of glutamate, and some tranquilizers, by boosting GABA. Exercise, even for as little as 20 minutes, seems to boost levels of both glutamate and GABA.)

Although glutamate and GABA govern an estimated 80 percent of brain activity, other, more famous, neurotransmitters are crucial, too, most notably serotonin, norepinephrine, and dopamine. They also regulate the flow of information around the brain.

Later in this chapter, we'll pay special attention to another brain chemical, BDNF (brain-derived neurotrophic factor). BDNF is such a hot focus of research that in recent years, scientists have published more than 5,000 papers on BDNF's effects.

DEMENTIA, MILD COGNITIVE IMPAIRMENT, AND SCHIZOPHRENIA

One of the most feared problems of later life is Alzheimer's disease, the most common form of dementia, along with mild cognitive impairment, which is a decline in memory and other cognitive abilities that raises the risk of Alzheimer's.

It's important to recognize that these cognitive decline diseases are *not* a normal or inevitable part of aging. But they are alarmingly common. The US Centers for Disease Control and Prevention deems Alzheimer's disease a "public health crisis," noting that in 2013, an estimated 5 million Americans over age 65 had Alzheimer's, with that prevalence expected to rise to 13.8 million by 2050.

Since most drug treatments have been disappointing, anything that could help prevent or slow the progression of these diseases would be an enormous boon.

Fortunately, exercise can do just that.

Indeed, if everyone who is currently inactive became physically active at the modest levels recommended by governmental guidelines, an estimated one in seven cases of Alzheimer's disease could be prevented, according to a 2013 estimate from the Ontario Brain Institute.

To be sure, a state-of-the-science meeting on Alzheimer's at the National Institutes of Health in 2010 came to a rather tepid assessment of the research on exercise and Alzheimer's risk reduction, saying the data are too preliminary to draw firm conclusions.

But a year later, when researchers from the Mayo Clinic looked at a broader range of both animal and human research—including 1,603 publications identified in a PubMed search—a far more encouraging picture emerged. Meta-analyses of prospective studies showed "significantly reduced later risks of dementia associated with midlife exercise," the Mayo team found. Exercise also reduced the risk of mild cognitive impairment.

When University College London researchers systematically reviewed 16 prospective studies of people without dementia at baseline, they, too, found that physical activity is inversely related to risk of dementia. In a five-year Canadian study of 4,615 men and women over age 65, physical activity—compared to no exercise—was also linked to lower risk of cognitive impairment, Alzheimer's, and dementia of any type.

Alzheimer's disease wreaks havoc in the brain in multiple ways, but one of the most important is that it attacks the synapses, the tiny structures that allow chemical signals to pass between neurons. In fact, Alzheimer's could be called "a disease of synaptic failure," says Cotman of the University of California, Irvine.

One of the ways Alzheimer's disrupts synapses is that the hallmark protein beta-amyloid, which causes the characteristic sticky plaques of Alzheimer's, binds to synapses, making them dysfunctional. A major benefit of long-term exercise is that, at least in animal models, it can reduce levels of beta-amyloid in the brain. Aerobic exercise may also improve levels of the tau protein, another marker of Alzheimer's. It's this protein that, when twisted, causes Alzheimer's characteristic tangles.

In addition to lowering the *risk* of Alzheimer's and mild cognitive dementia, exercise can also be a treatment. It's not known whether there is a window of opportunity past which exercise would not slow cognitive decline. But the research is encouraging.

In a 2010 study, researchers from the University of Washington randomized 33 people aged 55–85 with mild cognitive impairment to high-intensity aerobic exercise or stretching for six months. Aerobic exercise significantly improved cognitive function—especially for women, who showed improvement on a wider variety of tests than men.

The Mayo Clinic's analysis similarly concluded that people who already have cognitive problems but who exercise do better than sedentary controls in randomized controlled trials, with better cognitive scores after 6–12 months of exercise. Aerobic exercise for 6–12 months is also linked to better *connectivity* among different parts of the brain.

Similarly, in a 2012 New York study, people with Alzheimer's disease who did *some* physical activity had a lower risk of dying during the course of the five-year study than those who didn't, and people who did *a lot* of physical activity had an even lower risk. "Exercise may affect not only risk for Alzheimer's disease," the authors concluded, "but also subsequent disease duration: More physical activity is associated with prolonged survival in Alzheimer's disease."

And in a meta-analysis of 2,020 people with dementia and related cognitive impairments participating in 30 randomized studies, exercise once again increased cognitive function. A particularly compelling study in Australia randomized 170 older people who had "memory problems" (but did not meet criteria for frank Alzheimer's) to six months of moderate-intensity exercise or sedentary behavior. The exercise group had significantly better scores on a standard Alzheimer's test, and the benefit persisted for a year and a half.

In a different Australian randomized study of 100 people with mild cognitive dementia, six months of resistance (as opposed to aerobic) training significantly improved cognitive function, and the improvement lasted at least 18 months. In a 2016 randomized study from Wake Forest School of Medicine, researchers used a new MRI technique and showed that people with mild cognitive impairment who did aerobic exercise showed greater increases in brain volume than those who just stretched.

Researchers have long known that a particular gene variant called APOE-4 raises the risk of Alzheimer's. In a complex study at the Cleveland Clinic, researchers gathered almost 100 people aged 65–80. Many had a family history of Alzheimer's, and some carried the APOE-4 variant.

The researchers sorted the volunteers into four groups and did brain scans on all of them, focusing on the hippocampus, the brain's memory center. They then repeated the scans a year and a half later. People with the "bad" gene who did *not* exercise showed significant shrinkage of their hippocampi, a striking finding, given the short time span. But people with the "bad" gene who *did* exercise showed almost no hippocampal shrinkage, just like the people who did not carry the APOE-4 gene variant.

In a separate study, researchers studied 347 older Dutch men and found that those who exercised less than an hour a day were at higher risk of cognitive decline than those who exercised more. The risk of that decline was especially strong in men carrying the APOE-4 gene variant.

Other chemical messengers are also part of the story, including BDNF (brain-derived neurotrophic factor), which is responsive to exercise and is strikingly reduced in people with Alzheimer's. Interestingly, BDNF levels are also significantly lower in Alzheimer's patients who are declining rapidly than in those whose disease is progressing slowly.

Exercise may even aid cognitive functioning in people with schizophrenia, a thought disorder, and Parkinson's disease.

In a University of California, Los Angeles, study of people having their first episode of schizophrenia, researchers used MRI scans to assess gray matter volume in the prefrontal cortex and the hippocampus. Schizophrenic patients with a history of low levels of physical activity had greater losses of brain volume in these areas than people who had higher levels of exercise.

In a meta-analysis of studies involving 385 people with schizophrenia, University of Manchester researchers found that aerobic exercise improves cognitive function in a linear fashion.

Exercise, as we've seen in preceding chapters, has numerous effects all over the body. But one of the most important involves blood flow, and nowhere is that more crucial than in the brain. Indeed, reduced blood flow to key areas of the brain is one of the early signs of both vascular dementia (inadequate blood supply to the brain) and Alzheimer's disease. And giving "young" blood to older animals may rejuvenate aging brains.

In a Scottish study in mice, for instance, researchers found that reduced cerebral blood flow quickly led to an increase in the amyloid protein. In humans, Arizona researchers using MRI (magnetic imaging) brain scans found that cerebral blood flow was 20 percent lower in people with Alzheimer's compared to non-demented people. (Interestingly, in the early stages of disease, as the brain changes from normal cognition to dementia, the brain compensates by temporarily *increasing* blood flow to crucial brain areas, including the hippocampus.)

It's now clear that aerobic exercise can dramatically increase cerebral blood flow and capillary growth, even in older adults. Even more encouraging is the fact that exercise-induced increases in blood flow occur in precisely the areas where new neurons grow, the dentate gyrus part of the hippocampus, the sub-region most crucial for memory.

Unfortunately, it's also abundantly clear that *stopping* aerobic exercise *decreases* cerebral blood flow in at least eight key brain areas, including the hippocampus. In a clever but depressing study of 12 exceedingly fit Masters athletes (aged 50 or over), University of Maryland researchers persuaded the runners to cease exercising for 10 days. Blood flow to the left and right hippocampus dropped sharply, by 20–30 percent.

BOX 8.3 NEW NEURONS IN THE HUMAN ADULT HIPPOCAMPUS?

While animal studies clearly show that exercise induces new neuronal growth in the hippocampus, human studies have not been able to answer this question explicitly because it's difficult and normally unethical to experiment on living human brains. This has forced scientists to assess post-mortem tissues from humans instead. Some studies do show that exercise induces increased human hippocampal volume, but this could be due to factors other than new neuronal growth, such as the growth of glial (non-neuronal) tissue and increased vascularization. Other studies have come to conflicting conclusions.

Regardless of exercise as a trigger, scientists are struggling to figure out whether the hippocampus in adult humans can grow new neurons at all. One Swedish study, for instance, concluded that not only are new neurons formed in the human adult hippocampus, but they are formed at the rate of 700 new ones a day. The Swedish team also concluded that neurogenesis continues throughout adulthood and that the rate of formation of new neurons is comparable in mice and humans. Other researchers, too, have found evidence of new neuronal growth in the human hippo-campus throughout life. But other teams have not found clear evidence of new neuron growth.

On March 15, 2018, researchers from the University of California, San Francisco, dropped a bombshell on the field of neurogenesis. In a paper in Nature, the team, led by senior researcher Shawn Sorrells, studied brain tissue from macaque monkeys and 59 people from newborns to adults up to age 77. (The human tissue came from people who had died or who had had surgery for epilepsy.)

The researchers found that new neuronal growth in the hippocampus declines sharply after birth, leaving only a handful of new neurons by 13 years of age, and virtually none later on.

Perhaps, the authors speculated, the lack of new neurons has something to do with the larger brain size of humans compared to rodents. Or maybe, the stem cells from which new neurons grow stop self-renewing after birth. Or perhaps new human neurons take longer to mature than in rodents. Or maybe, the studies that do find new neuronal growth have been mistakenly finding new growth not in nerve cells, but in glial cells, the glue-like cells that surround neurons.

Not surprisingly, the paper evoked howls of disagreement, including from Fred "Rusty" Gage, one of the first scientists who, back in the 1990s, challenged the then-prevalent view that no new neurons were generated in adulthood. In a statement to NPR, Gage, interim director of the Salk Institute, said his results and others' "repeatedly confirm that neurogenesis can occur in the adult brain."

Roughly a month after the Sorrells paper, research scientist Maura Boldrini and her team at Columbia University published their own bombshell. They, too, looked at the brains of healthy people who had died between the ages of 14 and 79. Not only did they find, as dogma had long held, that healthy, human adults keep making new neurons in the hippocampus throughout life, but that, as the 2013 Swedish research had shown, their 2018 findings fit with the idea that people produce about 700 new hippocampal neurons per day.

Sorrells and co-investigator Mercedes Paredes say that their findings may not conflict as much with dogma as might appear. Neuronal growth in the adult hippo-campus might still happen, not by the generation of new neurons, but by adding new parts to existing neurons, specifically new synapses and dendrites.

"Think of a forest," says Sorrells. "There are two ways it can increase in size. One way is to plant more trees. The other is to wait for the trees that are there to grow in size."

Harvard psychiatrist John Ratey dubs it "Miracle-Gro for the brain." University of California, Irvine, neurologist Carl Cotman calls it a "miracle molecule." To *Science* magazine, it's simply a "crucial protein."

By whatever nickname, BDNF, which stands for brain-derived nerve growth factor, is arguably one of the most important molecules ever discovered. BDNF has long been believed to do two important things in a tiny part of the hippocampus called the dentate gyrus, at least in animals: boost the growth of existing nerve cells and the synapses between neurons, and trigger stem cells to become brand new neurons.

Back in the 1950s, Italian neurobiologist Rita Levi-Montalcini and a colleague discovered what would turn out to be a molecule related to BDNF, which she named nerve growth factor (NGF) because it does exactly that—it makes nerves grow. She won the 1986 Nobel Prize for her discovery. (She went on to become a senator in the Italian Senate and, in 2009, became the first Nobel laureate to live to 100.)

It would be decades before other scientists, probing the ways the body makes and nurtures new nerves, would eventually, in 1982, discover BDNF, the second member of this family of molecules. Over time, the discovery of BDNF would lead to an explosion of insights.

In lab after lab, eager scientists began unraveling BDNF's many tricks. They learned that light can trigger production of BDNF, and that simulation by whiskers and electricity can, too. They learned that BDNF lives all over the nervous system, but that it is especially high in the hippocampus. They learned that BDNF revs up excitatory currents in the synapses between brain cells, and that certain types of learning dramatically boost BDNF in the hippocampus. (They also discovered that BDNF levels rise sharply during epileptic seizures, and that blocking it may stop seizures.)

Over time, they would learn that low levels of BDNF are associated with Alzheimer's, Parkinson's, and Huntington's diseases, as well as depression. (In fact, lithium, a major treatment for bipolar disorder, appears to work in part by raising BDNF levels.) And they learned that increases in BDNF may offset age-related atrophy of the hippocampus, at least in animals.

But the real breakthrough came in the early 1990s when California neurobiologist Carl Cotman wondered, as he recalls, "Wouldn't it be cool if BDNF was induced by exercise?" Intrigued by that possibility, he proposed a study of exercise and BDNF to a post-doctoral student who, as Cotman jokes, "looked at me as though I had lost it." He tried other colleagues and finally found a grad student who enthusiastically agreed.

To Cotman's delight, his hunch panned out, and the "Eureka moment" soon followed. In 1995, he and his team published the first evidence of a BDNF–exercise connection—a letter to the journal *Nature* showing that exercise is linked to BDNF levels. In subsequent research, Cotman found that even just one week of exercise, at least in rodents, is enough to "turn on" the gene that controls production of BDNF. In other words, aerobic exercise, through genetic activation, boosts brain "plasticity"—the ability of the brain to change and grow.

The most dramatic evidence *in humans* that exercise directly boosts BDNF came in 2011 in an Irish study of male cyclists tested right after strenuous exercise. The researchers performed memory tests before and after intense exercise and found that an acute bout of exercise boosted both BDNF levels in the blood and recall. More important, the researchers said, it's likely that the increased BDNF came from the brain, not the rest of the body. A Boston University meta-analysis of 29 human studies involving 1,111 people also showed that exercise induces increased blood levels of BDNF.

To be sure, not all studies in humans show a rise in BDNF with exercise. A 2017 German study of cognitively healthy people aged 65 or older found no rise in BDNF with three months of aerobic training. A 2018 meta-analysis of 14 human studies involving 737 participants did not look at BDNF per se, but did look at hippocampal volume and found no significant effect of aerobic exercise on total volume, though this and other research suggests growth in *parts* of the hippocampus.

Still, it's clear that Cotman's original 1995 work set the research world on fire, prompting many researchers to try to figure out exactly what exercise was doing in the brain. One of most prominent is Henriette van Praag, who previously worked at the Salk Institute for Biological Studies and is now a neuroscientist at the National Institute on Aging.

Initially, van Praag, working in the late 1990s with her Salk colleagues Gerd Kempermann and Fred Gage, wanted to understand the link between "enriched environments" and the growth of neurons in the hippocampus of mice. At that time, scientists thought that things like larger cages, more social interaction, expanded learning opportunities, along with physical activity, were all linked to better brain function. Her question was, which of these was most important?

The answer? Running. In a pivotal 1999 paper, van Praag and her team showed, in animals, that running doubled the number of surviving nerve cells in the dentate gyrus of the hippocampus. Not only did the number of nerve cells increase, the newly created neurons were fully functional.

In 2005, van Praag's team divided middle-aged mice into two groups, one with a running wheel and one without. After one month, the running mice were much quicker at learning and remembering how to navigate a maze than similarly aged mice not allowed to run. Van Praag's team went on to show that exercise is "the critical factor" of an enriched environment that elevates BDNF levels and increases the growth of new neurons in the hippocampus. Even when running doesn't start until mid- to later life, it still can promote brain plasticity.

Other researchers have documented similar effects. In one study in Finland, for instance, researchers assigned male rats to different exercise groups and a sedentary control group. One group was given running wheels and allowed to run as much or as little as they wanted. Most ran moderately for several miles a day. Another group did a rodent form of resistance training, which involved climbing a wall with weights attached to their tails. The third group was put through a rat version of high-intensity interval training, required to run fast for three minutes at a time, then slowly for two minutes, and repeating that for a total of 15 minutes. All the groups were followed for seven weeks.

The rats that jogged at will showed the most gain in neurons in the hippocampus, and the more mileage a rat logged, the better the neurogenesis. And the weight-training rats? They got stronger, but showed virtually no neurogenesis.

Exactly how, at the molecular level, BDNF might trigger neuronal growth is an active research focus. But scientists have some clues. With exercise, brain waves change in a pleasant direction, that is, toward theta rhythm, a relaxed state often linked to creativity. This leads to the release of the neurotransmitters serotonin and norepinephrine, and more rapid firing of nerves. This in turn can result in activation of the gene that makes BDNF. In fact, if serotonin-producing nerve cells are damaged, BDNF production stops.

BDNF works by passing its signal to nearby cells by landing on a receptor called TrkB (pronounced "track B," for tyrosine kinase B). This receptor is key. When scientists block it with antibodies, BDNF signaling grinds to a halt.

BDNF turns out to be one of several exercise-induced growth factors for the hippocampus. If scientists block receptors for these growth factors, too, nerve growth also ceases. Estrogen, too, is increasingly recognized as playing an important role, in part because deprivation of estrogen has been shown to reduce BDNF gene expression. Contrarily, replacing estrogen at menopause seems to protect gray matter. And being fit can prolong the positive effect of hormone therapy.

Cotman, among others, is as excited today as he has always been: "BNDF definitely makes nerves grow in the hippocampus." In fact, he says, BDNF levels not only increase in the hippocampus after just a few days of exercise, but stay high for a week or two, before returning to baseline after three to four weeks. In other words, BDNF induces a kind of "molecular memory. . . . It doesn't wear off fast." To get this effect, though, physical activity has to be fairly vigorous and frequent, at least three or four times a week for at least 45 minutes per time. Stretching or weightlifting doesn't cut it.

Cotman and colleagues from Rush University have also explored just how persistent this effect is. They looked at autopsied brains of recently deceased people who died of non–brain-related causes. They correlated the autopsy findings with seven years' worth of data on how much or little the people had exercised. "We found enormous gene changes," says Cotman. The brains of the stalwart exercisers showed as many as "a couple of hundred" positive genetic changes in precisely the genes that would ordinarily become less active with aging.

In a similar study, Rush University researchers did annual cognitive assessments and tracked BDNF levels in 535 people, then did autopsy exams after the people died. Higher levels of BDNF were strongly linked to slower cognitive decline, and the link was strongest in people with dementia.

The bottom line? Exercise is the best thing going to protect the brain.

CHAPTER 9
Exercise and Mood

RUNNING HEALS

In the early 2000s, Abby Lee (aka Zoe Margolis to her fans) gained a public profile with her popular blog, "Girl with a One-Track Mind," and best-selling book of the same title. Her blog claims more than 250,000 visitors a month. In 2008, *The Observer* newspaper ranked her blog 24th among the world's most powerful blogs. Her book has been translated into 15 languages.

But in 2015, Margolis did her fans, and the world, a huge favor, which may have taken even more courage than writing about her sex life. She wrote a piece for *The Guardian* about her crippling depression—and how she healed herself with exercise.

"At the start of this year," Margolis wrote, "I was in the depths of the worst depression I have ever experienced. My public face was a mask of success, confidence and happiness, but privately, I was defeated. The long-term relationship that I had hoped would last the rest of my life and lead to children had ended, painfully. Work was at a standstill, and I was broke. I felt overweight and unhappy with my tired, sluggish body."

Her entire existence was miserable: "Every waking moment was filled with crushing anxiety and heavy sadness. . . . When you lack the energy even to get out of bed in the morning, the last thing you need to hear is that you should pull yourself together and go to the gym."

But she did—first, for walks in a nearby park, then for runs in jogging shoes that had lurked in her closet for years. Slowly, as the days and the miles ticked by, she began to feel better. Now, she says, "When I run, I know that at some point . . . positive brain chemistry happens, and

I feel brilliant." She's boiled it down to a simple equation: "I feel crap, so I run, and afterwards, sometimes for days, my depression lifts. . . . For me, it is truly a lifesaver."

In fact, not only is exercise now considered a proven way to help prevent depression and to treat it once you've got it, new research on exercise and mood is revolutionizing scientists' understanding of what depression is in the first place.

The brain chemistry that for years was assumed to be the main problem in depression—a deficiency of the neurotransmitter serotonin, for which drugs like Prozac were the supposed cure—is no longer the whole story.

The more important driver of depression may be a deficiency of our old friend from Chapter 8, BDNF (brain-derived neurotrophic factor). People who are depressed turn out to have too little BDNF in their brains. When they exercise, BDNF goes up, and they feel better. In fact, in depressed rats (yes, there are ways to make rats depressed), injections of BDNF directly into the brain reverse depressed behavior. Of course, it's not *quite* that simple in humans, but that's the thrust.

We're getting ahead of our story, though. In this chapter, we'll start with the *observational* evidence for exercise as a way to *prevent* depression, anxiety, and stress, then analyze the impressive body of *interventional* studies documenting exercise as a *treatment* for mood problems. Then we'll look at the new research on the molecular mechanisms by which exercise combats depression. Along the way, we'll see why running may have made the brains of early humans bigger, and what really underlies the "runner's high."

IT'S A SAD, SAD WORLD

Around the world, in rich countries and in poor, people are feeling ever more miserable. Between 1990 and 2013, the number of people suffering from depression and/or anxiety grew by almost 50 percent, from 416 million to 615 million, according to the World Health Organization. That's a significant 10 percent of the planet's population.

Worldwide, 800,000 people a year die from suicide. In the United States, it was 45,000 as of 2016 and rising. Anxiety is even more common than depression, affecting roughly 40 million American adults; depression in the United States affects more than 16 million.

In fact, depression is now the leading cause of disability worldwide, and is a major contributor to the overall global burden of disease, according to 2017 figures from the World Health Organization.

Depression, which can be mild, disabling, or severe, is characterized by feelings of sadness, loss of interest or pleasure, feelings of guilt or low self-esteem, disturbed sleep or appetite, feelings of tiredness, and poor concentration. According to the American Psychological Association, anxiety is characterized by feelings of tension, worried thoughts, and physical changes such as increased blood pressure.

We'll see in this chapter that as an exploding body of research shows, exercise can be worth its weight in gold, both as a preventive measure and as a treatment.

BOX 9.1 RUNNER'S HIGH

There's no question that exercise improves mood and reduces depression. But an actual high? Is it real? If so, what could trigger it?

The short answer is yes, it's real. And it's not just endorphins at work.

"Although a great deal of research data argue for the participation of endogenous opioids in mood regulation during and after exercise, most of the evidence is 'indirect,'" says University of Georgia professor of exercise science Rod Dishman.

Indeed, it would take an awful lot of painful exercise to trigger enough endorphins to explain the "runner's high," agrees Boston University psychologist Michael Otto.

It's true that blood levels of endorphins do rise in humans after exercise. But higher endorphin levels in the blood don't necessarily mean there are higher levels in the brain, where mood effects would occur, although one small study does suggest this. But if endorphins are truly the mechanism for the mood-enhancing effects of exercise, this effect should be blocked by injections of naloxone, an opiate (and endorphin) blocker.

It isn't.

The real trigger for the runner's high, according to current thinking, is a class of chemicals called endocannabinoids, marijuana-like substances produced naturally in the body.

Unlike endorphins, which are large molecules that can't easily cross into the brain from the blood, endocannabinoids are small, fatty molecules that can easily slip into the brain, producing feelings of transcendence and a genuine high.

The proof is in the ferrets. Unlike most animals, which love to run, ferrets balk at the mere prospect. They hate it, says David Raichlen, a University of Arizona biological anthropologist, who has spent many hours in the lab trying to get ferrets to run. They just won't, and the reason, he has concluded, is that they don't get high from running. They don't get increased levels of endocannabinoids if they run.

But people do, and that's the take-home lesson: Don't be a ferret. Run hard, swim hard, dance hard. With luck, you will trigger those endocannabinoids. You won't just ward off depression and anxiety and stress, but if you work hard enough, you may actually get high.

EXERCISE AS PREVENTION: OBSERVATIONAL EVIDENCE

In observational, as opposed to interventional, studies, there's a built-in dilemma: Do people who exercise feel better as a *result*? Or are people who feel better to start with more likely to exercise? Or both?

One of the first studies to document this link came out in 1988. It showed that the higher a person's level of exercise at the beginning of the study, the lower the risk of depression eight years later.

Six years after that study, groundbreaking research by exercise scientist Ralph Paffenbarger cemented that observation. Rates of depression were significantly lower among men who exercised regularly, according to his study, which tracked thousands of male Harvard alumni for 25 years.

Bolstered by those early results, researchers from around the world—Finland, Norway, Australia, Korea, Europe, the United States, and elsewhere—began tracking the exercise–mood connection, broadly confirming Paffenbarger's findings.

Even when researchers take into account every conceivable variable that could muddy the results—age, sex, ethnicity, financial strain, chronic conditions, disability, body mass index, alcohol consumption, smoking, social relationships—the exercise link holds up.

The same is true when researchers study the flip side—happiness—as opposed to depression. In one cleverly designed 2017 study, British researchers used smartphones and a new app that could track people's activity levels and send them questions throughout the day to report their mood.

They concluded that people were happier when they had been moving in the 15 minutes prior to being queried than when they had been sitting or lying down. People who moved around a lot were also happier with life in general.

A 2017 European study that followed nearly 34,000 men and women without depression or other mental health problems found that, 11 years later, regular leisure-time exercise was linked to a reduced incidence of depression, though not anxiety.

Finally, a 2016 systematic review of studies involving *more than 1 million men and women* showed that people with the lowest cardiovascular fitness were 75 percent more likely to develop depression than people with the highest fitness.

BOX 9.2 DID RUNNING MAKE OUR ANCESTORS' BRAINS BIGGER?

A long, long time ago, about 7 or 8 million years, we—or more precisely, our human ancestors—were still living a lot like our cousins, the chimpanzees. We kept up our simian habits, eating fruit and hanging out in a sedentary lifestyle.

Then suddenly, about 2.5 million years ago, the earth's climate cooled as the ice age set in. Prairies evolved where forests of fruit trees had been. We had to adapt— or starve. Out of necessity, we began to shift our diets toward animal protein. That meant hunting, and that meant running, a lot of running. Indeed, endurance running, as we saw in Chapter 1, allowed us to practice persistence hunting (chasing animals until they dropped from exhaustion), the newly discovered trick that would keep us alive. It also helped keep us out of the claws and jaws of predators.

But in truth, running may have done a lot more than just keep us fed. As we saw in this chapter, running induces a cascade of molecules, most notably, BDNF (brain-derived neurotrophic factor), which has long been believed to stimulate new neuron growth in the brain. Quite literally, running may make the brain grow.

"Hunting and gathering upped the amount of exercise per day," says biological anthropologist Raichlen of Arizona. And that, he thinks, could have been a stimulus (or at least one stimulus) for the growth of the disproportionately big brain that is the hallmark of our species today.

But here's the fascinating thing. "Food isn't always the only motivator" for running, Raichlen contends. Feeling good is, too.

For humans and many other mammals (though not ferrets), running triggers a cascade of molecular signals that improve mood, often significantly. It's not just the "runner's high." The larger point is that exercise is essential for maintaining and restoring mental health.

BLOOD, SWEAT, AND TEARS: EXERCISE AS TREATMENT

While it's possible to challenge causality in observational studies, interventional studies are harder to dispute. In interventional studies, one group of people is randomly assigned to exercise, usually aerobic, while a similar group is assigned to no exercise or something minimally demanding, like stretching. Both groups are tested before and after the study period for levels of anxiety, depression, or stress.

Overall, the evidence is overwhelming. It shows that exercise is an excellent treatment for depression, that it is often as effective as antidepressant medications, and that it works synergistically at the molecular level as an adjunct to medications.

The first study suggesting a link between physical activity and depression was published more than 100 years ago, in 1905, in the *American Journal of Insanity* [*sic*]. A pair of researchers from McLean Hospital, a psychiatric facility outside of Boston, managed to persuade two depressed patients to exercise. The researchers rather loftily extrapolated from this tiny sample to conclude that there must be "a large class of patients whose feeling of inadequacy, retardation, and mental depression are indications for exercise, both passive and active."

It took decades for other researchers to take the bait in serious scientific fashion. Finally, in 1979, University of Wisconsin researchers published the first *randomized controlled* study comparing exercise— favorably, as it turned out—with other types of depression treatment. In the mid-1980s, the Wisconsin team compared exercise with group psychotherapy for depression and found it to be at least equal in effectiveness.

By the late 1980s, other researchers had begun documenting the positive effects of exercise for depression treatment. In one of the first to look at resistance training as well as aerobic exercise, University of Rochester researchers showed in 1987 that both types of exercise can alleviate depression. Two years later, Norwegian researchers came to a similar conclusion. (Since then, Australian researchers have also shown that resistance training is an effective treatment for depression.)

But things really took off with the work of James Blumenthal, a psychologist at Duke University. Back in the 1980s, while studying the benefit of exercise for people with cardiovascular disease, Blumenthal noticed that exercise appeared to be a mood lifter as well.

Intrigued, the Duke team gathered 156 men and women aged 50 or older and randomly assigned them to aerobic exercise with a group, antidepressant medication (Zoloft), or both. After 16 weeks, the results were stunning.

All three groups got better. But while the group getting only Zoloft (sertraline hydrochloride) saw their depression lift quickly, by 16 weeks of treatment, exercise was *just as effective* in reducing depression.

This finding was all the more impressive because the patients had major depressive disorder—severe depression lasting two weeks or more. The study also cemented another thing: that exercise works just as well for older people as for younger.

The even better news? When the Duke team followed up with these 156 people 10 months after the study began, the people in the exercise group were *much less likely to relapse* into depression than the other groups. "For each 50-minute increment of exercise," Blumenthal found, "there was an accompanying 50 percent reduction in relapse risk."

The Duke team didn't stop there. In yet another study of 202 adults with major depression, exercise was *comparable* to medication (Zoloft) in relieving major depression. And the effect was dose-dependent, a finding confirmed by other researchers.

All of this led researchers to wonder what would happen if exercise were *combined with medication,* an important question because many people taking antidepressant pills get only partial relief. A Texas team took on the challenge, showing in a series of studies that adding exercise to medication brings significant benefits. A Scottish team came to similar conclusions, as did an Italian team and an American team from Rutgers University.

But it's when researchers pool data from numerous studies—in meta-analyses and systematic reviews—that exercise shows its true power. To cite just one of those analyses, in 2013 the Cochrane Collaboration, a prestigious group of international researchers who analyze the quality of medical evidence, examined 35 studies and concluded that physical activity was *comparable to psychological therapy and medication* at relieving depression.

The jury is clearly in. Exercise is such a powerful treatment for depression that older studies may actually have *underestimated* its effects. Indeed, researchers conducting a 2016 meta-analysis of 25 randomized controlled trials concluded that the data showing the effectiveness of exercise for depression treatment are so strong that "more than 1,000 studies with negative results would be needed to nullify the effects of exercise on depression."

EXERCISE FOR ANXIETY?

Unfortunately, there has been less research on exercise for anxiety, and the studies that have been done have had more mixed results.

In one early study of people with panic attacks, for instance, researchers found that regular aerobic exercise beat placebo, but was not as effective as medication. An early meta-analysis of 40 studies also found exercise had only a low to moderate effect on anxiety reduction.

More recently, anxiety researchers tested exercise and a popular non-drug therapy called "cognitive restructuring" (in which people learn to challenge negative thoughts). Both approaches produced significant reductions in anxiety sensitivity compared to the control group. (Anxiety sensitivity is the heightened responsiveness to sensations associated with anxiety.)

Researchers have also compared exercise, relaxation training, and the anti-anxiety drug Paxil (paroxetine) in 75 people with panic disorder. People taking Paxil did better than those getting a placebo pill. Unfortunately, people doing exercise training did not fare better than those doing relaxation.

Similarly, a University of Maryland study found that exercise and just sitting quietly were about equally effective against anxiety. But exercise does seem to be better than no treatment at all, as a University of Arizona team found when they pooled data from 49 randomized controlled trials.

In 2015, Australian researchers did the ultimate in research studies: a *meta-meta analysis*, that is, a meta-analysis of meta-analyses, all of which had high-quality data.

For this heroic effort, the researchers combined 92 studies on exercise and *depression* involving 4,310 people, and 306 studies on exercise and *anxiety* involving 10,755 people. Physical activity reduced both anxiety and depression, but had a much stronger effect on depression. The effect on anxiety may have been murkier because clinical anxiety can manifest in so many different ways (panic attacks, phobias, generalized anxiety disorder, etc.), all of which may respond differently to exercise.

Put bluntly, exercise seems to be somewhat but not dazzlingly effective at reducing anxiety.

MECHANISMS: WHY EXERCISE HELPS

At last, the nitty-gritty: How is it that molecules triggered by exercise can exert such potent effects on mood?

It's a fascinating story. In fact, the emerging insights on exercise and depression are revolutionizing the way in which brain scientists understand depression itself and are forcing a major rethinking of the ways that traditional antidepressant drugs work.

For decades, neuroscientists have believed in the monoamine hypothesis of depression. This is the idea that depression is caused, at least in part, by deficiencies of three important neurotransmitters (monoamines): norepinephrine, dopamine, and most notably, serotonin.

The "proof" of this theory lay in the observation that antidepressant drugs appear to relieve depression by raising brain levels of serotonin and norepinephrine. These drugs work by blocking the re-uptake of the neurotransmitters from the synapses between neurons, thus leaving more of the neurotransmitters available.

"In the '50s and '60s, the idea was that depression involved a deficit of serotonin, and that blocking reuptake of serotonin by drugs like Prozac remedied this deficit," says Yale University neuroscientist Ronald Duman, director of the Abraham Ribicoff Research Facilities. "But that never panned out. There is no strong evidence that depression is a serotonin deficiency."

Not all neuroscientists would put it quite that emphatically. But the new view, strongly bolstered by research on exercise and the brain, is that serotonin and its cousins are only part of the story.

The central player is now thought to be BDNF, brain-derived neurotrophic factor, the molecule that makes new brain cells grow. BDNF goes up with exercise and interacts in complex, bi-directional ways with neurotransmitters, especially serotonin.

It's now clear that both antidepressants and exercise trigger BDNF. And that BDNF and serotonin work as what scientists call a "dynamic duo"—serotonin stimulates the expression of BDNF, and BDNF enhances the growth and survival of serotonin-producing neurons.

BDNF, in other words, is a link between exercise and mood. High BDNF levels are strongly correlated with better mood and less depression. Exercise is a major, and by far the most practical, way to boost BDNF in the hippocampus.

The hippocampus, as we saw in the previous chapter, is a major brain center for learning and memory. Exercise is believed to trigger better memory and cognition by raising levels of BDNF, which in turn may cause the growth of new hippocampal cells or boost synaptic connections between existing neurons. (Recently, some researchers have questioned whether new neuronal grow actually occurs in the adult human hippocampus, the memory center of the brain, but many researchers still believe it does. See Box 8.3 in Chapter 8.)

But the hippocampus, which is strategically located in the limbic system, is not just involved in cognition. It is also a major center for processing emotions. And that, of course, makes it ground zero for depression.

"The basic idea is that depression is a neurodegenerative disease. With depression, there are fewer synapses and reduced neuronal growth in the hippocampus," says neuroscientist Carl Cotman, founding director of the Institute for Memory Impairment and Neurological Diseases (MIND) at the University of California, Irvine.

The good news, he says, is that "both exercise and antidepressants relieve that. BDNF stops the neurodegenerative pathways and builds the brain back up. The circuits become functional again."

In brain scan studies, major depression has been shown to lead to a shrinkage of the hippocampus. In fact, the degree of shrinkage correlates well with how long a person has been seriously depressed. Post-mortem studies also have revealed distinctly small hippocampi in the brains of people who were depressed.

In theory, two things could account for shrinkage of the hippocampus—destruction or death of hippocampal cells, or the failure of the hippocampus to generate new nerve cells. Researchers think it's primarily the latter at work in depression.

There's no question that exercise is a powerful way to boost BDNF levels in the brain. In fact, a meta-analysis of 29 studies found that *even a single session* of exercise was enough to boost BDNF levels. Chronic exercise is linked to even higher levels of BDNF.

Antidepressants like Prozac also work in part by raising BDNF levels, not just by keeping more serotonin around in the synapses between nerve cells. And more serotonin leads to increased expression of the gene that makes BDNF, which leads to creation of new nerve cells in the hippocampus, says Duman.

The clue that led to the revised view of depression was timing.

Researchers had long been puzzled about why it takes so long—four to five weeks—for traditional antidepressants to improve mood. Then they noticed a curious thing—that this amount of time, four or five weeks, is almost exactly how long it takes for new neurons to become fully functional.

That suggested that relief from depression could depend on the maturation of new hippocampal cells, which supports the idea that BDNF is a major player. (New, rapid-acting antidepressants such as ketamine work through different pathways—too fast to involve creation of new hippocampal cells.)

This revolution in the understanding of depression began in the late 1990s. In 1997, Duman discovered that antidepressant drugs trigger a chemical called c-AMP (cyclic AMP), which boosts production of BDNF in the hippocampus. This increase in BDNF occurred in precisely the areas of the hippocampus most depleted by stress. (Stress has long been suspected to be closely tied to depression.)

All of this suggested, as Duman puts it, the need for "an updated molecular and cellular hypothesis for depression." His idea is that both stress-induced vulnerability and the mechanisms by which antidepressants work occur because of specific chemical changes inside cells. These changes ultimately affect the survival and function of particular neurons.

One early clue was what happened in 1997 when researchers injected BDNF directly into the brains of depressed rats, right into areas of the brainstem where serotonin and norepinephrine are produced. Just as the emerging theory predicted, BDNF boosted activity in those areas and relieved depression.

(For the record, there are various ways to simulate depression in rats and mice. Researchers can give repeated electric shocks that the animals can't escape, or force them to swim in tiny pools that they can't escape from. The result is that the animals give up, a kind of "learned helplessness" that is believed to mirror depression in humans.)

In 1999, French researchers showed that depleting serotonin in a key part of the hippocampus (the dentate gyrus) decreased the production of new nerve cells, bolstering the idea that depression may be linked to shrinkage in the hippocampus, and, ultimately, to BDNF.

In 2000, noting that both physical activity and antidepressant medication independently increase expression of the BDNF gene, Cotman's team took it to the next step. By *combining* exercise with medications, the team found, the two approaches are synergistic at the cellular level, with both methods working together to boost BDNF levels and reduce depression.

In 2002, Duman's team confirmed that a single injection of BDNF into the hippocampus produced an antidepressant effect in rodents undergoing the learned helplessness and forced swim tests. In fact, just that one injection produced an antidepressant effect comparable to standard antidepressants.

The team went on to show that Prozac reversed the depletion of hippocampal cells caused by inescapable stress.

In 2006, Canadian researchers picked up the thread, further piecing together the evidence that exercise can alleviate even major depression and that different mechanisms converge to trigger new nerve growth in the hippocampus.

Although BDNF is now considered the star—at least at the moment—of the exercise–mood connection, scientists are finding other molecules that also appear to play key roles. One is VEGF (vascular endothelial growth factor). Secreted from the blood, VEGF acts on endothelial cells to make new blood vessels grow. But VEGF does more than that. It appears to make new nerves grow in the hippocampus. And it can be increased by exercise.

In 2000, researchers from Austria, Switzerland, and Germany tracked 13 ultra-marathon runners as they trained in the mountains near Davos, Switzerland. They found that VEGF rose sharply after the run, and stayed high for five days. In 2002, other researchers showed that injections of VEGF into the brain of rats triggered growth of new hippocampal cells. In 2003, Stanford University researchers showed that if VEGF is blocked, the new nerve growth in the hippocampus that normally occurs with running doesn't happen.

Meanwhile, at Yale, Duman was on the track of another potential factor. In 2007, his team compared the brain activity of sedentary mice to that of mice allowed to run as much as they wanted on running wheels. Within a week, the mice with access to wheels were voluntarily running more than six miles a night. Inside their brains, the team found that 33 genes in the hippocampus were turned on, 27 of which had never been identified before.

Among those genes, one in particular was dramatically increased: VGF (not to be confused with VEGF). When the team gave mice VGF, it acted as a powerful antidepressant. When they blocked VGF, the antidepressant effect of exercise disappeared and the mice showed signs of depression.

Other molecules, too, are now believed to be involved in the exercise–mood connection, including pro-inflammatory cytokines, that is, immune cells that promote inflammation. Exercise seems to change these molecules in a favorable direction in people with major depressive disorder.

As for those old favorites, the monoamines, exercise does raise their levels, too. But it's tricky to draw conclusions. To assess brain levels in humans, researchers would have to do highly invasive procedures such as spinal taps to obtain cerebrospinal fluid. In animals, on the other hand, researchers have shown that exercise can boost brain levels of norepinephrine and tryptophan, a precursor of serotonin.

Yet another molecule triggered by exercise, PGC-1 alpha, the molecule we met in Chapter 5, also seems to reduce depression. In 2014, researchers from the Karolinska Institute in Stockholm reported that mice with high levels of PGC-1 alpha were able to attack a nasty protein called kynurenine, which is found in high levels in the blood after stress.

This molecule can cross into the brain from the blood, potentially leading to depression. In the Swedish mice with high PGC-1 alpha, though, the nasty form of kynurenine was changed in such a way that it could no longer cross into the brain. This suggests that exercise-induced PGC-1 alpha may also help combat depression.

It's a complex story, becoming more so with every discovery. But the overall message is clear. For a plethora of biochemical reasons, exercise is one of the best antidepressants going.

It can help *prevent* depression. It is an effective *treatment,* often as effective as medications. It works *synergistically* at the molecular level with medications. It helps *prevent relapse* into depression. It works as well for *older people* as for younger ones. It is *dose-dependent*—the more, the better. And it even *reverses the loss of brain tissue* that is linked to depression.

WHAT'S A PERSON TO DO?

Abby Lee (aka Zoe Margolis) got it right.

So did Elizabeth Droge-Young, a 30-something Rhode Island science writer with a PhD in evolutionary biology. Her thesis at Syracuse University was a study of what she calls the "wacky" mating behavior of "promiscuous beetles." She is happily married and is "mom" to two cats and a cockapoo.

But, like Margolis, she has coped with severe depression. In fact, she has been repeatedly hospitalized for depression so awful it wasn't clear she would survive. For her, things started to go downhill while she was still a student. "Life was going well," she remembers. She had passed her exams. She got married. Then depression hit.

"I had no energy to do things," she said. "I had trouble concentrating, trouble writing, my cognition was severely impacted. I was just sleeping a lot, lying on the couch, not even enjoying movies. It was hard to see a future that looked enjoyable or fulfilling."

Nowadays, she does it all—psychotherapy, medications, meditation, and psychological skills such as "distress tolerance." But exercise, she has found, is crucial. She rides a stationary bike while chatting with friends via Skype. "It's fun," she says. "All of these help me on the path to healing."

Still, for Margolis, Droge-Young, and millions of others with depression, some questions remain.

For instance, how long does the mood boost from exercise last? In a 2010 meta-analysis and systematic review of 13 randomized trials, a Danish team concluded that exercise is primarily a short-term remedy, which means that, to keep feeling better, you have to keep exercising regularly.

It's also been unclear whether seriously depressed people will stick with an exercise program. But a 2015 meta-analysis of 40 randomized trials by researchers from the United Kingdom, Belgium, Australia, Italy, and Brazil found that the dropout rate for depressed people in exercise trials was actually *lower* for those assigned to exercise than those in control groups.

Yet another issue is whether there's an optimal time of day for exercise to produce the biggest antidepressant effect. It's still an open question, but evidence suggests exercise later in the day works best for depression.

As for what's most important to get the anti-depressive effect of exercise: frequency, duration, or intensity? It's frequency, at least until exercise habits are well-established.

As for the most important practical question, how much exercise does it take to effectively treat depression? That is still a somewhat open question.

Some studies suggest that just 30–45 minutes three times a week may be enough. Others suggest a bit more, three to five 45–60-minute sessions a week of moderately intense aerobic exercise. Still others recommend high-intensity interval training, or HIIT.

The bottom line, though, is clear: "Exercise is medication," as Cotman of the University of California, Irvine, puts it. "Basically, you have to keep taking it on a regular basis—at least three times a week, for at least half an hour per time."

CHAPTER 10

It Takes Guts: Exercise and the Microbiome

BURLY IRISH LADS

They were burly, young lads, members of a professional Irish rugby team—perfect physical specimens, exactly what the researchers needed for the first study of its kind in humans. The researchers, from the Teagasc Food Research Centre in Ireland, were interested in, well, the men's poop.

With a little coaxing, the athletes agreed to supply the necessary material, along with some blood. They also agreed to be interviewed by a nutritionist about their diets, to keep daily logs of what they ate, to get DEXA (a type of X-ray) bone scans, and to have their waist-hip measurements recorded.

The researchers also recruited two groups of non-athletes to serve as controls: one group, men who were reasonably active, was matched for size and BMI (body mass index) with the husky athletes; the other was also reasonably active but had higher BMIs.

The researchers' hunch, triggered by previous research in animals, was that healthy bacteria in the athletes' guts would be more plentiful and diverse than the bacteria from the control groups. Large, diverse communities of bacteria, viruses, fungi, and other microbial life that live in the gut are increasingly recognized as a key marker of human health. What nobody knew yet was whether exercise could increase the vigor of these microbial communities, or at least be correlated with it.

In 2014, the Irish team reported its findings. Sure enough, at least according to relatively simple tests, the athletes had significantly more diverse bacteria than the other two groups, including higher levels of a bacterial family named *Akkermansia*, which has been linked with a lower risk of both obesity and chronic inflammation.

What the researchers *couldn't* tell was how much of a role the athletes' diet also played. The rugby players tended to eat more protein, especially whey protein, than the control groups, and protein is known to correlate with microbial diversity.

In subsequent, more sophisticated tests published in 2017, the researchers discovered even greater differences in the microbes living in the guts of athletes compared to the control groups, though it was still unclear how diet fit in. In ongoing studies, they're now trying to see if people who start out in sedentary lifestyles improve their microbial diversity if they start going to the gym and eating more protein.

To be sure, it's long been known that exercise has multiple effects on the GI (gastrointestinal) tract, including the fact that intense exercise reduces the amount of time fecal material stays in the system, a substantial benefit since this minimizes the amount of time that potentially carcinogenic compounds can penetrate deeper into the system. When transit time gets too short, though, the result can be the non-beneficial, and definitely not popular, phenomenon dubbed "runner's diarrhea."

But that's old news for today's researchers. The hot topic now is what effects exercise—separate from diet—may have on the microbiome.

MICROBES MATTER

Until recently, if we bothered to think at all about the bugs living in our guts, noses, mouths, vaginas, and other intimate nooks and crannies, it was only when those bugs made us sick—at which point we zapped them with antibiotic, antiviral, or antifungal drugs and went merrily on our way.

Now, thanks to new research, things are more complicated. And that's a good thing. We now know that in addition to the "bad" microbes that make us sick, there are trillions of "good" bacteria, fungi, viruses, and other tiny critters inside us that keep us healthy. These microbes evolved along with us over the eons; some estimates say the microbes outnumber mammalian cells by about 10 to one. Others suggest it's closer to one to one. Regardless of their numbers, they play a major role in our immune system, digestion, and overall health.

Collectively, these microbes are called the *microbiota*. Their genes comprise the *microbiome*. It's not just humans who live in close proximity to these bacteria, by the way. All living creatures do. Microbial communities are also found in a number of environmental niches, including the soil, seawater, and glacier ice.

The microbiome is now deemed so important for health that, more than a decade ago, the National Institutes of Health kick-started research into the human microbiome, documenting, among other things, that each of us carries thousands of species of microbes and millions of microbial genes within us. By 2016, that initial investment had led to the $121 million government-wide research project called the National Microbiome Initiative. This effort is also supported by private funding, including the Bill and Melinda Gates Foundation, which is investing $100 million over four years.

Scientists and doctors have become so conscious of the microbiome's role in human health that they're more cautious than ever about antibiotics, which indiscriminately wipe out hordes of beneficial as well as harmful bacteria, much as herbicides destroy weeds and desirable plants—the entire garden.

A healthy microbiota has been shown to play a key role in providing energy, producing vitamins, nutrients, and a strong immune system. By contrast, a poorly functioning microbiota, or one with less microbial diversity, has been linked with a number of diseases, including ulcerative colitis, Crohn's disease, colon cancer, diabetes, cardiovascular disease, allergies, asthma, eczema, and autism, although these links are correlations, not cause and effect. Indeed, a low-diversity microbiome is strongly linked to nasty colon infections with the *Clostridium difficile* bacterium.

Poor microbial functioning is also linked to metabolic syndrome—a cluster of conditions including high blood pressure, insulin resistance, large waist, and abnormal cholesterol levels that raise the risk of heart disease, stroke, and diabetes. The gut microbiome is different between obese and lean people, too, with less microbial diversity in obese people.

Aging significantly changes the gut microbiota, too, making it less vibrant and diverse. Older microbiota have been shown to promote intestinal permeability and systemic inflammation.

In fact, researchers have found that the more frail an older person is, the more likely it is that the gut microbiota has low diversity. Older people living in long-term care facilities tend to have even less microbial diversity than older people still living in the community.

On the plus side, it's clear that people (and animals) with abundant, varied gut microbes are healthier, are less prone to obesity, and have better immune systems than those with less diverse microbiota. The gut microbiota is now deemed so crucial to health that it's been dubbed the "forgotten organ," comparable in metabolic importance to the liver.

Probing the exercise–microbiome connection is tricky in part because our live-in microbes are such an amazingly diverse bunch. Not only is each person's microbiota distinct from another's, but each part of the body—gut, nose, skin, mouth, vagina—has its own distinct community of bugs. In one forensic study, scientists examining bacteria left on computer keys were able to determine which person had touched the keys.

One of the most intriguing aspects about our microbiota is where it comes from: Mom.

Babies acquire their first microbes during birth, as they pass through the mother's vaginal microbiota. For that reason, babies born vaginally have higher gut bacterial counts than babies born by cesarean section, which turns out to be a significant advantage. The inherited microbiota helps babies develop better immune systems and lower risk for a number of diseases, including asthma.

Such is the importance of these microbes to newborns that babies born by C-section are sometimes given microorganisms artificially. That's exactly what Rob Knight, a microbiome expert at the University of California, San Diego, did when his daughter was born by emergency C-section. He and his wife took samples of her vaginal microbiota and spread them on their baby's skin, ears, and mouth, the sites that would have taken in these microbes had it been a vaginal birth.

And it's not just the vaginal microbiota that's good for babies. Breast milk has its own, separate microbiota. In fact, breast milk is not so much food for the baby per se as "the sugars in breast milk are food for the baby's developing microbiome," says Lita Proctor, director of the Human Microbiome Project at the National Institutes of Health.

In recent years, scientists have been teasing apart the myriad ways in which this elaborate microbial system influences health. One of the most important is that the microbiota "teaches" our immune systems to recognize friend and foe and to temper its reactions appropriately. For example, if you are exposed to a potential pathogen like salmonella, it's important that the immune system recognize and get rid of the bug;

but it's also important that the immune system not over-react to normal microbes living in a healthy gastrointestinal tract, lest we end up with frequent inflammation and disease.

The gut, though we don't often think about it this way, is one of the first places where things from the outside world—food as well as toxins—meet the inner world of the body. It's there, deep in our guts, that immune cells have to learn to tell the good guys from the bad guys. Indeed, the gut microbiota regulates not only local intestinal immune function, but systemic immune function as well.

The microbes in our gut also help regulate hormones, damp down inflammation, and generally keep the metabolism humming smoothly. And, strange as it may seem, the microbes in the gut are part of what's known as the gut-brain axis, a two-way link involving hormones and nerve signals that connects the central nervous system, the gastrointestinal tract, and the enteric nervous system. (The enteric nervous system, dubbed "the second brain," is a web of nerves that controls the gut.)

The gut microbiota is actually seen today as an endocrine organ, which secretes hormones and other chemicals that travel into the bloodstream and act in distant parts of the body, including the brain. Perhaps that's why microbes in the gut have been shown to influence emotional behavior, mood, stress and pain responses, and neurodevelopmental disorders such as autism. Irish researchers have even shown that the microbiota has a role in the regulation of fear responses by acting on the amygdala, a fear center in the brain.

More obviously to most of us, the gut microbiota is essential for digestion. Our human genome contains genes for only about 20 digestive enzymes, which means we have to rely on enzymes made by gut bacteria to digest much of our food. Gut bacteria, especially the strain called *Bifidobacterium*, also make important vitamins, including vitamin K, B$_{12}$, biotin, folate, and thiamine.

Gut bacteria also make important short-chain fatty acids by fermenting dietary fiber. Some fatty acids travel to the lungs, where they provide protection against allergic inflammation. The short-chain fatty acid butyrate travels to the blood–brain barrier, where it helps maintain the barrier's integrity. (The blood–brain barrier is a membrane that keeps blood from the circulation from entering the brain.)

Given that gut bacteria are so important for digesting food, it's no surprise that changing one's diet has a huge effect on the gut microbiota. (Artificial sweeteners, by the way, change the gut microbiota in potentially dysfunctional ways, though more research is needed.)

If you eat mostly protein and animal fat, your gut will have a lot of bacteria called *Bacteroides.* If you eat more fiber and carbohydrates, on the other hand, your gut will be dominated by a different bacterium, *Prevotella.* (Healthy people in general tend to have lots of *Bacteroides* and *Firmicutes.*) For bacteria living in our guts, dietary fiber from fruits and vegetables is the best diet of all. The more fiber available, the more the bacteria chomp happily away, keeping the microbiota flourishing.

Nowhere is this more apparent than in studies comparing traditional, rural people with those who live in fruit-poor, fiber-poor Western cultures. In one clever study by researchers from the University of Helsinki and others from the United States, Europe, and South Africa, a group of African-Americans who normally ate a lot of animal protein, fat, and very little fiber were switched to the low–animal protein, low-fat, high-fiber diet typical of rural Africans, and a group of rural Africans were switched temporarily to the American diet. The microbiomes of both groups changed markedly—in a healthy direction for those switching to a high-fiber diet, and in an unhealthy direction for those decreasing their fiber.

In another fascinating study, researchers from Stanford University examined the microbiota of the Hadza, a group of about 1,300 hunter-gatherers in western Tanzania near the Serengeti. Their microbiota changes starkly with the seasons, as their food supply changes. The year-round staple of the Hadza diet is fruit from the baobab trees. But in the dry season, when it's easier to hunt, they eat a lot of animals and dig for tubers. In the wet season, they live on berries and honey from beehives, and their microbiota changes accordingly. Overall, the Hadza microbiota has been shown to be significantly more diverse than that of people in a control group in Italy.

PROBIOTICS, PREBIOTICS, AND, LESS APPEALINGLY, FECAL TRANSPLANTS

Let's get the ick factor out of the way right off the bat.

One approach to a healthier microbiota is fecal transplantation, that is, artificially introducing microbiota from one person to another. This technique is used to treat diseases, most notably the bacterial infection called *Clostridium difficile.* Fecal transplants are done through tubes down a patient's throat or via enemas, and in the future, probably by pills—not a pleasant thought.

Far more pleasant are probiotics and prebiotics. Probiotics are supplements containing various strains of beneficial bacteria. Prebiotics are nutrients that support the growth of beneficial gut bacteria. Researchers are exploring both as ways to create healthier gut microbiota.

Though widely hyped in the press, probiotics had not until recently been shown to produce clear health benefits, aside from assuaging irritable bowel syndrome and, in a study of athletes, reducing the number of sick days. But that is changing, bolstered by studies like a dramatic 2017 experiment in India.

Indian physicians had long been concerned, especially in rural areas, about sepsis, a serious infection of the blood that kills a million newborns a year worldwide. The researchers gathered 4,556 healthy infants and randomly gave some, but not others, an oral probiotic containing *Lactobacillus plantrum*. Stunningly, they achieved a 40 percent reduction in sepsis among the babies getting the microbiota boost—impressive, to say the least. But exercise matters, too.

EXERCISE AND THE MICROBIOTA

In animals, University of Colorado researchers have demonstrated that exercise pays off, if started early. After six weeks of exercise, the Colorado team found, juvenile rats wound up with healthier gut microbiota—and a higher likelihood of being lean—than rats that only exercised as adults.

Other researchers have shown that in rats allowed to run voluntarily, exercise improves gut microbiota, in particular increasing short-chain fatty acids. Still other researchers have shown that exercise can change the gut microbiota no matter what kind of rat they studied—skinny rats, fat rats, even hypertensive rats. Not surprisingly, mice benefit, too.

More important, in 2016, a study of 39 healthy people with varying levels of cardiorespiratory fitness showed that higher fitness was correlated with increased microbiota diversity and increased levels of the short-chain fatty acid butyrate.

In 2017, Spanish researchers reported on a study of 40 premenopausal women in which they compared the gut microbiota of women who were at least minimally active with the microbiota of those who were sedentary. Overall, exercise was not linked, as the team had hoped, to better microbiota in active women. But it did promote the bacterial strains known to be the most important for health.

And here's the most impressive finding so far.

Researchers at the University of Illinois at Urbana-Champaign set out to see if they could separate the effects of exercise and those of diet on microbiota in mice and people. In the human experiment, they designed a study that involved tracking 32 men and women who were not regular exercisers.

Half of the people were obese and half were of normal weight. The researchers took blood and fecal samples and tested each person's aerobic fitness. They then put all the volunteers into supervised exercise workouts of gradually increasing intensity and duration. All the volunteers were asked *not* to change their diets.

The tests were repeated six weeks later, then another six weeks later. Everybody's microbiome changed to some extent, with some microbial genes increasing in activity, and others decreasing. Importantly, exercise increased the microbes that make short-chain fatty acids (in particular, butyrate) that are crucial for reducing inflammation both in the gut and in the rest of the body. The biggest increases were in people who were lean to start with.

The crucial take-home lesson is this: Exercise *alone,* without dietary changes, can alter gut microbiota. Even just a few weeks of exercise can change the microbiota in a positive direction.

Quitting exercise, sad to say, wipes out these beneficial effects.

CHAPTER 11

Immunity, Inflammation, and Exercise

THINK GOLDILOCKS—OR MAYBE NOT

Let's cut to the chase. Exercise, done regularly and in moderation, is terrific for the immune system. It reduces chronic inflammation, an underlying cause of aging and many conditions including diabetes, heart disease, atherosclerosis, and arthritis. It also protects the immune system from being suppressed by mental and physical stress. Too little exercise, on the other hand, is linked to more inflammation and poorer immunity.

To scientists, this fits a classic J-shaped curve. Moderate amounts of exercise are linked with better immune function, and extreme amounts (very high or very low) have been linked with worse—kind of like Goldilocks.

All this makes intuitive sense, in part because healthy immune function is a system in balance: too weak an immune response to a germ and you wind up sick. But an excessive response is the underlying problem with allergies and autoimmune diseases, in which immune cells attack the body's own tissues.

"What you want is an optimal, robust but not exaggerated immune response," says Monika Fleshner, a professor of integrative physiology at the University of Colorado. Young people, whether they exercise or not, have pretty good immune responses—adequate but not excessive. Unfortunately, she says, older people tend to have poorer immune function.

The notion of a nice, neat J-shaped curve is intuitively appealing. But new research is throwing a monkey wrench into this formulation. It turns out that the idea that *too much* exercise—like training for or running a marathon—suppresses immune function and raises the risk of infection may not be true. This long-standing dogma, as we'll see in a moment, is now under attack.

The first hint that there even was such a thing as immunity came with the Greek historian Thucydides, who survived the plague of Athens (430–426 BC). He looked around at the survivors and wondered why people who survived the epidemic could nurse the sick without getting sick again themselves. Something about having had an infection, he reasoned, must be protective.

But it would be centuries before physicians began to unravel the complexities of the immune system, much less think about potential links between exercise and immune function. It wasn't until the 20th century, for instance, that doctors began wondering why some elite athletes seemed to get sore throats around the time of competitions. It took even longer to document that immunity declines with age, a process called immunosenescence, and longer still to realize that exercise may attenuate this process.

Today, the field of exercise immunology has exploded, with more than 2,000 scientific papers published just since the formation of the International Society of Exercise and Immunology in 1989.

In this chapter, we'll focus first on exercise and inflammation, then on the benefits of exercise beyond reducing inflammation, and finally, on the mechanisms that produce changes in immune function with exercise and how these may—or may not—influence susceptibility to infection.

BOX 11.1 PLAYING DEFENSE

The immune system is a network of defenses against invading microorganisms. It's not the only defense—the skin, and even eyelashes, act as mechanical barriers to invaders. Mucous membranes, saliva, tears, and respiratory membranes also flush out invaders. Stomach acids kill pathogens in food.

But once an invading organism makes it past those barriers, it's up to the immune system, whose cells are made in the bone marrow, to do battle.

The first step is activation of the innate immune system. This is a generalized, non-specific response—carpet bombing, not sniper fire. It's immediate and doesn't confer long-lasting immunity, as vaccinations do.

It starts with inflammation. Cells of the innate immune system that respond to tissue damage from pathogens release chemicals called cytokines that attract blood to the area, making it red, swollen, painful, and hot. Inflammation can occur with or without infection, that is, without any pathogens present, as happens with autoimmune diseases.

The innate immune system involves many types of white blood cells (leukocytes), including macrophages, mast cells, neutrophils, eosinophils, basophils, natural killer cells, dendritic cells, and something called complement (proteins that work with other parts of the immune system).

Dendritic cells link the innate immune system to the fancier part of the immune system, the "adaptive" or "acquired" immune response. First, a pathogen is gobbled up by an immature dendritic cell. The cell then places antigens (specific markers) from the invader onto its outside membrane, showing it—like a sommelier presenting a fine wine—to white cells called T cells. At this point, the dendritic cell becomes an antigen-presenting cell.

The T cells then recruit B cells, each of which is genetically endowed with receptors that can spot one specific antigen. This means that, collectively, B cells are capable of recognizing millions of different antigens.

When a B cells spots the antigen it is capable of recognizing, that B cell makes antibodies against that antigen, and then copies itself in the next few days (clonal expansion), creating a huge pool of B cells that can now make antibodies against that particular invader. This adaptive immunity is also what happens with vaccination, or when you fight off an infectious disease. It's also the basis for immunological "memory."

With acute exercise, the first response is a big burst of neutrophils, followed by a second, slower increase. Other immune cells rise a few hours after acute exercise, too, including monocytes and natural killer cells.

INFLAMMATION

The link between exercise and inflammation is complex. But it's clear that there are several interconnected pathways by which exercise damps down harmful, chronic inflammation. In essence, exercise shuts down inflammation after it has accomplished its beneficial effects and before it becomes chronic and harmful.

The take-home lessons are clear: Aerobic exercise provides the biggest anti-inflammatory effects, though resistance training helps, too. The ideal prescription, as a major, 10-year study showed, is to make exercise a permanent part of daily life. You don't have to kill yourself in the process: Even one 20-minute session of moderate exercise can produce anti-inflammatory effects.

In a nutshell, inflammation, which is primarily part of the innate immune system (see Box 11.1), is both good and bad. It's good when it's localized and short term, as when resistance training causes micro-tears in muscle cells. In this scenario, inflammation helps heal those tears, which helps muscle cells get bigger and stronger. Inflammation is bad when it doesn't shut off—when it becomes chronic and systemic, occurring all over the body.

(For the record, exercise can sometimes cause problems *not* by depressing the immune system, but by *revving* it up too much, as with exercise-induced asthma, a narrowing of the airways. In rare but dramatic cases, exercise can even trigger anaphylaxis, a potentially life-threatening allergic reaction.)

The first, and most obvious, link between exercise and inflammation is that exercise helps prevent obesity. Fat tissue, especially visceral fat—the deep adipose tissue that surrounds organs—used to be thought of as an inert lump. But visceral fat is now known to be highly active metabolically.

"When people gain weight," says Connie Rogers, associate professor of nutritional sciences and physiology at Penn State University, "their adipose tissue swells and gets bigger." As visceral fat cells swell, some of them rupture—in essence, creating a kind of injury.

As with other injuries, the immune system quickly swings into action, sending immune cells called macrophages to the area. There, macrophages do two things—they not only repair the tissue damage, but also pump out pro-inflammatory cytokines, molecular signals that trigger inflammation all over the body.

The cascade of unhealthy events goes like this: Physical inactivity (sedentary behavior) leads to increased visceral fat accumulation, which leads to chronic systemic inflammation, which leads to insulin resistance (a precursor of diabetes), atherosclerosis, neurodegeneration, and even tumor growth. In other words, sedentary behavior, by raising the risk of chronic inflammation, raises the risk of all the diseases linked to inflammation. Indeed, compared to folks who exercise regularly and moderately, couch potatoes are clearly more prone to infections.

Consider one of the main consequences of inflammation: insulin resistance, which is triggered by an increase in inflammatory molecules, including a pro-inflammatory cytokine called TNF-alpha. In obese people, cells in fat tissue secrete too much TNF, which changes a signaling pathway inside cells that results in insulin no longer being effective. This means that sugar gets left in the bloodstream. "In essence," says University of Memphis assistant professor of nutrition Brandt Pence, "TNF messes up the signaling, which leads to insulin resistance, a precursor of diabetes."

Exercise helps *prevent* chronic inflammation in a number of ways—by increasing adrenaline, cortisol, growth hormone, and other factors that modulate the immune system. It also directly triggers an increase in *anti-inflammatory* cytokines. Indeed, evidence of the direct, *anti-inflammatory* powers of exercise—and the *pro-inflammatory* effects of sedentary behavior—has been pouring out of research labs for the last two decades.

In 2001, a study of nearly 6,000 men and women aged 65 or older found that the most active had dramatically lower levels of an important inflammatory marker called C-reactive protein, or CRP. In 2002, a study of 3,638 middle-aged men and women similarly found that those who exercised regularly had substantially lower CRP than sedentary folks.

That same year, researchers analyzing US government data on nearly 14,000 adults again found that the *less* people exercised, the *higher* their C-reactive protein. This pattern—more exercise, lower CRP levels; less exercise, higher CRP—has held up consistently, among older as well as younger people. It doesn't take much exercise to get the benefit—moderate activity for just 2.5 hours a week can keep CRP in the healthy range, regardless of a person's weight.

Even in people who already have inflammatory-based conditions like type 2 diabetes and coronary artery disease, exercise can help control that chronic inflammatory state. In fact, the anti-inflammatory effect of exercise on CRP may be as good as or even better than medications.

Italian researchers, for instance, wondered what an exercise intervention could do for people with type 2 diabetes and metabolic syndrome. (Metabolic syndrome is a dangerous cluster of problems including high waist circumference, high triglycerides, low HDL ["good" cholesterol], high blood pressure, and high blood sugar.)

They randomized 82 patients into an exercise group or a no-exercise control group. The exercisers achieved significant decreases in CRP and other inflammatory markers, *whether or not they lost weight*. The effect was strongest in people who combined high-intensity aerobic training with resistance exercise, as other research confirms.

In another study, Brazilian researchers gathered 34 people with coronary artery disease who had not been exercising. (Arterial disease occurs when white blood cells in artery walls become chronically inflamed.) At the outset, the researchers put the patients through a 50-minute bout of reasonably strenuous exercise on a stationary bike, then measured their CRP and other inflammatory markers. The markers rose sharply.

The researchers then randomized the patients to a four-month regular exercise program or general lifestyle recommendations. After that, all the participants had another 50-minute cycling test. Those in the exercise group were superstars—their inflammatory response was nice and low. But the non-exercisers pumped out high levels of inflammatory proteins, just as before.

All this becomes even more important as a person ages. Luckily, exercise turns out have its most dramatic anti-inflammatory effects in older people. Indeed, in a systematic review of 13 randomized controlled studies of exercise interventions in sedentary people, Irish researchers found that the biggest and most consistent anti-inflammatory benefits were in older people.

BOX 11.2 EXERCISE FOR A YOUTHFUL IMMUNE SYSTEM

Consider this hardy bunch of British cyclists, aged 55–79.

These riders, male and female, had been active all their lives, cranking out about 400 miles a month, though none of them was a competitive athlete. The researchers began by studying cognitive and physical attributes of the cyclists and compared the results to those of sedentary older people and to young folks. In that 2014 study, the team found that the cyclists had reflexes, memory function, balance, and general metabolic health more similar to 30-year-olds than to sedentary older people.

But the researchers didn't stop there. They embarked on another round of research to look in more detail at the older cyclists' muscle cells and immune function, specifically T cells, a major infection-fighting component of the immune system.

In the older, sedentary people, the researchers found, the thymus gland pumped out only low quantities of T cells. But in the cyclists, the thymus gland was as active as ever, pumping out almost as many new T cells as in younger people. Since, as we saw in Chapter 6, contracting muscle cells put out hormones that protect the thymus, this may be one reason why exercise keeps T cells—and the immune system in general—functioning well.

In other words, exercise can make an old immune system young, including allowing older people to generate better responses to vaccinations. It protects against the damaging effects of stress, too.

And consider these American folks.

In a paper published in 2004, Colorado physiologist Fleshner put humans through the same protocol that had already been shown effective in rats. First, she recruited 46 men: Some were young (aged 20–35), and of these, some were physically active and some sedentary; the other men were older (aged 60–79), and some of these were active and some sedentary.

Fleshner then gave all the men shots of a substance dubbed KLH, a protein known to trigger immune responses in lab tests, but a substance that most people would not have encountered in real life.

The result? The young men, as expected, all had optimal, healthy immune reactions to the novel substance—they made appropriate numbers of antibodies but did not have an excessive, runaway immune response. But older men who exercised had immune responses just as good as the younger men. Only the sedentary older men had poor immune responses.

In 2008, Fleshner and researchers from the University of Illinois at Urbana-Champaign carried the idea further. They took 50 previously sedentary people in their 60s or older and randomly assigned them to either moderate aerobic exercise or simple stretching. Eight months later, they gave all the volunteers injections of KLH. The older folks who received exercise training had markedly robust levels of key antibodies. Those who received flexibility training did not.

EXERCISE VERSUS INFLAMMATION

For years, scientists were baffled about the mechanisms by which exercise exerts its effects on inflammation. Today, they have important new clues.

Researchers now know that the cytokines that are triggered by *infection* are different from cytokines induced by *exercise*. (Cytokines, as we noted earlier, are small proteins made by immune cells that carry signals from one cell to another, ramping up or down immune response.)

With *infection*, especially bacterial infections, the immune system pumps out both anti- and pro-inflammatory cytokines, chemicals with clunky names like TNF-alpha, IL-1B, IL-Ira, TNF-R, IL-6, and IL-10.

With *exercise*, by contrast, not only do pro-inflammatory cytokines like TNF-alpha and IL-1B *not* go up, but IL-6 goes up, then rapidly declines. In essence, exercise damps *down* the cytokines that increase chronic inflammation, and *boosts* those that suppress it. Put differently, exercise improves our responses to infection and facilitates the resolution, that is, the shutting off, of the inflammatory response, says Fleshner of Colorado.

Let's pause here for a fascinating, albeit geeky, moment.

A major player in the inflammatory response is IL-6 (interleukin-6), which is both a pro-inflammatory and an anti-inflammatory cytokine and is made by both immune and muscle cells. When triggered by infection, IL-6 is produced largely by immune (not muscle) cells and is pro-inflammatory. When triggered by exercise, IL-6 comes mostly from muscles and reduces inflammation.

In essence, IL-6 is a double agent. If chronically elevated, it is linked to bad outcomes such as obesity, diabetes, cancer, neurodegenerative problems, and depression. But when released short term from muscles during exercise, IL-6 boosts anti-inflammatory cytokines and speeds healing. Exercise-induced IL-6 also helps destroy fat, which independently reduces chronic inflammation.

In a dramatic study of IL-6, Danish researchers asked male volunteers to rest, ride an exercise bike for three hours, or get infusions of IL-6. All were given a substance called LPS, which comes from bacteria such as *E. coli* and signals the immune system that a pathogen is present. This signaling triggers a low-grade inflammatory cytokine response. In the resting state, volunteers produced high levels of pro-inflammatory TNF-alpha in response to the LPS. But with exercise, this inflammation was blocked, a clear demonstration of exercise's anti-inflammatory effect.

In a different Danish study in mice, researchers showed that exercise can suppress cancer growth by activating IL-6, along with adrenaline.

Of course, it's not only IL-6 that is affected by exercise. Exercise has other ways of reducing inflammation. Exercise *reduces* markers on immune cells called toll-like receptors. Their job is to signal immune cells that pathogens are present and trigger an inflammatory response. Exercise reduces these receptors, which lowers production of pro-inflammatory cytokines.

Exercise also raises levels of a protein called PGC-1 alpha. PGC-1 alpha is best known for driving creation of new mitochondria. But it also damps down chronic inflammation. Exercise also boosts proteins called MAPK and NF-kB, which are linked to inflammation. And it can have beneficial effects on the microbes in the gut, the microbiota.

For years, scientists have thought that *extreme* amounts of exercise could suppress the immune system. After all, competitive athletes often complain of sore throats, prompting concern that there could be an "open window" of vulnerability to infection after strenuous exercise, a time when the immune system seemed to dip.

This window was thought to be about three to four hours, but potentially, a week or more. Even more depressing for extreme athletes, there seemed to be a high risk of getting an infection at the worst possible time—right around an ultra-marathon.

Genetics may explain some of this supposed excess of sore throats among competitive athletes, in particular a genetic predisposition to produce more pro-inflammatory cytokines. And some research has showed that prolonged, intense exercise such as marathon cross-country ski races can decrease levels of an immune component found in saliva called IgA. This, researchers thought, might explain a higher prevalence of respiratory infections in elite athletes.

But in the last several years, exercise immunologists began taking a closer look at this window of vulnerability and sore throats in heavy exercisers. It has turned out that many athletes complaining of sore throats didn't have infections at all. They had localized swelling and scratchiness, probably caused by breathing hard and inhaling irritating particles.

In 2018, the putative link between strenuous exercise and immune suppression was challenged further by researchers in Bath, England, who reviewed studies in both humans and rodents. At least in rodents, the Bath team found, immune cells don't die off after intense exercise, as had been thought, but migrate into the bloodstream and on to peripheral tissues, a potential infection-fighting benefit. (It's not known whether this migration happens in humans.)

The Bath team also concluded that rather than suppressing immunity, an acute bout of exercise improves immune "surveillance," the detection system by which immune cells are on high alert for bacterial and viral invaders. The team also concluded that even a single bout of exercise enhances the body's response to vaccination, prompting their conclusion that people should not fear that exercise will suppress their immune systems.

Perhaps most important for most of us, the Bath team found that it is a "misconception to label any form of acute exercise as immunosuppressive" and that "exercise most likely improves immune competency across the lifespan"—to which we can only say, Amen.

CHAPTER 12

Exercise and Cancer

FINDING THE LUMP

Five days before Christmas in 2015, Marcia Bailey, a 54-year-old ordained American Baptist minister and assistant professor at Temple University, went for a routine gynecology appointment, just another "to do" notation in the calendar that tracked her busy life.

During the academic year, Bailey teaches undergrads to think critically, using ancient and modern literature to get them to analyze statements and take apart arguments. She's also a "transitional minister," working with church congregations in the midst of changing ministers, with all the complicated feelings of loyalty, anger, and trepidation that such changes engender: "I am there to help them put their past in perspective and help them envision the future with the new person."

Married for more than 30 years—"to the same person," she adds, "you have to say that these days"—she has three grown children, all in their 20s. Life was—and still is—full. But—"My doctor found a lump," she says matter-of-factly. Four days later, it was confirmed as breast cancer, Stage II. Then came chemotherapy for six months, then a lumpectomy, then radiation—the nightmare familiar to so many people with cancer.

"The chemo was supposed to help shrink the tumor. It wasn't effective, but they were able to do a lumpectomy anyway," she says. The tumor turned out to be invasive in some parts and noninvasive in others, with tentacles that reached out from the center: "They couldn't find the ends of those."

Bailey is done, at least for the moment, with standard treatment and has turned her energies to doing everything she can, most notably exercising and losing weight, to increase her chances for survival. She has lost 35 pounds, down from 170 when she was diagnosed, and says she feels "amazing."

Inspirational, for sure. Yet Bailey is also part of a gathering storm of people whose lives have been turned upside down by cancer.

Worldwide, more than 14 million people like Bailey were newly diagnosed with cancer in 2012, the latest year for which figures are available. More than 8 million died. And it's getting worse. In 2030, almost 22 million people are expected to receive a cancer diagnosis. And 13 million will die.

To be sure, some of this dramatic increase is due to the worldwide growth of the aging population. And some of it is just plain bad luck—random errors in DNA as stem cells replicate. But much of it, the American Cancer Society says, stems from our unhealthy Western lifestyle—smoking, bad diets, and, no surprise here, an appalling lack of exercise.

In Europe alone, an estimated 165,000–330,000 cases of six major cancers could have been prevented in one year alone by sufficient exercise. Worldwide, an estimated 25 percent of all cancers are caused by being overweight or obese and having a sedentary lifestyle, according to the International Agency for Research on Cancer (IARC), part of the World Health Organization.

Even sitting for too many hours a day can raise cancer risk, despite regular exercise. (See Chapter 3.) And that is particularly a problem for women. In a large study of 69,260 men and 77,462 women, the more time women spent sitting, the higher the overall risk of cancer, especially multiple myeloma and breast and ovarian cancer.

The flip side of all this—the good news—is that exercise can substantially lower the risk of getting cancer in the first place, can reduce fatigue and improve quality of life if you already have cancer, and, perhaps most important, can lower the risk of recurrence and boost chances of survival.

A caveat here, though. There's a strong *association* between exercise and cancer risk reduction, but so far, it is just that—an association, not proven cause and effect. It's possible that people who exercise also eat better, weigh less, are more compliant with their medications, and are generally healthier overall—the "healthy person" effect.

In this chapter, we'll highlight the evidence for the links between exercise and cancer and, in the last section, explain the biochemical reasons why exercise can be so beneficial.

In the spring of 2016, an international team of researchers released findings from the largest-ever study of exercise and cancer risk—a study so big it allowed, for the first time, an assessment of the benefits of exercise for preventing not just the most common cancers, but for less common cancers as well.

Prior to this research, hundreds of studies had shown the benefits of exercise for reducing the risk of breast, colon, and endometrial cancer. But studies on other cancers had involved too few people to draw firm conclusions.

For the massive 2016 study, researchers pooled data from 1.44 million men and women aged 19–98 to examine the link between moderate to vigorous exercise and the risk of 26 different types of cancer. (The exercise included walking, running, swimming—at least 150 minutes a week.)

When the study started, none of the participants had cancer. By the end of the follow-up period—a median of nine years—nearly 187,000 did. The 32-person research team was a blue-ribbon group from the National Cancer Institute, the American Cancer Society, and academic institutions in the United States, Norway, Sweden, and France.

The results were crystal clear. Higher levels of exercise were linked to lower risk of 13 types of cancer. For seven of these cancers (esophageal, liver, lung, kidney, stomach, endometrial, and myeloid leukemia), regular exercise reduced cancer risk by 20 percent or more. For all kinds of cancers combined, higher levels of exercise reduced risk by 7 percent.

Close on the heels of that landmark study, another large international effort led by a team from Harvard Medical School reported their findings on nearly 90,000 women and more than 46,000 men, all participants in the Nurses Health Study and the Health Professionals Follow-up Study, respectively.

In this study, the researchers lumped exercise together with other lifestyle variables—not smoking, drinking moderately, and being of normal weight. The results? Between 20 and 40 percent of cancer cases and half of cancer deaths could potentially be prevented by lifestyle modifications.

In yet another large study, this one involving 79,000 Japanese men and women, daily physical exercise was again linked with a significantly decreased cancer risk in both sexes, though exercise seemed to benefit women more.

Overall, the link between exercise and reduced cancer risk seems to be dose-dependent—the more exercise you do, the better your chances of escaping cancer. Curiously, though, exercise has different protective effects for different cancers. There is strong evidence for the protective effects of exercise for breast and colorectal cancer, for instance, but less strong evidence for prostate, endometrial, and lung cancer.

With colorectal cancer, some research suggests that 12–14 percent of cases could be avoided with regular, vigorous exercise. But the benefit may actually be bigger. A 2009 meta-analysis, which pooled data from 52 epidemiological studies, found that the most physically active people had a 24 percent lower risk of colon cancer than the least active. Interestingly, the exercise benefit is stronger for colon cancer than for rectal cancer. One possible reason is that physical activity reduces the amount of time potentially carcinogenic substances in food waste remain in the colon.

For breast cancer, it's clear that more active women are less likely to get cancer than less active women. A 2013 meta-analysis of 31 prospective studies showed that being physically active reduced breast cancer risk by about 12 percent. Other studies show that women who exercise 30–60 minutes a day have as much as a 20–30 percent reduced risk of breast cancer. Exercise is especially important in adolescence because it can delay the onset of puberty and, hence, reduce the number of ovulatory cycles in which estrogen is produced.

Even in women who do get breast cancer, those who exercised as teenagers get breast cancer later in life than those who didn't exercise as teens, even if they have the genes BRCA1 and BRCA2, which raise breast cancer risk. Exercise also reduces body fat. Since body fat makes estrogen, which can drive breast cancer, reducing body fat reduces estrogen levels.

For endometrial (uterine) cancer risk, a meta-analysis of 33 studies showed that women who were very active physically had a 20 percent lower risk of the cancer than less active women. For ovarian cancer, the data are slightly weaker, but still encouraging. Cervical cancer risk declines with exercise, too.

Prostate cancer is a bit more puzzling. But scientists think there is a "probable" 10–30 percent reduction in prostate cancer risk with exercise, possibly because exercise can increase a protein that binds free testosterone, thus reducing levels of this hormone, which can drive prostate cancer.

Just as exercise is associated with a reduction in the chance of *getting* cancer, it is also linked to *living longer* once you've got it, by reducing both the risk of recurrence and death from the cancer itself, and by reducing the risk of other fatal diseases.

The good news, at least in the United States, is that mortality after a cancer diagnosis has been falling steadily. Between 1991 and 2014, it fell 25 percent. This is in contrast to the world as a whole, for which cancer deaths are projected to rise by 60 percent by 2030.

Obviously, earlier diagnosis and better treatment have been keys to improved survival. But exercise may play a vital role as well, thanks to a new field called "exercise oncology." To be sure, it's still a matter of debate exactly what doses and which types of exercise are best for which type of cancer. But the data are encouraging.

Let's start with breast cancer.

Marcia Bailey is one of more than 3.1 million American women who are currently being treated or who have completed treatment for breast cancer.

But unlike Bailey, many women *decrease* their physical activity after a breast cancer diagnosis. In a way, that's not surprising. Chemotherapy and radiation take a huge toll on the body. And cancer that has metastasized to the bones can make bones too fragile to risk fractures from exercise. But for those like Bailey who can manage it, exercise is a powerful weapon.

To be sure, a few studies have come to puzzling conclusions. One found that exercise boosted survival only if women ate lots of fruits and vegetables. Another found that exercise was linked to a reduction in both breast cancer mortality and all-cause mortality, but not to the risk of recurrence. And another found that exercise had no benefit in terms of recurrence or cancer death, but did have a benefit in terms of death from other causes.

In general, though, research shows that exercise is clearly linked to a survival benefit.

The first evidence came in 2005 research that was part of the Nurses Health Study in which researchers followed 2,987 female nurses who had been diagnosed with Stage I, II, or III breast cancer for an average of eight years. Women who walked three to five hours a week at a 20-minute-per-mile pace reduced their risk of dying from their cancer.

Women whose tumors had receptors for estrogen and progesterone got the biggest benefits.

In 2006, University of North Carolina researchers found that women who were already exercising before diagnosis had a survival advantage. In 2008, Yale University researchers reached the same conclusion, although women who took up exercise after a diagnosis benefited, too. (On the flip side, the Yale study showed, *decreased* exercise after diagnosis was linked to a fourfold increase in the risk of death.)

In 2015, British researchers confirmed the big picture, analyzing 22 studies involving 123,574 breast cancer patients. Women who had been exercising before their diagnoses had lower risks of all-cause and breast cancer mortality, though again, exercising after a diagnosis helped, too.

Exercise may be linked to better survival in other cancers as well.

Harvard School of Public Health researchers tracked 2,705 men with prostate cancer and found that exercise was linked to better survival rates both from the cancer itself and from other causes. In fact, for the most vigorous exercisers, exercise was associated with a 49 percent lower risk of death from all causes, and a 61 percent lower risk of death from prostate cancer. These findings have been replicated in other studies.

The same goes for colorectal cancer. In a 2006 study, researchers at Boston's Dana-Farber Cancer Institute followed 573 people with Stages I–III colorectal cancer. Once again, exercise was linked to increased survival both from the cancer itself and from other causes. More research is underway, including an interventional trial by Canadian researchers that will randomly assign some patients to an exercise program and others to a control group for three years.

EXERCISE DURING TREATMENT: FATIGUE AND QUALITY OF LIFE

In the not-so-old days, doctors believed that chemotherapy and radiation were so debilitating that cancer patients should get all the rest they could and avoid exertion at all costs. But that notion changed dramatically with a spate of encouraging studies beginning in the late 1980s.

In 1989, researchers at the College of Nursing at Ohio State University reported on a randomized trial of 45 women getting chemotherapy for Stage II breast cancer. Ten weeks of interval-based aerobic exercise not only did no harm, but reduced nausea and improved physical functioning. Exercise, in other words, was not only safe, but beneficial, even in the throes of chemotherapy.

Spurred by that finding, other researchers took up the challenge, finding over and over that moderately intense exercise was a powerful weapon against fatigue and helped improve quality of life during and after treatment.

One of those researchers is exercise physiologist Karen Mustian, a cheerful, athletic-looking woman who has worked with Olympic athletes. She is an associate professor at the University of Rochester and a pioneer in the study of aerobic and resistance exercise, as well as Tai chi and yoga, for cancer patients.

Mustian, director of the PEAK lab at the University of Rochester, remembers vividly how, as a young woman in North Carolina, she watched helplessly as her two beloved grandmothers battled cancer. "I was shocked," she recalls. "At that age, I was naïve. I thought doctors had the answers. I could not wrap my head around why my grandmothers were getting worse, not better."

Around that time, the American Cancer Society was organizing a Relay for Life, in which teams of participants pledged to keep at least one member walking or running for 24 hours. Mustian leapt at the chance to chair it. Soon, women battling breast cancer who had been on the relay teams began coming up to her and telling their stories.

"They would say things like, 'If it weren't for exercise, I wouldn't be getting out of bed.' Or, 'Without exercise, I wouldn't have the will to live.' They were anecdotally attributing things to exercise. I had this 'Aha!' moment." She has been studying the effects of exercise on cancer patients ever since.

"For most people, man or woman," she says, "when you get a diagnosis of cancer, you feel that your body is failing you, that you have lost control over it. Exercise is one of the biggest tools we have to help people feel more empowered, to feel they have some control over their body."

Of all the side effects cancer patients face during treatment, fatigue is the most common and often the most distressing. In fact, it tends to have a more negative impact on daily life than vomiting, nausea, pain, and depression. Worse yet, it may not get better with rest, and can linger for years, even after treatment is over. But, as Mustian and others have shown, exercise can be even more effective than medications at combatting cancer-related fatigue.

In a 2017 meta-analysis of 113 studies involving 11,525 participants, Mustian's team found that exercise and psychological therapy (each alone and in combination) improved fatigue better than drugs. Exercise and psychotherapy were linked to a 26–30 percent reduction in fatigue, drugs to only a 9 percent decline.

To be sure, not all studies have shown such a benefit. To their surprise, Canadian researchers found that neither aerobic exercise nor resistance training improved quality of life, though it did improve self-esteem.

But like Mustian, other researchers in Canada, Norway, Switzerland, Australia, Italy, the Netherlands, India, and the United States have found that exercise has, as one team put it, a "nearly universal quality of life benefit for people with cancer."

And it's not just women with breast cancer who benefit.

In one Australian study of 57 men with prostate cancer, men randomized to aerobic and resistance exercise reported less sexual dysfunction and more interest in sex. This is especially important because the men were all getting hormonal treatment, which can dampen libido and cause fatigue. Other studies in men with prostate cancer have similarly shown a benefit for exercise in reducing fatigue and improving quality of life.

For people with colorectal cancer, on the other hand, the role of exercise in improving quality of life is less well documented, and less encouraging. In a 2014 systematic review and meta-analysis, researchers found no evidence for improvement in quality of life or fatigue, at least in the short term.

Surprisingly, some research shows a benefit from exercise even toward the end of life in people with advanced cancer. A randomized trial of 231 cancer patients expected to survive for two years or less, for instance, found that eight weeks of exercise helped with overall physical functioning, though it did nothing to combat fatigue. A review of six other studies suggested a benefit of exercise for 84 palliative care patients, but there were not enough data to draw firm conclusions.

HOW EXERCISE FIGHTS CANCER

One might assume that enhanced blood flow, which occurs with exercise, would make tumors grow even faster. But, paradoxically, the exact opposite turns out to be true. It's when tumors are hypoxic, that is, when they *don't* get enough oxygen from the blood, that they go into high gear, secreting growth factors that ultimately trigger metastasis (cancer spread). Moreover, increased blood flow to tumors has another beneficial effect—it brings more chemotherapy to the cancer.

Essentially, tumors don't like it when they're not getting enough oxygen. "It's as if the tumor says, I can't breathe here, so let's pick up and move somewhere else in the body," as Kansas State University exercise physiologist Bradley J. Behnke puts it.

"When a tumor lacks oxygen, it releases just about every growth factor you can think of, which often results in metastasis," he says. "Oncogenes are turned on with lower oxygen pressure." On the other hand, when there's lots of oxygen around, the tumor is more quiescent and the microenvironment around it becomes less conducive to aggressive spread.

In 2010, Duke University researchers injected female mice with human breast cancer, then allowed some to run as much as they wanted on running wheels, while others were confined to a sedentary life. The team regularly measured the blood flow around the tumors. They found, as expected, that blood flow was significantly higher in the exercising group, so much so that the microenvironment around the tumors became normalized, meaning that there would be less spreading of the tumors.

In 2013, Behnke led a team of researchers that randomized some rats with prostate cancer to live in cages with running wheels and others to a sedentary lifestyle. The rats allowed to run wound up with tumors that were in a far less hypoxic (oxygen-deprived) state than the sedentary rats. The team followed up with a 2014 study that demonstrated that acute exercise led to a huge—200 percent—increase in blood flow to prostate tumors in rats and to an increase in the number of blood vessels around the tumor.

In a 2015 study, researchers from Duke University, Massachusetts General Hospital, and Memorial Sloan Kettering Cancer Center confirmed that aerobic exercise, by increasing blood flow, slowed tumor growth.

This team surgically implanted breast cancer cells into female mice and then divided them into two groups, one that was allowed to run on wheels in their cages and another that was not. The runners had slower tumor growth and healthier blood vessels surrounding the tumors. Then the researchers introduced chemotherapy. The mice that exercised *and* got chemotherapy had the best outcomes, with significantly smaller tumors.

But increasing tumor blood flow is not the only way exercise combats cancer. One of the most important other ways is by reducing excess fat.

Adipose tissue, as we've seen, increases chronic inflammation, which can drive tumors. Fat also triggers higher levels of insulin and IGF-1, hormones that can spur tumor growth. Fat tissue also makes estrogen, another driver of breast cancer growth. Fat tissue makes androgens, too, which can drive prostate cancer.

"We know from more than 100 studies that women who are overweight or obese at the time of diagnosis have a higher risk of mortality," says Jennifer Ligibel, who is running a large research project called BWEL, the Breast Cancer Weight Loss study, in 1,000 centers nationwide. Ligibel is a medical oncologist and head of the Leonard P. Zakim Center for Integrative Therapies at the Dana-Farber Cancer Institute in Boston.

A 2014 meta-analysis of 82 studies involving an impressive 213,075 women, for instance, concluded that obesity and being overweight were both associated with poorer overall and breast cancer-specific survival. The same holds for other types of cancer, too. Overweight and obesity contribute to 14 and 20 percent of all cancer-related deaths.

What scientists are now trying to figure out, says Ligibel, is "whether *losing* weight will reduce the risk of recurrence," that is, whether the negative effects of being heavy can be reversed by exercise and weight loss. "We still have an incomplete understanding of the molecular pathways that connect body weight and breast cancer. There are a lot of missing pieces. If exercise and weight loss improve survival, we want to know why."

Marcia Bailey wants to know, too, which is one reason she has joined the more than 3,000 women being enrolled in Ligibel's study. After less than a year on the study, Bailey had lost the 35 pounds she needed to lose. "People say, 'Oh, my gosh. You look fabulous,'" she says, joy in her voice. She herself can barely recognize the thin woman in the mirror.

"I don't look like the old me," she says. "I had colored my hair for years and it used to be down to my shoulders. Now it's white and as short as I can get the stylist to do it. I've had to buy new clothes because the old ones don't fit. When I went back to work, I had to introduce myself to my old colleagues."

Weight loss for cancer patients like Bailey is crucial in part because it helps normalize insulin levels. Both insulin and its related hormone, IGF-1, are "growth factors" that can trigger the malignant transformation of cells. They also drive the growth of existing cancer cells and help cancer cells spread. Not surprisingly, people with diabetes and high insulin levels have a higher-than-normal risk for certain cancers.

Encouragingly, in a randomized trial of 82 previously sedentary women with breast cancer, Ligibel's team found that a 16-week program of resistance and aerobic training substantially reduced insulin levels, while insulin levels did not fall in women assigned to the non-exercise group. Other researchers are also studying the insulin connection to cancer.

Beyond weight loss and insulin, exercise acts in other ways to slow cancer growth. One is by activation of the stress hormone adrenaline.

In a 2016 study, Danish researchers randomly assigned some mice with cancer to live in cages with running wheels and others to cages without the wheels. The mice that were allowed to run wound up with increased adrenaline and increased natural killer cells, which attack cancer cells. The running mice had a 60 percent reduction in both the incidence and growth of five different types of cancer.

To make sure that adrenaline was a key factor, the researchers took another step. They blocked adrenaline production in some of the running animals. As hypothesized, these animals did not show a reduction in cancer growth. And when the researchers gave the sedentary animals large doses of adrenaline, those animals *did* do better at fighting off their tumors than sedentary mice not given an adrenaline boost.

Another way that exercise may slow cancer is by nudging cancer cells to commit suicide, a process called apoptosis. In one study, researchers from the Duke Cancer Institute, Massachusetts General Hospital, and Memorial Sloan Kettering Cancer Center randomized mice with breast cancer to exercise or a sedentary life. Exercise significantly reduced tumor growth and boosted apoptosis. In fact, adding an exercise regimen to standard chemotherapy was more effective at delaying tumor growth than chemotherapy alone.

Exercise also affects cancer outcomes by reducing levels of sex hormones.

Researchers have long known that the hormone estrogen can drive breast cancers. Similarly, it's long been known that androgen can drive prostate cancer. Since adipose tissue can make these sex hormones, reducing fat tissue by weight loss and exercise can lower the levels of sex hormones.

In one 2003 study of older women with breast cancer, researchers from the Fred Hutchinson Cancer Research Center showed that, compared to thinner women, obese women had 35 percent higher concentrations of an estrogen called estrone and a 135 percent higher concentration of another estrogen, estradiol. This helps explain why heavier women have poorer prognoses than thinner women. Other studies have come to similar conclusions.

There's yet another reason why heavier women produce more estrogen. Fat tissue also makes an enzyme called aromatase, which converts androgen into estrogen. (Drugs called aromatase inhibitors, which block this conversion, have long been used to combat estrogen-driven breast cancers.)

In a randomized 2016 study, researchers gathered women with breast cancer who were being treated with aromatase inhibitors. The 121 women in the study were randomized to a year of usual care or aerobic plus resistance exercise. Women who exercised wound up with a significant increase in lean body mass, a decrease in body fat, and a decrease in body mass index, all signs that exercise may improve survival.

YOU DON'T HAVE TO LOVE EXERCISE

For people like Marcia Bailey who already have cancer and are willing to do anything to boost their chances for survival, the details of these mechanisms don't matter. Whether it's better insulin control, normalized hormone levels, or less tumor hypoxia, the take-home message is that exercise and weight control can help.

Bailey already feels she's one of the lucky ones. In the BWEL trial, she was randomized to the weight-loss intervention, which means she received intense coaching on nutrition and exercise.

"We act like exercise is a choice," says Bailey. "But I don't choose to brush my teeth. I just do it. I don't question it. The same with exercise. You don't have to love exercise, you just do it.

"I am invested in this body in a different way than I was before. I know that exercise alone isn't going to keep a recurrence from happening, but it's something I can do. One of the realities of having cancer is that you become disempowered, so I can choose this. I can't control whether it comes back or not, but exercise is one of the things that people know can help."

So Bailey has made plans for a hiking trip with her daughter, and more racquetball, weights, stretching, and stair climbing on an exercise machine.

"My coach says, 'You haven't even imagined some of the physical things you can do.' He's right. Maybe I'll run a marathon, or do something wild like that. That is one of the ways I have to frame it to keep being excited. I got another chance at this. Some people don't get another chance."

CHAPTER 13
Those Tiny, Telltale Telomeres

THE "AHA" MOMENT

Back in the mid-1970s, biologist Elizabeth Blackburn, then at Yale University and now president of the Salk Institute for Biological Studies, was in her lab cultivating pond scum, of all things, in big glass jars. She was determined to extract DNA from the tiny critters that she calls "almost adorable."

One day, holding a dripping X-ray film up to the light in a darkroom, "excitement surged through me as I understood what I was seeing," she recalls. "At the ends of chromosomes was a simple, repeated DNA sequence. The same sequence, over and over and over."

She knew exactly what she had found: telomeres, little caps on the ends of chromosomes, much like the plastic tips at the ends of shoelaces. "I had discovered the structure of telomere DNA," she remembers. "The telomeres were sending a message: There is something special here at the ends of chromosomes."

There was indeed something special about the DNA in telomeres, as earlier work by a previous generation of geneticists, notably Barbara McClintock and Hermann J. Muller, each a Nobel Prize winner, had hinted at. Blackburn and her colleagues Carol Greider and Jack Szostak went on to win their own Nobel Prize in 2009 for their discoveries about telomeres.

Telomeres are now one of the hottest, and most controversial, areas of aging research, crucial not just to our understanding of the biology of aging but to the development of cancer as well. Even in usually austere academic circles, different assessments of telomere research are prompting fierce scientific debate.

One issue is whether things like exercise can impact telomeres in a beneficial way, as some studies suggest, and whether other things, like stress or being overweight or being depressed, can damage them, an association also reported in some studies.

Another is the questionable ethics of commercial testing of telomeres, including online advertisements aimed at people hoping to find their supposed biological, as opposed to chronological, age.

Yet another is the tendency of the media to hype encouraging findings, and perhaps of some scientists to be too cautious. In a meta-analysis of studies involving more than 43,000 people, for instance, having very short telomeres was associated with an 80 percent increased risk of having cardiovascular disease. But the researchers held back from suggesting a causal link, perhaps because something else could have caused both short telomeres and heart disease independently.

Telomeres, the little chunks of matter at the center of all this, are made of DNA and proteins. They act like the aglets on shoelaces, keeping chromosomes intact so that cells can divide properly. The length of DNA in these caps can determine the life span of a cell.

As we age, though, telomeres fray, shrinking a bit with every cell division. This is a normal, natural process. But when telomeres shrink below a certain critical threshold, the cell can't replicate its DNA because the cell division machinery can't copy the full length of the chromosome all the way to the end.

At this point, the cell either becomes "senescent" (too old to divide normally) or dies, *unless*—and this is a huge "unless"—the cell manages to activate an enzyme to *restore* telomere length. This sounds like a good thing, and often is, but it is also a step that can contribute to cancer.

Intuitively, you would think that shortened telomeres might be not just a potential *sign* of aging, but a *cause*, albeit not the only cause. You might also think that simply measuring the length of a person's telomeres would be a clue to a person's biological (as opposed to chronological) age. After all, telomeres get shorter with age, so why wouldn't short telomeres show how fast a person was aging?

Alas, things are not that simple, for a number of reasons. Among other things, telomere shortening does *not* seem to correlate in expected ways with the epigenetic clock (see Chapter 1). If all the biological clocks in the body were running at the same pace, in theory, the telomere clock and the epigenetic clock should be in sync. It's possible that telomeres and the epigenetic clock are simply independent markers of aging. But it could also be that aging can't be influenced by reversing the telomere clock alone.

It's that intrinsic complexity that makes it difficult to evaluate studies suggesting that healthy lifestyle habits like exercise may be linked to longer telomeres, that stress may be linked to shorter telomeres, or that commercial tests measuring telomeres are anything more than a scam.

"While it's true that telomeres do decrease in length as a person ages and that longer telomeres are associated with better health, it's not clear whether the length of telomeres per se is the important variable, or whether it's the *change* in telomere length over time that counts," says Matt Kaeberlein, a geneticist and researcher on aging at the University of Washington.

Moreover, when scientists measure telomere length, they usually do it in immune cells taken from the blood, not from cells all over the body. Shorter telomeres in immune cells can indeed be evidence of a declining immune system, which can, of course, be linked to a higher risk of death. But it's declining immune function that causes most of the correlations with health or the risk of death, Kaeberlein says, not telomere length per se.

In addition, there's a huge range of normal telomere lengths, which means that "small changes are meaningless," says Mary Armanios, clinical director of the telomere center at Johns Hopkins University School of Medicine.

Jay Olshansky, a bio-demographer at the University of Illinois, Chicago, is emphatic: "Unless your telomeres are so short you are about to die, this whole thing is almost complete nonsense. . . . The telomere story has failed miserably as an explanatory variable for human aging."

But other researchers take a very different view, among them Eli Puterman, assistant professor in the school of kinesiology at the University of British Columbia. "We shouldn't throw out the baby with the bathwater," Puterman says, arguing that telomere length is a real biomarker of aging. True, he says, "there's no cutoff point where you can say that when you are at X telomere length, that's so short you will die early. It's not like blood pressure where you can say that if you're at a certain level, that's predictive of heart disease." But that doesn't mean telomere length isn't a genuine biomarker of aging, he says.

Indeed, some recent studies "take us as close as we can get to showing a causal relationship in humans," argues Elissa Epel, a professor in the department of psychiatry at the University of San Francisco. "It's important to see the strengths and weaknesses of any one biomarker."

BOX 13.1 CELL DIVISION

DNA consists of two parallel, twisting strands made up of four building blocks called nucleotide bases. The four building blocks are called, in biological shorthand, A, T, G, and C, and they always pair up in the same fashion. The nucleotide called A always "holds hands" through a chemical bond with its partner T, and C always pairs up with G. Put differently, each A on one strand of DNA always pairs up with a T on the parallel strand, and a C on one strand with a G on the other. Before a cell divides, it has to make a new copy of each chromosome; to be copied, a chromosome's two strands of DNA must unwind and separate from each other so that each strand can be copied for the "daughter" cell.

TELOMERASE

Telomeres are ubiquitous—almost all cells have them, except bacteria, whose DNA is circular and hence doesn't have ends that need to be protected.

But the DNA in a telomere is different from regular DNA. Unlike "coding" DNA, the DNA in telomeres does not contain a genetic blueprint for making proteins. It just sits there, a physical buffer protecting the rest of the DNA. (Just as telomeres protect the ends of chromosomes, other molecules comprise the so-called shelterin complex that protects telomeres.)

In humans and other vertebrates, the DNA in telomeres is a repetitive sequence of the nucleotides TTAGGG, along one strand of DNA, which pairs up with AATCCC on the other strand. The more of these repeating sequences a person has, the longer his or her telomeres.

As Blackburn's team discovered, telomeres can change in length. The key turned out to be an enzyme that restores the correct sequence of DNA at the ends of chromosomes. Unlike most enzymes, which consist entirely of protein, this one, telomerase, is weird—a combination of a protein (hTERT) called reverse transcriptase, and hTR, a chunk of RNA that can act as an enzyme.

Telomerase is most active when cells are dividing the most vigorously, that is, during fetal development and later on, in stem cells, egg and sperm cells, lung cells, cells lining the intestinal tract, hair follicles, and, unfortunately, cancer cells.

In the lab, when scientists add a telomerase gene to normal human cells, it dramatically extends the cell's ability to replicate. (Recently, Texas scientists were able to boost production of telomerase in cells from children with progeria, a rare genetic disease in which aging is vastly accelerated.)

But boosting telomerase can also drive cancer. Indeed, it's in part because cancer cells have so much telomerase that they can keep dividing forever, in essence becoming "immortalized." (Many types and stages of cancer also involve *shortened* telomeres, a puzzle we'll explore in a moment.)

The discovery of telomerase was one of those "Eureka" moments in science, and Blackburn remembers it vividly. In 1983, Greider, her then-new graduate student, reasoned that the only thing that could restore DNA to telomeres must be an enzyme. On Christmas Day, 1984, Greider developed an X-ray film that showed just such an enzyme.

"The next day, her face alight with suppressed glee in her anticipation of my reaction, she showed me the X-ray film," recalls Blackburn. "We looked at each other. Each of us knew this was it. Telomeres could add DNA by attracting this previously undiscovered enzyme, which our lab named telomerase."

That moment is engraved in Greider's memory, too. "It was exactly what we were looking for. But we both realized it looked too good to be true, so we spent nine months trying to disprove what we thought we were seeing. When we did the experiment that was the clincher, I went home, put on Springsteen and danced!"

That clincher? "When we removed telomerase in pond scum, their cells wore down and they died," Blackburn recalls.

TELOMERES AND AGING

The decline of telomere length over the human life span is striking: A newborn baby starts off with telomeres that are 10,000 nucleotide base pairs long. (Nucleotide bases are the building blocks of DNA.) By age 35, a person has telomeres that are 7,500 base pairs long, and by 65, only 4,800 base pairs long.

Telomere length at birth can somewhat predict adult telomere length, but individuals also have different rates of telomere attrition. A number of genes are known to lead to very short telomeres and a higher risk of certain diseases.

But how you live your life may also play a role in telomere length, with the emphasis on "may." Bad lifestyle habits such as smoking, being obese, stress, lack of exercise, exposure to pollution, and poor diet all may increase the pace of telomere shortening and aging. Good lifestyle habits, on the other hand, including exercise, stress reduction, and a diet rich in antioxidants and fiber, may slow the pace of telomere attrition.

Indeed, some studies suggest that telomere length can actually predict survival. A small but influential 2003 study created a buzz when it focused on people older than 60: People with shorter telomeres were found to be three times more likely to die from heart disease and eight times more likely to die from infectious diseases.

But since then, studies of varying size and quality have come to inconsistent findings. A 2011 review of telomere length as a biomarker of aging, for instance, found that five out of 10 studies found a significant relationship between shortened telomeres and increased risk of mortality, while the other five studies did not. But that review came out *before* a large study of more than 64,000 people that *did* find an association between shorter telomeres and mortality.

STRESS: DO TELOMERES KEEP THE SCORE?

Some researchers have found that chronic emotional stress, usually defined as a combination of anger, irritability, anxiety, and depression, is linked to shortened telomeres.

Adversity in childhood may even predict shorter telomeres later in life, though a causal link in humans has yet to be shown. In a small 2016 study in adult rhesus monkeys, though, those who had been reared by their own mothers in social groups had longer telomeres than those reared without their mothers. In wild seabirds, those exposed to early postnatal stress (handling by humans) had more telomere shortening than those not exposed.

In humans, there may be a complex relationship involving psychological stress, telomere shortening, and psychiatric disorders, a relationship that unfolds over a lifetime, say University of California, San Francisco, researchers Elissa Epel and Aric Prather.

In a prospective Duke University study, for instance, researchers tested children's telomeres at the age of five years, then again at age 10, and correlated this with exposure to violence at home. The children who experienced two or more kinds of exposures to violence had significantly more telomere erosion than children who didn't, regardless of sex, socioeconomic status, or weight. Recent meta-analyses have also shown that childhood adversity is associated with telomere shortness.

In a 2017 meta-analysis including 16,238 people, for instance, researchers found a significant association between childhood stressors and shorter telomere length at age 42, although the size of the effect was small. In another 2017 meta-analysis of 41 studies, researchers found a significant association between early adversity and telomere length, and a larger effect size. In a 2017 meta-analysis involving 30,919 participants, though, researchers found a significant association between childhood trauma and faster telomere erosion in adulthood, but again, the effect size was small.

Precisely why chronic stress might shorten telomeres is still a puzzle, but it's clear that stress triggers higher levels of hormones, including cortisol, adrenaline, and noradrenaline, as well as increased oxidative damage from free radicals, all of which can lead to shorter telomeres.

Interestingly, the DNA that comprises telomeres is more susceptible to oxidative damage than regular DNA. Blackburn and Epel, in fact, argue that the effects of stress on telomeres start in the womb. It's as if the "baby's telomeres are listening to Mom's stress," as they put it in their 2017 book, *The Telomere Effect*.

The first suggestion of a link between stress and telomere length came in 2011, when researchers from the University of California, Irvine, teamed up with Blackburn and Epel to study 94 healthy young adults, half of whom were the offspring of mothers who had experienced severe stress during pregnancy, and half, children of mothers with non-stressful pregnancies. Exposure to severe stress *in utero* was associated with shorter telomeres in the adult offspring. In 2013, the team found that maternal stress during pregnancy was associated with shorter telomeres right from the get-go, in newborns.

Other researchers have similarly found that babies born to mothers who never completed high school had shorter telomeres than those born to mothers who did. Older kids whose parents were less educated were also found to have shorter telomeres. If telomere length is a biological marker of aging, this difference might be equivalent to six years less of life.

And the more adverse conditions a child lives with, some studies suggest, the shorter his or her telomeres may be in adulthood. (Adverse conditions include living with an alcoholic parent or depressed family member, sexual or physical abuse, and other dysfunctional situations.)

In a major 2016 study, Puterman, Epel, and others examined 4,598 men and women from the US Health and Retirement Study. A single adverse event in a person's life was not associated with telomere shortening in adulthood, nor was childhood poverty. But lifetime *cumulative adversity* did predict a 6 percent greater likelihood of shorter telomere length, an effect mostly due to the adversity in childhood. In this study, each additional adverse event in childhood raised the likelihood of shorter telomeres in adulthood by 11 percent, suggesting, as the authors put it, "that the shadow of childhood adversity may reach far into later adulthood in part through cellular aging."

These findings fit with a number of other studies, including a European study of 4,441 women aged 41–80 that found that adverse events in childhood were associated with shorter telomeres in adulthood. The Puterman findings also fit with a 2013 study from Butler Hospital in Providence, Rhode Island, a 2013 Duke University study, and a 2016 systematic review of other studies by Brazilian researchers.

On the other hand, a 2015 cross-sectional study found the opposite—that while *recent* stressful events may be associated with shorter telomeres, psychosocial stressors earlier in life were not. A 30-year New Zealand study also found no association between telomere length and life stresses from birth to early adulthood, again, in a cross-sectional study.

Depression, which is not the same as stress but often overlaps with it, has also been reliably linked in many studies to shorter telomeres. In fact, a 2016 meta-analysis that included 34,347 people suggested a solid link between depression and shorter telomeres. Some researchers hypothesize that depression may be a state of accelerated aging in which chronic stress leads to increases in cortisol, more oxidative stress, more inflammatory cytokines, and shorter telomeres.

In one study of Latino preschoolers, for instance, children growing up with severely depressed mothers had significantly shorter telomeres than children growing up in happier homes. Similarly, a study of 97 daughters aged 10–14 showed that even before they had any signs of depression themselves, the daughters of depressed mothers had shorter telomeres than the daughters of non-depressed mothers. The daughters' shorter telomeres were associated with higher emotional and physiological reactivity to stress.

Living without any parents at all, of course, is highly stressful, too, and may be similarly hard on telomeres, as the plight of children in Romanian orphanages years ago suggested. American researchers found that the children who spent the most time in the extreme social deprivation of the orphanages had the shortest telomeres. Children who were lucky enough to eventually be adopted showed remarkable recovery, though their telomeres were still far shorter than those of never-institutionalized children.

Even when psychological and social stress is delayed until adulthood, it can be linked with shorter telomeres, although the magnitude of the effect is small. Telomere shortening has also been found in psychiatric disorders as a whole, according to a 2016 meta-analysis involving 14,827 people.

In one 2014 study, American, British, and Welsh researchers gathered 333 healthy men and women aged 54–76 and put them through standard mental challenges designed to induce acute stress. The researchers measured cardiovascular, neuroendocrine, and inflammatory responses. In many of the participants, the acute stress challenge elicited a normal response—a rise in reactivity, followed by a rapid decline when the stress was over.

But in men with shorter telomeres, recovery from the stress challenge was blunted. Interestingly, these men also showed higher levels of telomerase, suggesting that their bodies may have been trying to repair the damaged telomeres. (Inexplicably, however, women did not show this pattern.)

In a different study, adult women who reported the highest levels of stress had telomeres that were shorter. In a meta-analysis of nearly 4,000 people, those who had PTSD (post-traumatic stress disorder) had shorter telomeres than those who didn't, although curiously, this effect showed up with sexual assault and childhood trauma, but not combat.

Of all the stresses of modern life, being the caregiver of a person with Alzheimer's disease ranks among the highest. In a major study of 41 caregivers and 41 age- and gender-matched controls, the chronic stress of caregiving was associated not just with altered immune function but with excessive telomere loss as well. The stressed caregivers also showed increases in telomerase, once again a possible hint of the body's attempt to stop telomere shortening.

It's tempting to come away from such studies convinced that stress really does shorten telomeres and thereby accelerates aging and increases the risk of death. It's tempting, too, to conclude that healthy behaviors and lack of stress may be able to mitigate this effect of stress. But others caution that the science isn't quite there yet.

Almost as soon as scientists began to understand the power of telomerase to lengthen telomeres, a horrible realization dawned: Like so many other molecules in the body, telomerase has a Jekyll and Hyde personality.

The ability of telomerase to restore the telomeres at the tips of chromosomes is wonderful—it prolongs cellular life by keeping chromosomes intact and allowing cells to divide normally. But that very trick also drives cancer. In fact, 90 percent of all malignant cells use telomerase to prolong cellular life, making telomerase more widely expressed by cancer cells than any other marker.

By allowing cancer cells to replenish their telomeres with every cell division, telomerase allows cancer cells to become "immortalized," that is, to be able to avoid cell senescence and keep dividing. One result of all this runaway cell division was that nearly 600,000 Americans died of cancer in 2016 alone, the latest year for which figures are available.

Blackburn put the idea succinctly in her 2009 Nobel Prize speech: Telomerase "promotes cellular immortality by providing cancer cell telomeres with the means for continuous replenishment."

Importantly, this does not mean that telomerase actually *causes* cancer. What it does is allow cells that are already turning cancerous to keep dividing forever, unlike normal cells, which eventually run out of steam.

This fact is not lost on pharmaceutical developers: A drug that could block telomerase sounds like the perfect anti-cancer therapy. Since telomerase is highly active in cancer cells and barely active in most normal cells, an anti-telomerase drug could in theory target cancer cells and spare normal cells. And research does show that blocking telomerase kills cancer cells.

But, unfortunately, things have turned out to be much more complicated than that. In the past decade, at least two clinical trials of telomerase drugs had to be stopped because there was no survival benefit in cancer patients getting the drugs, although other small trials, including on a drug called Imetelstat from Geron, have yielded somewhat more encouraging results.

One problem, as researchers from the MD Anderson Cancer Center discovered, is that when telomerase is blocked, cancer cells develop alternate ways to keep telomeres long. Indeed, other researchers have shown that a surprising 5–10 percent of cancer cells are able to maintain their telomeres by these alternate pathways.

Worse yet, telomerase-blocking drugs may actually help cancers resist chemotherapy. (Resistance to chemotherapy is one of the main causes of cancer death.) Blocking telomerase can also have adverse effects on stem cells, which are crucial for regenerating tissues.

As if that were not bad enough, researchers studying yeast cells have found that when telomerase is removed, cells increase the activity of their energy-providing mitochondria (see Chapter 5). That's a good thing in normal cells, but a decidedly bad thing if it energizes cancer cells.

There may someday be a way to get the best of both worlds—a telomerase drug that could make longer telomeres in healthy cells without boosting cancer. Recently, Stanford University scientists led by stem cell biologist Helen Blau did find a way to temporarily tweak telomerase in human skin cells in a way that it allowed those cells to divide 40 times more than un-tweaked cells.

Because the stimulation of telomerase was short term, it didn't raise the risk of promoting cancer. (Spanish researchers have also found a way, using gene therapy, to boost telomerase in mice in such a way that it increased life span without promoting cancer. Unfortunately, some human research suggests such an approach could *drive* cancer.)

There is some encouraging news in all this, though. Despite slow progress on telomerase-blocking cancer drugs, scientists' fascination with telomeres and telomerase has led to a more sophisticated understanding of how cells become cancerous and "learn" to live forever.

For years, they grappled with this puzzle: Long telomeres drive cancer. But short telomeres are also associated with cancer—in fact, short telomeres, which occur when there is not enough telomerase around, are an early sign of cancer.

Scientists now have a better idea of what happens. When a cell is on the verge of becoming cancerous, telomeres shorten. In fact, short telomeres are a good predictor both of getting cancer and of dying from it.

Two meta-analyses illustrate the point. In one, University of Texas researchers pooled data on more than 24,000 people and found that short telomeres were a marker for cancer risk. In the other, by researchers at the National Institutes of Health, short telomeres detected in blood (immune) cells were linked to an increased risk of cancer elsewhere in the body.

But here's the key: Cells don't become cancerous overnight. It takes multiple steps—or "hits"—such as mutations or genomic changes in specific genes to nudge a cell to become cancerous. These hits can result from exposure of DNA to toxic chemicals, free radicals, radiation, or cancer-causing viruses. During the initial stages of this process, the cell goes into crisis.

"Normally, short or dysfunctional telomeres in a cell in crisis cause activation of signals that lead to that cell's 'programmed' death, essentially cell suicide," says Masood Shammas, lead scientist in the medical oncology department at Dana-Farber Cancer Institute in Boston.

"But if, because of certain mutations, the cell manages to survive this crisis and continues to divide, its DNA then becomes unstable, which can lead both to transformation of that normal cell into a cancer cell *and* to activation of telomerase, the telomere lengthening enzyme. The result is that most cancer cells have elevated telomerase activity but also shorter telomeres," says Shammas.

"It's confusing," admits Greider, now director of molecular biology and genetics at Johns Hopkins University School of Medicine. "Cancer cells have short telomeres, but elevated telomerase. And once telomerase is activated, the telomeres in cancer cells don't go back up to their normal length, but are long enough that the cells can keep dividing. This is a growth advantage for cancer cells."

Shammas puts it this way: "Telomerase does not make cells turn into cancer but it does increase their life span. Once a cell is transformed into a cancer cell, telomerase increases the life span of that cell, making it immortal."

Which is just what Greider and Blackburn had theorized back in 1996: Telomerase "becomes active after a cell has already lost its brakes on proliferation."

TELOMERES AND EXERCISE

In early 2017, an exercise science professor at Brigham Young University named Larry Tucker stunned the community of researchers exploring the potential effect of exercise on telomeres.

Tucker's study wasn't the first time anybody had shown a positive association between exercise and longer telomeres in people, not just lab rats. Nor did it prove cause and effect. And it didn't settle the question of whether exercise just *maintains* telomere length or might *increase* it.

But Tucker's study of 5,823 adults aged 20–84 made headlines nonetheless. In his analysis of a large, random sample of US adults, Tucker showed that people who habitually exercised had much longer telomeres than sedentary folks—a difference that, if telomere length is a biomarker of aging, would be equivalent to 9 years less cellular aging.

That year, 2017, turned out to be a banner year for studies on exercise and telomere length. In one study of women whose average age was 79.2, researchers from the San Diego School of Medicine found that those who did more leisure-time physical activity had longer telomeres. In another San Diego study that tracked activity levels by accelerometers (Fitbit-like devices), older women who did at least two and a half hours a week of moderate physical activity had longer telomeres than those who did less. In a third San Diego study, researchers found that higher sedentary time, as measured by accelerometers, may be associated with shorter telomeres.

Not surprisingly, research suggests that people who exercise *a lot*—like marathon runners—also have long telomeres. In one 2013 Australian study, ultra-marathoners (whose races are longer than a 26.2 mile marathon) had telomeres that were 11 percent longer than age-matched sedentary folks. If telomeres are a biomarker of aging, this would translate to a biological age 16 years younger than the runners' chronological age.

A number of other studies also support a link between exercise and longer telomeres, and between lack of exercise and shorter telomeres. Some studies correlate telomere length not just to physical activity but to aerobic fitness, as measured on a treadmill test. These studies, too, suggest a link between fitness and telomere length.

To be fair, not all studies have lined up as expected. A South African study of marathoners found no difference in telomere length between marathoners and sedentary folks. A Connecticut study came to similar conclusions. Even a 2015 meta-analysis of more than 30 studies involving 41,230 people came up empty.

The real test of the potential effect of exercise on telomeres, of course, would be to randomly assign some people to exercise and others not and see what happens to their telomeres—an interventional study. "So far, nobody has really done the right study," contends Jay Olshanksy, the Chicago bio-demographer. Such a study, he says, "would be to take a group of people and have each person serve as his or her own control. Measure everybody's baseline telomere length. Then do an intervention that tests both favorable (exercise) and unfavorable (stress) risk factors. Then reverse the intervention. Measure the rate of change in telomere length during both time periods in each person during the experimental conditions and under controlled conditions. No one seems to have done this simple experiment."

But some researchers have come close.

At the Fred Hutchinson Cancer Research Center in Seattle, researchers randomized 439 middle-aged overweight or obese women to one of four programs: dietary weight loss alone, aerobic exercise alone, combined exercise and diet, or no intervention. Unfortunately for telomere theorists, there was no change in telomere length between the intervention groups and the controls.

In another interventional study of obese middle-aged Korean women, one group was put through six months of aerobic training and the control group was not. Again, there was no change in telomere length.

But a randomized interventional study suggests that six months of moderate-to-vigorous physical activity can actually *lengthen* telomeres in 68 previously inactive 50–75-year-old men and women. The participants were highly stressed family caregivers.

Finally, some studies are just plain heart-warming, even if they are not interventional. In a study of women aged 60 or older, some of whom were caretakers of spouses or parents with dementia, reasonable vigorous exercise was enough to wipe out the damaging effect of stress on telomeres. Put differently, even highly stressed caretakers did not show shortened telomeres so long as they exercised, while stressed but sedentary caretakers did.

BOX 13.2 BREAKTHROUGH OR SLOPPY SCIENCE?

Some studies of exercise and telomere length are music to the ears of some telomere researchers and sloppy science to others.

Case in point? A small, non-randomized 2013 study that purported to show that comprehensive lifestyle changes can not only protect telomeres from shortening, but can actually lengthen them. The study, led by physician/diet guru Dean Ornish, focused on men with low-risk prostate cancer. Ten of the men chose to follow a diet/ exercise/stress reduction program, while 25 others did not. All were followed for five years.

At first glance, these results seem impressive: A combination of a diet involving plants and unrefined grains, stress reduction by yoga and meditation, a weekly support group, and walking 30 minutes a day six days a week yielded a significant, 10 percent increase in telomere length. And the more of these healthy behaviors the active men adopted, the more their telomeres lengthened. By contrast, over the five-year period, the men who didn't change their lifestyles showed a 3 percent decrease in telomere length.

But it's tough to conclude much from this study. It lumped all lifestyle changes together and allowed the participants to choose whether or not to change their life-styles, so it's impossible to say what effect, if any, exercise alone might have had.

MECHANISMS: HOW EXERCISE MIGHT AFFECT TELOMERES

If exercise does in fact protect telomere length—and, as we've just seen, that's still an open question—there are several theoretical ways that this could happen: by boosting telomerase, by reducing oxidative stress, by reducing inflammation, and by preserving muscle satellite cells. So far, though, research on all these potential mechanisms is scant.

In 2009, a team of German scientists compared telomerase activity in middle-aged track and field athletes to that in non-exercisers. The athletes showed a significant increase in telomerase activity, as well as beneficial changes in at least two other factors. The athletes wound up with longer telomeres than the non-exercisers.

(In case you're worried that if exercise increases telomerase, it might increase your risk of cancer, take heart. Telomerase triggered by exercise is short term, while increased telomerase in cancer cells is permanent. Besides, as we saw, telomerase doesn't *cause* cancer; it just drives cell proliferation in already transformed, cancerous cells.)

The effect of oxidative stress on telomeres is tricky to assess. It has been known for years to lead to DNA damage in general and, more recently, to damage in the specific DNA sequence in telomeres. But while exercise does temporarily increase free radicals and oxida-tive damage, it simultaneously triggers enzymes that gobble up free radicals, so the net effect is a good one. In fact, *mild* oxidative stress may actually lengthen telomeres, though *severe* oxidative stress may shorten them.

This delicate balance was illustrated in a 2015 Italian study. The Italian researchers studied athletes running the Tor des Geants (Tour of Giants), an extreme race of more than 200 miles. They found that while chronic endurance training is linked to longer telomeres, during and right after the race, the athletes had temporary oxidative damage to DNA in telomeres.

As for chronic inflammation, it is obviously an unhealthy state of affairs. But, as we saw in Chapter 11, exercise is a powerful way to combat inflammation, through a variety of complex mechanisms.

And satellite cells in muscle tissue? This is iffy territory, but it's possible that exercise might increase a person's pool of satellite cells, which might help maintain length in the telomeres of these cells.

I TAKE THE TELOMERE TEST

Telomere research is among the most exciting areas in aging research, in part because of the tantalizing but still evolving links between telomere length and exercise, telomere length and stress, and telomere length and cancer.

In fact, many people, including me, are intrigued by simple, commercial blood tests of telomere length, despite the fact that this test is not approved by the US Food and Drug Administration. The idea that such a test might reveal one's true biological, as opposed to chronological, age has made online telomere testing a thriving business.

And that concerns some scientists.

"I don't know why this is happening," Armanios told me. "It's interesting that people psychologically want to hang on to a medical test to tell them how old they are . . . despite the fact that [online testing] is not rigorous."

Jay Olshansky, the University of Illinois researcher on aging, told me much the same thing: "Telomere testing is almost an entire waste of time . . . it's just a gimmick."

Among the problems, says Nobel Laureate Greider, is that different labs use different methods to measure telomeres. Some commercial labs use a cheaper, less accurate test, while academics often use a more expensive, more accurate test. Some commercial labs, for instance, use a technique called PCR (polymerase chain reaction) to increase a small sample of DNA into a larger sample that can be more easily studied. This test is easy to use, but there can be so much variation that test results are unreliable, she says. "In a medical setting, with robust clinical testing, for someone who might have short telomere disease—and that's less than 1 percent of the population—telomere testing is useful," says Greider. "For the general population, it's completely worthless."

Despite such strong caveats, I couldn't resist checking out the website of a telomere testing company. The first thing I noticed was that the people who wrote bad reviews for the website were those who had gotten "bad" news, that is, that their telomere age was *older* than their chronological age. They slammed the test, calling it invalid and not worth the money. Those whose tests suggested they were *younger* than their chronological age raved about the test.

Nonetheless, curiosity won the day. I sent away for the $89 test kit. When it arrived, I read the instructions, dutifully stuck my finger with the needle, dabbed a drop of blood onto the collection stick, put the stick in the bottle with the "stabilizing fluid," and sent it off.

Several weeks later, I got the results: I was 10 years younger than my chronological age.

Too bad I can't believe it. The commercial tests are just too unreliable.

CHAPTER 14

Exercise and Anti-Aging Pills

EXERCISE PILLS, SERIOUSLY?

Like it or not, exercise pills are poised to take off, potentially a boon to humankind, but also, unfortunately, a way to tempt even more Americans to stick with their unhealthy ways—most notably, their sedentary lifestyles.

Propped up by sensational headlines and the promise of a sweat-free way to get the benefits of exercise without actually doing it, some of these drugs are already available online, used by bodybuilders and other athletes willing to tamper with sporting rules—and their bodies.

Many, if not most, of these substances are *not* approved for these purposes by the US Food and Drug Administration, and many are on the list of banned substances by the World Anti-Doping Agency (WADA). Many, many more of these drugs, technically called "exercise mimetics" (exercise mimicking), are in the pipeline.

Anti-aging pills are in development, too, potentially a way to stave off the effects of a lifetime of sitting and eating too much, and even to tinker with our basic metabolism.

To be sure, the *economic* rationale for both exercise mimetics and anti-aging drugs is unarguable. A safe, effective exercise mimetic would be a gold mine for drug companies. So would an anti-aging drug, especially if it prolonged not just the life span, but the "health span" as well. "It would change all of life," a leading FDA official told POLITICO. "If there was something that really slowed the aging process, wouldn't everyone want to be in on it?"

The *scientific* logic is powerful, too. As we've seen in chapter after chapter in this book, exercise has multiple, diverse molecular effects all over the body, which means that artificially boosting the right molecules could, in theory, mimic *some* of these beneficial effects, though certainly not all.

Similarly, scientists who study aging have unraveled a number of the key molecular changes that underlie aging, which suggests that, again in theory, drugs to block these changes could be useful, too.

Cellular senescence, for instance, is a biological process, much like an emergency brake, that cells use to stop dividing. This is good in that it can prevent cancer cells from dividing out of control, but it's harmful in that these stalled cells remain in the body like debris, emitting chemicals that can damage other cells. A drug to kill senescent cells could be useful, indeed.

Moreover, in the big scheme of things, anti-aging researchers argue, research funds might be better used to target the basic processes of aging, rather than trying to cure one disease at a time. At least so far, the FDA approves drugs based on their ability to target a specific disease. In the view of the FDA, the biological process of aging is not a "disease."

But some argue it should be considered one. "I would love for the US Food and Drug Administration to regard aging as a condition that's worth treating," says anti-aging researcher David Sinclair, a professor of genetics at Harvard Medical School. "The reason is that aging is a decline in function. That, to me, is exactly what a disease is."

In the fall of 2018, the World Health Organization agreed, changing the language in a document called the ICD-11, thus opening the door for therapies directed against age-related diseases.

The business world is not waiting on such philosophical matters. A number of companies are betting their investors' money, and lots of it, on drugs to mimic exercise, slow aging, or both. A partial list includes Calico, CyteGen, Human Longevity, Inc., Unity Biotechnology, MetroBiotech, resTORbio, PureTech Health, Insilico Medicine, Mount Tam Biotechnologies, Sierra Sciences, and Mitobridge.

In California, the Palo Alto Institute has set up a $1 million "longevity" prize to "hack the code" of aging, and 30 companies are now in the race. Peter Thiel, the billionaire cofounder of PayPal, has teamed up with anti-aging researcher Aubrey de Gray to start the Methuselah Foundation, which is dedicated to regenerative medicine that could extend healthy life spans. Craig Venter, the genomics pioneer, is in the game, too.

As for exercise pills, many scientists who study the molecular biology of exercise are deeply skeptical, among them the authors of a landmark 2014 paper in the journal *Cell*.

"Although the concept of taking a pill to obtain the benefits of exercise without actually expending any energy has mass appeal for a large majority of sedentary individuals, such an approach is likely to fail," wrote Australian exercise and nutrition researcher John Hawley and his team. "Exercise training provokes widespread perturbations in numerous cells, tissues, and organ[s], conferring multiple health-promoting benefits," they said, "and it is the multiplicity and complexity of these responses and adaptations that make it highly improbable that any single pharmacological approach could ever mimic such wide-ranging effects."

True, they acknowledge, a "polypill" with multiple effects might work. But even such a pill could have unacceptable side effects, which means, as they put it, that "exercise itself remains the best 'polypill.'" A Spanish and American research team agrees that exercise is the "real polypill" because our genome has been shaped by evolution to respond to exercise, not pills.

"I am absolutely skeptical," adds Bruce Spiegelman, director of the Center for Energy Metabolism and Chronic Disease at the Dana-Farber Cancer Institute in Boston. "The notion of exercise mimetics sets off bells and whistles. It's bad for the lay public. Patients will say, 'This is a way to avoid exercise.'"

"I have nothing but scorn for people just trying to make a fast buck based on false narratives. I view it as an existential threat to serious scientists working in this area. It makes it look as though the goal of research is to make it so that lazy people who don't exercise can be fit, as opposed to research to discover molecules for people who really can't exercise, like Christopher Reeve after his riding accident," he says.

Indeed, during the years I have worked on this book, the thing that has impressed me most is how many *different* effects exercise has on the body, and how deep are its effects on the basic molecules in our cells. Some scientists, for instance, estimate that a *single* bout of high-intensity exercise generates more than 1,000 molecular changes. What happens to the other 999 effects if you modify just one? As we saw in Chapter 6, one organ alone—muscle—produces a torrent of hormones that have beneficial effects all over the body.

Think of it this way: Exercise *is* a drug. It *is* medicine. In fact, it's the best medicine going. It's also free. In other words, the only time it makes sense to take a pill instead is if you are too sick, injured, or disabled to move.

So, let's take a closer look at the emerging drugs being studied as exercise mimetics and/or anti-aging pills.

MTOR-INHIBITING DRUGS

For years, scientists have known that the most sure-fire way to extend life span is to restrict calories. Caloric restriction works in part by turning *down* the activity of a gene called mTOR, which stands for mammalian (or sometimes "mechanistic") target of rapamycin.

Rapamycin is an antifungal agent that was discovered on Rapa Nui, better known as Easter Island. It was by studying rapamycin that scientists discovered mTOR itself. Rapamycin, called an mTOR inhibitor, a drug that blocks mTOR, turns out to be a master regulator of cellular growth and metabolism. It is now under intense study as a life-extension drug.

The discovery that rapamycin increased life span was deemed one of the top scientific breakthroughs of 2009 by the journal *Science*. Today, many scientists believe that mTOR inhibitors to slow aging "are a matter of 'when' rather than 'if.'"

Luckily for researchers, and potentially the rest of us, rapamycin is already on the market to treat lung cancer and combat organ transplant rejection. The drug stops cell division in immune cells called T cells, which is why it works as an immunosuppressant. But, paradoxically, mTOR inhibitors, including rapamycin derivatives such as everolimus (RD001), can also *boost* immune function, even in humans. Other rapamycin mimics under study include epigallocatechin gallate, withaferin, and isoliquiritigenen, though so far, there's no good evidence that these compounds inhibit mTOR effectively.

Anti-aging researchers are fascinated by mTOR for other reasons, too. It is part of the pathway by which insulin and IGF-1, or insulin-like growth factor, act. Insulin regulates cell metabolism, while IGF-1 boosts cell growth, cell differentiation, and tissue repair, all potentially beneficial things.

But IGF-1 can also trigger age-related diseases by turning *up* mTOR. In other words, when mTOR levels are high, aging is accelerated; when levels are low, the rate of aging is slowed down.

Interestingly, exercise *increases* both IGF-1 and mTOR in certain tissues. This could have adverse effects, except that the exercise effect is short term and localized to specific tissues. In other words, the danger appears to come when IGF-1 and mTOR are increased all the time and all over the body, not just in muscles and not just for a short time. Some call this the "IGF trade-off" between exercise performance and longevity.

DIABETES DRUGS TO COMBAT AGING: METFORMIN

This FDA-approved drug, which is sold as Fortamet, Glucophage, Glucophage XR, Glymetza, and Riomet, has long been on the market to treat diabetes. It has also been shown to delay aging and extend health span in animals, and it may in humans, too. A new study called TAME (Targeting Aging with Metformin) aims to see if metformin works in humans to delay the onset of cancer, cardiovascular disease, and Alzheimer's. Another drug used to treat diabetes, acarbose, extends life span in mice.

Interestingly, metformin, which is used primarily to increase insulin sensitivity, also activates an enzyme called AMPK (more on AMPK in a moment) and indirectly inhibits mTOR, another potential benefit.

But some data suggest that in healthy people, metformin may *lower* maximal exercise capacity, prompting some scientists to reject metformin as a potential exercise pill. Metformin mimics include allantoin and gensenoside, though the evidence for them so far is weak.

HORMONES, MITOCHONDRIAL BOOSTERS, AND HEAT PRODUCERS

As we saw in Chapter 5, exercise triggers an important molecular cascade that ultimately produces more mitochondria, the energy factories inside cells. It goes like this: Exercise raises levels of an enzyme called AMPK, which works with another protein called SIRT1 to increase levels of yet another molecule, PGC-1 alpha, which in turn helps cells make more mitochondria, which ultimately produces energy (ATP). Exercise, in short, boosts mitochondria, while the process of aging does the opposite—it reduces mitochondria. So, drugs that affect the molecules in the mitochondrial cascade are important targets for drug developers.

AICAR-AMPK

AICAR is a peptide (a small protein) that *artificially* stimulates AMPK, the enzyme that is *naturally* triggered during exercise. The job of AMPK is to sense when a cell needs more energy. To do this, AMPK works with a molecule called PPAR-delta to increase levels of PGC-1 alpha. PGC-1 alpha is the master controller for creating more mitochondria.

In a 2008 study in *Cell*, researchers found that oral AICAR increased the body's ability to burn fat and increased endurance running in mice by 44 percent. AMPK can also increase a beneficial process called autophagy, by which damaged parts of cells are destroyed and life span may be prolonged.

Both AICAR and AMPK are for sale online. AICAR is not approved by the US Food and Drug Administration and is on the list of banned substances of the World Anti-Doping Agency. It is in clinical trials to treat some heart diseases and may help with problems like muscular dystrophy and diabetes. AMPK is not under discussion at WADA at the moment.

GW501516

GW501516 can boost levels of PPAR-delta, part of the mitochondria-building cascade, and increase endurance in mice. Endurance exercise is partly a function of muscles' ability to switch from burning glucose to burning fat. PPAR-delta is believed to tell cells to use fat instead of sugar. In mice, PPAR-delta also helps transform muscle fibers toward the slow-twitch type, which burn fat and fatigue more slowly. PPAR-delta activators are on WADA's banned list.

Glaxo Smith Kline, the maker of GW501516, put the drug on hold, after toxicity tests showed that mice given long-term, high doses of the drug developed cancer at a higher rate than untreated mice. An updated version of "516" is now under development. GW501516, also known as "endurobol," is on WADA's list of banned substances.

GSK4716

This is a synthetic small molecule that can boost levels of ERR (estrogen-related receptor), which in turn boosts creation of mitochondria. It also helps muscles shift toward slow-twitch type and helps new blood vessels form. It is sold online. It is not FDA approved and is under review by WADA.

SR9009

This man-made protein acts on a molecule called REV-ERB to control circadian rhythms; it also seems to increase the amount of energy mice expend without actually exercising. It may boost creation of new mitochondria and increase autophagy. It is sold online as Stenabolic. It is not FDA approved and is on WADA's prohibited list.

MOTS-c

This is a so-called mitokine, a hormone released from mitochondria that, at least in worms, seems to extend life. It appears to act on AMPK and helps maintain metabolic stability (homeostasis) and insulin sensitivity. It is under review by WADA.

Irisin

Irisin is an especially important myokine, a hormone pumped out by contracting muscles. While there had been debate about whether exercise boosted irisin in people as well as in mice, Spiegelman's lab confirmed that it does. Irisin not only stimulates the cells that build bones, but also helps turn white fat into brown fat, the kind that produces heat. It acts in part by activating PGC-1 alpha. It is produced in the body from a precursor protein, FNDC5. It is sold online, but is not FDA approved. It is under review by WADA, but currently is not banned.

Meteorin-like

This oddly named hormone is stimulated naturally by exercise in cold environments and regulates chemical interactions between the immune system and fat tissue. Artificially increasing levels of this hormone stimulates energy expenditure, improves glucose tolerance, and increases heat production. Meteorin-like is not under discussion at WADA.

BAIBA

When exercise increases levels of PGC-1 alpha, that, in turn, triggers secretion of BAIBA (beta-aminoisobutyric acid), a hormone made in muscles and secreted into the blood. BAIBA travels to white fat tissue, where it acts on PPAR-alpha receptors to ramp up activation of genes that turn white fat cells brown.

(–) Epicatechin

This is a plant-derived substance found in cocoa, tea, and grapes that acts on cardiac and skeletal muscle to increase mitochondria and blood vessels. It also appears to act on VEGF, a molecule that stimulates blood vessels to grow, and on nitric oxide. It is under review by WADA.

RESVERATROL, SIRTUINS, AND NAD+

Resveratrol

Resveratrol, a plant-derived chemical found in blueberries, the skin of grapes, and red wine, has long been controversial. It is sold legally as a dietary supplement and therefore does not need prior FDA approval, although manufacturers are not supposed to make false health claims, as some have.

Resveratrol was initially believed to trigger enzymes called sirtuins, especially one called SIRT1, and to improve exercise capacity, increase insulin sensitivity, create new mitochondria, protect against diet-induced obesity, boost blood flow to muscles, and improve lung function in mice. (Humans have seven sirtuins.) Dietary resveratrol may also mimic beneficial aspects of caloric restriction.

In 2004, David Sinclair, the Harvard genetics professor, founded a company called Sirtris Pharmaceuticals in Cambridge, Massachusetts, to develop resveratrol products (chiefly SRT501) and sirtuin-based anti-aging drugs.

But the initial scientific—and popular—excitement for resveratrol has faded, at least for a while. In 2008, GSK, a major drug company, bought Sirtris for $720 million. In 2010, some research suggested that resveratrol did, as claimed, trigger SIRT1. And Sinclair currently believes the doubts about resveratrol have been satisfactorily resolved.

Other researchers, however, have questioned whether resveratrol truly activates SIRT1 and whether resveratrol is as effective as claimed. In one study, mice and rats given resveratrol did not, as expected, show an increase in mitochondria in muscle cells or in life span. It also did not activate AMPK and SIRT1 and PGC-1 alpha and lead to better running endurance. In fact, at high doses, resveratrol was toxic. On the other hand, one SIRT1 activator (SRT2104) has extended life span in mice and may be safe and potentially effective in humans. That same drug has also improved psoriasis in humans.

Recently, there's been some good news. Resveratrol has been shown to inhibit a molecule called PDE4 that, through a series of steps, boosts production of AMPK, PGC-1 alpha, and SIRT1, which increase energy production in mitochondria. A PDE4 inhibitor that is 30,000 times more powerful than resveratrol has been approved by the FDA for chronic obstructive pulmonary disease (COPD) and is now being studied for type 2 diabetes. Resveratrol is under WADA review, but is currently not banned.

SIRT and Sirtuins

The SIRT genes make signaling enzymes called sirtuins that play a key, albeit complex, role in the aging process. Sirtuin activators seem to improve health span and life span in mice. Preliminary research shows SIRT1 activators may be safe for humans. SIRT1 is believed to remove a molecule called an acetyl group from PGC-1 alpha, the master molecule for mitochondria creation. This process, called deacetylation, changes PGC-1 alpha from an inactive form to an active one. Sirtuin research, however, has had a rocky history, with intense controversy and conflicting results, "a steep winding road," in the view of some researchers.

NAD+

This enzyme (nicotinamide adenine dinucleotide) is made in mitochondria and controls metabolic processes all over in the body, including

DNA repair and circadian rhythms. Since NAD+ levels decline with aging, replacing NAD+ with a drug makes scientific sense.

NAD+ is believed to work as a sirtuin activator. Without NAD+, sirtuins simply don't work. In mice, NAD+ improves the health span and muscle aging and helps prevent cognitive decline. Levels of NAD+ can be increased by a chemical called NMN (nicotinamide mononucleotide), which is found in broccoli, cabbage, cucumber, edamame (soybeans), and avocado. NAD+ can also be increased by another chemical, NR (nicotinamide riboside).

As with resveratrol and the sirtuins, there's been controversy about the aggressive marketing of NAD+-based products, including Basis, made by Elysium Health. Elysium is led by MIT biology professor Leonard Guarente and boasts Nobel Prize winners and other leading scientists on its advisory board. Basis combines two supplements, NR and pterostilbene, a molecule similar in structure to the resveratrol found in blueberries. In one human trial of Basis, the drug appeared safe. (Elysium was sued in 2017 for not paying its supplier.) Basis will be reviewed by WADA in connection with resveratrol.

MYOSTATIN SUPPRESSORS

Myostatin is a hormone made by muscle cells that *stops* muscle growth; therefore, drugs to inhibit this could *increase* muscle growth. The pharmaceutical giant Novartis has been conducting a clinical trial of a myostatin-inhibiting drug called Bimagrumab/Bym338, but tests of the drug have so far not proved successful. All myostatin inhibitors are banned by WADA.

Telomere Extenders

TA-65 is a nutritional supplement said to boost telomerase, the enzyme that restores length to telomeres (little protective caps on the ends of chromosomes that shrink with aging). One company claims to have used gene therapy to increase telomere length in its CEO. But drugs to restore telomere length could promote cancer. TA-65 is not banned by WADA based on current scientific literature.

Young Blood

The idea that transfusing an older person, or animal, with young blood can restore lost youth is appealing—and controversial, though that's not stopping some aggressive entrepreneurs. But there is some evidence in favor, including research that shows human umbilical blood transfused into old rodents can improve the animals' memory.

SO, THERE WE HAVE IT

At least part of it. Will one of these drugs "cure" aging? Will it be a new class of drugs called senolytics that target senescent cells (which are still alive but can no longer divide), perhaps with substances like dastinib and quercitin?

Will an exercise mimetic one day let paraplegics be as metabolically fit as marathoners?

Probably not. But one thing is certain: Scientists will learn even more about aging and about exercise's myriad effects on the body in the process.

CHAPTER 15
The Nitty Gritty: Q & A

1. **What's the basic exercise recommendation for adults?**
   At least 150 minutes a week (two and a half hours) of moderate-intensity exercise or 75 minutes (one hour and 15 minutes) of vigorous-intensity aerobic activity a week. Aerobic activity should be performed in episodes of at least 10 minutes at a time. For more extensive health benefits, five hours of moderate-intensity activity or two and a half hours of vigorous activity. In addition to the aerobic stuff, muscle-strengthening activity (resistance training) at least twice a week.

2. **What is "moderate" activity? What's "intense"?**
   The subjective way to distinguish these is simple: With moderate activity, your breathing quickens, but you're not out of breath. You break a light sweat after about 10 minutes. You can talk, but not sing.

   With vigorous activity, your breathing is rapid and deep. You sweat after only a few minutes. You can only say a few words without pausing for breath.

   More objectively, you can use your heart rate to gauge activity level. First, figure out your maximum heart rate. The simplest way is to subtract your age from 220. If you're 74, for instance, your maximum heart rate is 146—that's the maximum number of times your heart should beat in a minute during exercise. Moderate exercise activity gets you to 50–70 percent of your maximum heart rate; vigorous activity gets you to 70–85 percent.

3. **How can you determine your "fitness age"?**

Short of having a cardiac stress test on a treadmill at a medical institution, you can make some reasonable estimates with a few simple measurements at home. One way is to use the online methodology developed by researchers at the Norwegian University of Science and Technology. You can also follow the procedure on the Mayo Clinic website.

See the Appendix for links.

4. **What is VO2max?**

VO2max is a commonly used measure of aerobic fitness that basically shows the highest rate at which your body can supply oxygen to your contracting muscles. The American Heart Association believes that this measure is so important it should be considered a "vital sign," just like blood pressure, heart rate, temperature, and respiration rate.

5. **If you stop exercising, how fast do you lose fitness and strength? And how fast can you regain it?**

Unfortunately, maintaining fitness is truly a case of "use it or lose it." How fast you lose it, of course, depends on how fit you were to start with, how old you are, how recently you stopped exercising, and how long you had been exercising before you stopped.

For most of us, cardiovascular fitness starts to decline with just a week or two of inactivity, while losing muscle mass and strength takes an extra week or so. Athletes and serious long-term exercisers tend to lose fitness more slowly than those who haven't trained as long.

In one classic study from the 1980s, volunteers trained hard for nine weeks, then stopped for the next nine. When training stopped, VO2max and the "anaerobic threshold" both dropped rapidly. (The anaerobic threshold, also called the lactate threshold, is the moment during exercise when lactic acid builds up faster than it can be cleared away.)

In general, endurance (aerobic) conditioning can decline by as much as 25 percent after just three to four or five weeks of detraining.

Some reports suggest that even just two weeks of detraining can lead to a significant decline in cardiovascular fitness, though once you get back into exercise, aerobic capacity rebounds faster than muscle strength. And some data suggest that adverse metabolic changes can occur with as few as 10 days of exercise cessation. On the other hand, the enlargement of the heart from exercise declines fairly slowly—even complete bed rest only causes about 1 percent of heart muscle loss per week.

As a basic rule of thumb, to maintain cardiovascular fitness gains, you have to avoid breaks of longer than two to three weeks. On the plus side, if you have to temporarily cut back on how often you exercise and how much, you can maintain some gains by *not* cutting back on how hard you train, that is, on intensity.

Once you really lose fitness, it takes time—and patience—to regain it. After two to eight months of not exercising, you can lose all of your fitness gains. In fact, if you've really been inactive for a very long time, it can take a year to get into as good shape as you were in before you quit. (Bed rest, as we've seen, is particularly dangerous, leading to rapid losses of fitness.)

As for muscle strength, as opposed to cardiovascular fitness, things are a bit rosier—you don't lose the muscle mass you gain from resistance exercise as fast as you lose cardiovascular fitness. In part, that's because strength training triggers formation of new nuclei in muscle cells.

In a 2017 analysis, researchers found that muscle strength can be maintained without training for as long as three to four weeks, after which it declines, though it can be rapidly restored when you start up again. Other data support this idea. Some studies suggest that muscle mass gained from resistance training can last for months, even years. (Prolonged detraining, of course, does lead to muscle loss.)

Even for people who do very serious strength training—"lifters" who have been doing resistance training for more than three years and who compete at the collegiate or professional level— maximum strength levels can also be maintained for up to three weeks without training, though after that, things do fall apart.

With detraining, muscles do look smaller, but that's because they contain less glycogen (a stored form of carbohydrates) and water.

And it's not just aerobic and strength gains that you lose when you stop exercising, but improvements in blood pressure, cholesterol, and blood sugar levels, as well as muscle strength.

In a Spanish study of obese people with metabolic syndrome who did four months of aerobic interval training, just one month of no exercise led to the loss of many of these improvements, especially aerobic fitness.

6. What is high-intensity interval training (HIIT)?

This kind of training alternates short bursts of very vigorous exercise with rest or slower activity, a pattern that is repeated multiple times. The idea is that you can get many of the benefits of a longer, continuous workout in much less time.

The most famous test is the Wingate protocol, developed in the 1970s in Israel. It calls for a 30-second all-out effort, followed by four minutes of recovery. This pattern is repeated four to six times during one workout session. This amounts to three to four minutes of hard exercise per session, with three sessions a week for two to six weeks.

7. So is HIIT better than continuous training?

"Better" is a tricky word. At the very least, HIIT is highly effective and more time efficient, though, of course, any exercise is better than none at all. Before embarking on HIIT, check with your doctor if you haven't exercised in a while, are sick, or have hypertension or other cardiovascular problems. (For more on HIIT, see Chapter 5.)

8. Can you be both fit and fat?

The debate is still raging, and obviously, both fitness and healthy body weight are important. Some data suggest that fitness may be as important as weight, that is, that fitness strongly predicts mortality, regardless of body size. Put differently, some data show that higher levels of exercise can attenuate the mortality risk at all levels of adiposity. On the other hand, fatness or obesity does substantially reduce fitness, and other data suggest that you can't be both fit and fat.

Part of the problem comes in measuring fatness. In many studies, weight is gauged by BMI (body mass index). For the vast majority of people, BMI is a good measure of body fatness. But some people, such as weightlifters, can have a high BMI, suggesting they are overweight even when they are not. That's in part because muscle weighs more than fat.

In a study of nearly 117,000 women followed for 24 years, the lowest mortality, not surprisingly, was in physically active, lean women. Higher levels of physical activity *did* reduce mortality risk but did not eliminate the high risk associated with obesity. And being thin did not counteract the increase in mortality risk from inactivity.

A 2017 study of more than a half million Europeans followed for more than a decade found that there is no such thing as "fit but fat," as the leader of that study told *Fortune* magazine. This study found that being overweight raised the risk of coronary heart disease by up to 28 percent, even if a person was otherwise healthy. The study adds "to a growing body of evidence that suggests that being 'fat but fit' is a myth," the researchers from the Imperial College London noted in a statement.

The biggest and most recent study, a British analysis of 3.5 million people published in 2017, also found that people who are obese are at an increased risk of heart failure and stroke *even if* they are "metabolically healthy," that is, they don't show obvious warning signs such as high blood pressure or diabetes. As long as these folks were obese, the study showed, they were at a modestly increased risk of stroke, a nearly 50 percent increased risk of coronary heart disease, and a nearly doubled risk of heart failure compared to those who were not obese and were in similar metabolic health. The leader of this study put it bluntly to the *New York Times*: "The bottom line is that metabolically healthy obesity doesn't exist." Or at least, is a state of affairs that can't be maintained for long.

9. **Can you target exercise to control where your body loses fat?**
   It's not entirely clear. In general, exercise burns fat all over the body, but does not work as a "spot reduction" strategy. In other words, no matter how many sit-ups you do, you don't actually change belly fat into muscle; to lose fat, you have to expend more calories than you take in. But a 2015 study did show that weight training is particularly beneficial for reducing belly fat.

10. **Is more exercise better than less for extending longevity?**
    Yes, to a point. A large study of 16,939 Harvard alumni showed that death rates declined steadily as exercise increased up to the point of expending 3,500 calories a week, after which there is no reduction in mortality risk. Being physically active reduced mortality rates regardless of hypertension, smoking, and extreme gains in body weight. By age 80, habitual exercisers were likely to have an extra one to two years of life, compared to sedentary men.

    A 2015 analysis of pooled data from six studies involving 661,137 men and women in the United States and Europe aged 21–98 showed that people who do one to two times the recommended minimum of moderate physical activity have a 32 percent lower mortality risk than those who do none. At two to three times the minimum recommendations, there is a 37 percent lower risk. The upper threshold for reducing mortality risk occurs at three to five times the activity recommendations.

11. **Is there a level at which exercise is harmful if you're healthy?**
Mostly, no. That study of 661,137 people found that even at 10 or more times the recommended exercise dose, there was no evidence of harm. Other studies agree. On the other hand, a 2017 study did find that white men who exercised more than seven hours a week had a significantly higher risk of having plaque buildup in their arteries, though this does not necessarily translate into problems such as heart attacks.

Ultrasound studies done at the end of marathons have shown potentially worrisome changes in both left and right ventricles of the heart, though these changes are usually transient. Certain biomarkers are also elevated right after a marathon in some runners. Atrial fibrillation (an irregular rhythm in the top chamber of the heart) is also five times more likely in middle-aged men who are endurance athletes.

That said, a 2012 analysis of 10.9 million marathon runners showed a low overall risk of cardiac arrest and sudden death. When cardiac arrest does occur during long-distance running events, it does so rarely in half marathons (13.1 miles), but more often in full marathons (26.2 miles).

12. **Okay, but isn't exercise dangerous for some people?**
Yes, and obviously, if you're in doubt, check with your doctor, especially if you have heart or lung problems, including hypertension. Also, if your blood counts are low and your immunity is compromised because of cancer or cancer treatment, it may be wise to wait to exercise until your counts are normal.

In a major review of the benefits and risks of exercise for people with one or more of 26 conditions, Scandinavian researchers generally found few contraindications for exercise. Spanish scientists agreed.

However, there are some caveats. For people with ischemic heart disease, in which blood flow to the heart is compromised, it may be wise *not* to do short, high-intensity workouts. (See Chapter 4.) For people with hypertension, weight training should focus on lighter weights; if your blood pressure is over 180/105, you should consider drug treatment to control blood pressure before exercising.

For people with type 2 diabetes, overall, exercise is more a benefit than a risk. But you should postpone exercise if blood sugar levels are too high or too low; if you have hypertension or diabetic eye problems, including advanced retinopathy, it may be wise to avoid high-intensity training. If you have nerve pain or foot problems, weight-bearing exercise can lead to ulcer and fracture.

If you have an acute exacerbation of asthma, take a temporary break from training. Ditto if you have an infection—wait until it's gone. If you have cystic fibrosis as well as an infection, wait until you're better.

If you have osteoarthritis with an acute joint inflammation, rest that joint until it's improved, but exercise other joints. If you have osteoporosis, avoid exercises that increase your risk of falling. Don't exercise a body part with a recent fracture. If you have rheumatoid arthritis, use low weights for strength training and be careful with your neck. If you have bone metastases from cancer, don't lift heavy weights.

And then there's the common-sense stuff. Exercising an acutely injured body part is silly—as is doing things like biking on busy roads, especially without a helmet.

13. **Should you exercise if you're sick?**
That depends on what you're sick with and how sick you are.

Don't exercise if you have a fever over 101° Fahrenheit. If you've got a cold and your symptoms are mostly above the neck (minor sore throat, runny nose, sneezing, etc.), it's okay to exercise, moderately. If your symptoms are below the neck (chest congestion, stomach pain, etc.) wait until you're better. If you do exercise, reduce the intensity and length of your workout. Don't exercise if you have severe fatigue or widespread muscle aches.

In general, regular aerobic exercise strengthens the immune system. (See Chapter 11.) But immunity can decrease slightly about 90 minutes after exercise, at least in elite athletes, then bounces up again. After a marathon, it can stay a bit low for 72 hours. Wash your hands a lot if you work out in gyms during cold and flu season.

Light exercise if you're mildly sick can even make you feel better, and can bring oxygenated blood to an area of infection, potentially helping to fight the infection. But stay hydrated. And don't do dumb things, like rock-climbing if you have vertigo or diving if your ears are plugged up!

14. Should you exercise while pregnant?

If you're healthy and your pregnancy is normal, the American College of Obstetricians and Gynecologists and the Centers for Disease Control and Prevention recommend exercising for at least 30 minutes at moderate intensity for most, or all, days of the week.

It used to be thought that exercise during pregnancy could increase the risk of preterm birth, perhaps by increasing levels of the stress hormone, norepinephrine. But an analysis of nine studies involving more than 2,000 women found no significant difference in preterm births in women who exercised aerobically for 35–90 minutes three or four times a week during pregnancy compared to those who didn't. In fact, the women who exercised had a better chance of a vaginal delivery.

How long and hard you exercise depends on your previous activity levels. Exercise during pregnancy can reduce risk of gestational diabetes. Exercise, including low- to moderate-intensity weight training, can also help prevent excess weight gain, reduce back pain, and ease constipation.

Hormonal changes during pregnancy will make your joints more flexible, which can raise the risk of joint injury. Your balance may be off, too, because of your growing belly. Your need for oxygen increases as well.

Try to avoid contact sports in which you could get hit in the abdomen or activities like skiing that increase your risk of falling. "Hot" yoga is probably a bad idea, too, because you can overheat. Exercising at altitudes more than 6,000 feet is also unwise, unless you're used to it.

Also, don't exercise without asking your doctor if you have certain types of heart or lung disease, cervical "insufficiency," if you're carrying multiple fetuses, or if you have severe anemia or pre-eclampsia (pregnancy-induced high blood pressure).

Exercise during pregnancy can reduce the risk of giving birth to a baby with serious heart defects, too. In one experiment, mice allowed to run during pregnancy bore far fewer babies with heart defects than mice not allowed to run, even if the mothers-to-be were old.

Exercise is also important after pregnancy. Granted, time and sleep are at a premium with a new baby, but exercise is key because it can help strengthen your abs and help prevent postpartum depression. You can start a few days after childbirth, but check with your doctor if you've had a cesarean delivery.

15. **Does exercise help with menopausal symptoms?**

It's not clear. Some research finds that exercise does not help ease hot flashes, though it does help with sleep quality, insomnia, and depression.

Other research suggests that regular, moderate-endurance exercise may reduce the frequency and intensity of hot flashes, though it's not clear how. In a 2016 interventional study of 21 women with hot flashes who underwent a 16-week exercise training program, exercise was linked with fewer hot flashes. But to get this effect, women had to build up to working out vigorously four or five times a week for 45 minutes each time. No one is sure how exercise might affect this, but it may be by improving the body's heat-regulation processes.

16. **Should men and women exercise differently?**

By and large, no, but there are some caveats, and responses to exercise may differ. With weight training, for instance, men, with their higher levels of testosterone, tend to bulk up more than women. But the difference is small.

On the other hand, women, thanks to lots of estrogen, often have looser joints, which can raise the risk of joint damage with sudden twisting movements, as in basketball. Women's knees are more vulnerable than men's because the "Q-angle," the angle between the hip and the knee, is greater because women's hips are wider, which is great for childbearing, but not so good for landing from a jump and twisting. The extra torque in women's knees can more easily shred the ACL (anterior cruciate ligament).

Men tend to have stronger tendons than women because they synthesize more collagen after exercise, making their tendons less susceptible to injury. Men also tend to have somewhat higher VO2max levels than women.

A caveat, though—some bodybuilding coaches, among them Menno Henselmans, a business consultant turned fitness coach, contend that there are some differences in the way men and women should train, noting, among other things, that women may be less subject to fatigue and may be able to handle more training.

17. **Can you be allergic to exercise?**

Yes. It's rare, but it can be life-threatening, in which case it's called exercise-induced anaphylaxis (EIA), a kind of shock. In some cases, the allergic reaction is triggered by a combination of certain foods followed by exercise, in which case it's which called FDEIA, or food-dependent exercise-induced anaphylaxis. Usually, the reaction happens during or right after exercise and can be manifested by hives, swelling, digestive problems, respiratory problems, and other signs of shock. The most common food triggers are crustaceans and wheat flour. The cause appears to be changes in immune cells called mast cells, which release histamine. Immediate treatment involves epinephrine and antihistamines, as well as airway maintenance and cardiovascular support.

18. **What causes muscle cramps?**

Believe it or not, nobody is quite sure.

Historically, lots of things have been postulated to contribute to exercise-induced muscle cramps, including overuse of a muscle, dehydration, holding a position for too long, nerve compression, inadequate blood supply to a muscle, imbalances of electrolytes such as magnesium, potassium, and sodium, and accumulation of lactic acid. But science hasn't supported much of this.

Current thinking is that muscle cramps, generally thought to be harmless, occur because of hyperactivity of the nerve-muscle reflex arc—in other words, overuse of feedback communication involving nerves and muscles. Prolonged sitting or bad posture may predispose these reflexes toward malfunctioning. Stretching, for 15–30 seconds, may help get rid of the hyper-excitability of a cramping muscle.

During a muscle cramp, the spinal cord may actually—mistakenly—tell the muscle to keep contracting. Inadequate conditioning also contributes to cramps because untrained muscles are more prone to fatigue. Exercising in intense heat may also trigger cramps. Severe muscle cramps can be extremely painful; if cramps are severe and frequent, it makes sense to see a doctor.

19. **Why do muscles feel sore after exercise?**

It's called DOMS, for delayed-onset muscle soreness, and it usually strikes a day or two after a big workout. The main culprit is eccentric exercise, that is, exercise that involves lengthening a muscle while it is contracting, like lowering your arm after a biceps curl. (Eccentric movement seems to trigger DOMS more than other motions.) Technically, DOMS is seen as a "Type I muscle strain injury."

As we saw in Chapter 6, exercise triggers tiny tears in muscle tissue, which lead to painful inflammation and, ultimately, repair and stronger muscles. There are other theories, too, including lactic acid buildup, muscle spasms, connective tissue damage, and enzyme changes. But no single theory is likely to explain the entire process.

Although some exercisers contend that free radicals (toxic forms of oxygen created during exercise) are to blame and that therefore antioxidants are the answer, that's not true. (See Question 22.) Icing the affected area may not help, either.

What may help is massage or the do-it-yourself version, using a foam roller on the sore muscles. NSAIDs (non-steroidal anti-inflammatory drugs) can help. So can exercising non-sore parts of the body for a few days until DOMS disappears.

20. **Does exercise change the kind of fat you have?**

Though most of us assume all our body fat is pretty much the same, there are actually several different kinds. There's subcutaneous fat, which lies just under our skin and is basically harmless, and visceral fat, which covers our internal organs and in excess amounts can be metabolically harmful, in part because it secretes biochemical signals that increase chronic inflammation and insulin resistance. Muscles can use fatty acids from fat as fuel.

But fat also comes in different colors. Brown fat is considered "good" because it can generate heat. In general, lean people have more brown fat than obese people, and kids have more brown fat than adults.

Exercise can transform white fat into brown fat, which is desirable in part because it is metabolically more active and burns more calories. A hormone called irisin, produced in working muscles, can turn some white fat cells into brown. People who exercise tend to have higher levels of irisin than sedentary folks. Exercise may also stimulate production of proteins that lead to growth of more blood vessels.

21. **Does exercise alone help you lose weight?**

Yes, but it takes an awful lot of exercise. Olympic swim champ Michael Phelps, for instance, consumed 12,000 calories a day during peak training, but as he put it himself, all he did was "swim, eat and sleep."

But most of us ordinary mortals don't exercise that much. And, as we saw in the obesity section of Chapter 4, the math is against you. In theory, since weight gain results from too much food and too little exercise, you *could* lose weight just by increasing exercise and keeping food intake constant. But for most of us, that doesn't work because we tend to *underestimate* the calories we ingest in food and *overestimate* how many calories we burn in exercise. A 160-pound person walking at a 20-minute-per-mile pace burns just 255 calories in an hour—the calories in one small muffin!

Just by itself, without dietary changes, exercise usually won't help you lose weight. In fact, some data show that Americans have actually been exercising more in recent years, even as the obesity epidemic has worsened. Diet alone even edged out diet-plus-exercise in one study of weight loss. But in general, combining exercise with diet seems to work best.

22. **How does exercise affect appetite?**

It's complicated. Most research shows that exercise suppresses appetite, at least for a couple of hours. But not in everybody. Go figure.

Exercise, particularly strenuous exercise, can act as an appetite suppressant by lowering levels of the hormone ghrelin, an appetite stimulant often called the "hunger hormone," and boosting levels of blood lactate and blood sugar, which lessen the need to eat.

One study, for instance, found that vigorous *aerobic* exercise—60 minutes on a treadmill—lowered levels of ghrelin and also raised levels of peptide YY, an appetite suppressor, although *resistance* exercise had a more mixed effect. The hunger-suppressing effect of vigorous exercise lasted about two hours. In a subsequent study, the same researchers confirmed that exercise intensity and, to a lesser extent, duration were linked to lower ghrelin levels. Exercise can also increase levels of leptin, according to a Spanish research review. Leptin is an appetite suppressor.

But exercise can sometimes stimulate appetite. While appetite does go down immediately after exercise, as body temperature cools down again, appetite may increase.

Bottom line? It really is complex. But overall, it's easier to regulate appetite if you're expending a lot of energy, one of the big benefits of exercise. In essence, exercise makes for better "coupling" of energy intake and energy expenditure. Besides, when you're sedentary it's harder to control appetite.

23. **Is caffeine a performance enhancer?**

Yes. Caffeine can act as a performance enhancer (or "ergogenic aid") during exercise and competitions. Caffeine doesn't actually boost maximum oxygen capacity, but can improve speed and power during races. Interestingly, this effect holds true in events lasting 60 seconds to those lasting two hours. There's no evidence that caffeine leads to dehydration or ion imbalances. The bad news, at least in one study, is that drinking coffee may not work as well as "doping" with pure caffeine.

Moderate to high doses of caffeine (5–13 milligrams per kilogram of body weight) have profound effects on exercise. Low doses (less than or equal to 3 mg per kg of body weight) don't change the whole-body response to exercise, but can improve vigilance, alertness, mood, and cognitive processing during exercise. The effects of caffeine probably stem from changes in the central nervous system.

Caffeine may also help keep dopamine levels high in the brain areas needed for concentration and reduce the perception of pain and effort during exercise, potentially helping maintain effort longer.

24. **Do antioxidant vitamins offset the benefits of exercise?**

It's fair to say that, at the very least, antioxidant vitamins don't enhance the benefits of exercise. Exercise does create free radicals, toxic forms of oxygen. And free radicals do cause "oxidative stress." But exercise also triggers formation in the body of antioxidants, which can counteract the effect of some free radicals. If you take supplementary vitamin C or E, for instance, you may wind up with fewer of the enzymes that trigger what you want—an increase in mitochondria (the energy factories) in muscle cells. In other words, antioxidant supplementation may actually retard the expected increase in fitness and strength from exercise. This seems to hold true whether exercise is aerobic or resistance training.

To be sure, antioxidant supplements, which have been vigorously promoted by the supplement industry, have long been popular among athletes eager to improve performance. But the current thinking is that free radicals are not as "bad" as once thought, nor antioxidant supplements as "good." In fact, an imbalance—too many antioxidants compared to free radicals—can result in its own problem, dubbed "antioxidant-induced stress," in part because antioxidants themselves become highly reactive after they donate their electrons to free radicals. Antioxidants that occur naturally in food appear to be much safer than large doses of supplements.

25. Is it safe to exercise if you take beta-blockers?
Beta-blockers are cardiac medications that block the effects of adrenaline, the "fight-or-flight" hormone. They are used to lower heart rate and blood pressure. In general, it's fine to exercise while on beta-blockers, but don't push it in an attempt to get your heart rate up to the level you attained without beta-blockers.

Check with your doctor to find out what target heart rate you should aim for while on these medications. If you can't talk while exercising, back off a bit. There are also other drugs that your doctor might consider switching to.

26. Are "accelerometers" and other "activity trackers" accurate?
Somewhat. These devices are a great way to guard against deluding yourself about how many steps you actually get per day. Because they are so much better than just asking people to remember how much they exercised on a given day, accelerometers are the coming wave of exercise research.

They're also great when exercise researchers use them (notably, the research-grade devices such as ActiGraph GT3X+) to track what you do, as opposed to what you say you think you did.

But accelerometers and other movement sensors such as Fitbit, Jawbone, Nike Fuel, Garmin, Samsung GearFit2, TomTom, and Apple Watch, while pretty good at counting steps, are not so good at calculating caloric expenditure and heart rate, especially during higher-intensity workouts.

Research studies have shown mixed results. In one court case against Fitbit, a non–peer-reviewed study commissioned by the plaintiffs and vigorously denounced by Fitbit found that the device was highly inaccurate during intense exercise. (For what it's worth, I wear a Fitbit and have found it very inaccurate for heart rate with vigorous workouts, but better step-counting, except on elliptical machines.)

In another study of different Fitbit devices and Jawbone UP24, the devices were good at counting calories for sedentary activity, but overestimated energy expenditure during exercise, including walking. In this study, one device, the Fitbit Flex, was more accurate than the others at judging energy expenditure and steps.

On the other hand, a Stanford University School of Medicine study of seven wristband activity trackers came to completely different conclusions: that six of the devices were fairly accurate for heart rate, but none of the seven was accurate for calories burned.

27. Can exercise improve vision?

Surprisingly, yes, especially aging-related vision problems such as AMD (wet age-related macular degeneration), cataracts, and glaucoma.

Among other things, exercise, as we saw in Chapters 8 and 9, triggers production of BDNF (brain-derived neurotrophic factor), which may boost the number of brain cells, including cells in the retina. (The retina is technically part of the brain.) Some vision problems stem from high blood pressure and cholesterol, which can be lowered via exercise. Exercise also helps control type 2 diabetes, which can damage the retina.

One 2013 study found that moderate walking and vigorous running are both linked to a lower risk of cataracts. A massive 2015 Swedish study of 52,660 people followed for an average of 12 years found that those who exercised the most had a 13 percent reduced risk of cataracts compared to people who exercised the least.

As for BDNF, dubbed "Miracle Gro" for the brain, exercise may do as much for the eyes as for the rest of the brain. In a clever 2009 study of more than 40,000 middle-aged distance runners, researchers found that the runners who logged the most miles were the least likely to get macular degeneration, regardless of weight, cardiorespiratory fitness, and smoking.

In an interventional study in mice, researchers from Emory University assigned half of a group of mice to a sedentary lifestyle and allowed the others to run on little treadmills for an hour a day. After two weeks, half of the mice in each group were exposed to very bright light for a few hours, a way of experimentally inducing retinal degeneration. All the mice then went back for two weeks to whatever condition they were in before, either sitting or running. Then the scientists looked at all the animals' retinas—the mice that didn't exercise had lost 75 percent of their retinal neurons and their vision was failing. The mice that had exercised were able to maintain twice as many neurons as the unexercised mice, despite exposure to that bright light.

In a separate experiment, the researchers took another batch of mice and had half exercise and half not for two weeks, then measured the levels of BDNF in their bloodstream and in their eyes. The exercising mice, as expected, had more BDNF. Then, the researchers injected still other mice with a substance that blocks BDNF before they exercised and were exposed to the bright light. Bingo! Without BDNF, these animals' retinas were not protected by exercise.

But there is a potential shadow over all this positive news. A 2017 Korean study that tracked 211,960 middle-aged and older men and women found that those who exercised vigorously five or more days a week had a 54 percent increased risk of macular degeneration. But, as the authors themselves note, there is no strong biological rationale for this finding, and no association was found for women. So this has to be taken with a large grain of salt.

28. **Does exercise benefit the skin?**
Yes.

At a minimum, improved circulation is just as good for the skin as for every other organ in the body, bringing freshly oxygenated blood to skin cells and taking away cellular waste products. Since exercise can also ease stress, it can help reduce stress-related skin problems such as acne and eczema, too.

But recent research suggests that exercise may even reverse skin aging. As we hit midlife, the layers of the skin begin to change, most notably the outer layer of the skin called the stratum corneum, which thickens, while a deeper layer of the skin, the dermis, gets thinner, explains *New York Times* fitness columnist Gretchen Reynolds.

It's been known for a number of years now that exercise is good for mitochondria, the energy factories inside cells (see Chapter 5). In fact, in 2011, McMaster University researchers showed that in mice bred to age prematurely, exercise restores sagging mitochondria and prolongs life.

With that in mind, the McMaster team then set out to see what effect, if any, exercise might have on the aging of human skin. In a meticulous 2015 study, they showed that endurance exercise does indeed slow aging-induced changes in the skin. It does so by increasing levels of hormones called myokines, which are made in contracting muscle cells. Specifically, the researchers found that a myokine called IL-15 triggers the exercise-associated improvements in the skin of older people. Indeed, they found higher levels of IL-15 in the skin of exercisers compared to non-exercisers.

29. Does exercise affect the teeth?

Well, maybe, and perhaps not for the better. But don't let that stop you from exercising.

The data are preliminary, and potentially flawed. Working out long and hard may temporarily change saliva in a more alkaline direction, which could interfere with a protein in saliva whose job is to prevent tooth decay.

A 2013 study in the *British Journal of Sports Medicine* looked at 278 athletes participating in the London 2012 Olympic Games. Their oral health was remarkably poor, despite their stupendous overall fitness. In fact, a majority had high levels of tooth decay, and some also had gum disease and erosion of tooth enamel. It wasn't clear why these ultra-healthy folks had such bad dental health, but nearly half had not had a dental exam or hygiene care in the previous year. The athletes studied were not a random sample, but were recruited from a free dental care clinic, and many of the athletes were from Africa, where dental care can be less available.

In 2015, German researchers compared the teeth and saliva of 35 competitive triathletes and 35 healthy people who were not athletes. Fifteen of the athletes also volunteered for an experiment in which they did an increasingly strenuous run, during which their saliva was collected several times. Overall, the athletes showed more erosion of tooth enamel than the controls. They had more cavities, too—and the more hours they exercised, the more cavities they had.

When both the athletes, who trained hard (nine hours a week on average), and the non-exercisers were at rest, their saliva was chemically similar. But during the running part of the experiment, runners produced less and less saliva (even if they were hydrated) and their saliva became more alkaline, a process that can lead to the buildup of plaque.

Surprisingly, the researchers found no direct link between sports drinks and nutrition and dental decay. But stay tuned on this one—it may be that athletes drink more sugary drinks than reported.

30. Why should you "surprise" your muscles?

Believe it or not, your muscles get "bored" if you do the same workout over and over. After six to eight weeks of the same routine, your neuromuscular system adapts and goes on cruise control. You'll still build muscle, but not as much as with a tougher workout. To prevent plateauing, you can increase the intensity of training and/or substitute new exercises for old ones every couple of months.

Many factors contribute to the beneficial effects of varying your exercise routine. At the molecular level, the body doesn't perceive easy exercise as a stress. (In this case, "stress" is a good thing.) But when exercise is hard enough, the sympathetic nervous system pumps out catecholamines (the "fight-or-flight" hormones, adrenaline and norepinephrine). These hormones act on a protein called CRTC2, which in turn improves the body's ability to use sugar and fatty acids, ultimately yielding bigger, stronger muscles. If there's insufficient exercise stress, some researchers say, this catecholamine cascade never gets cranked up. In other words, there's some truth in the "no pain, no gain" theory.

31. **Does exercise affect circadian rhythms? Does it help remedy jet lag?**

Yes, and yes.

Circadian rhythms, which exist in animals, plants, and some microbes, are physical, mental, and behavioral changes that follow a daily cycle. In fact, many of our organs—the heart, liver, and brain—even have their own distinct circadian rhythms.

A hot topic these days, "circadian" (which means "about daily," or roughly, 24-hour) rhythms, were the subject of a 2017 Nobel Prize. These biological patterns are triggered when light hits a tiny part of the brain called the suprachiasmatic nucleus. (During our evolutionary history, the light that controlled this was sunlight; now, artificial light, especially in the evening, often disrupts these natural rhythms.)

These natural rhythms have powerful effects on sleep, alertness, hunger, activity, and many other functions. Indeed, one study showed that the risk of having a car accident goes up 8 percent in the week after the spring shift to daylight saving time, which causes people to lose one hour of sleep. In the fall, when the shift provides an extra hour of sleep, there's a similar reduction in accidents.

Young people tend to move around a lot during the day and not so much at night, but this pattern becomes somewhat less regulated as we age. (Older people tend to move less during the day and to be restless at night.)

But, crucially, exercise, by pumping out important biochemicals that act on various organs, can help keep circadian rhythms synced properly, while lack of exercise can do the opposite. Exercise can even restore an out-of-sync circadian rhythm to a more normal, healthy one.

In studies in mice, carefully scheduled exercise was able to re-set dysregulated circadian rhythms, in part by changing gene expression in the suprachiasmatic nucleus in the brain. In other studies, exercise seems able to affect circadian rhythms, especially those linked to activity and moving around, and lack of exercise can disrupt these rhythms. Exercise can shift the molecular circadian clock in muscle tissue, too.

As for jet lag, scientists are trying to see if exercise, as well as exposure to sunlight, in the new time zone helps re-set the circadian clock. In one study, researchers simulated jet lag in hamsters by altering the normal day-night lighting in their cages, then allowed some animals to run on little wheels. The animals allowed to run adjusted to "jet lag" much faster than non-exercising animals. Humans, too, can benefit from exercising, especially exercising outdoors, to reduce jet lag. Some researchers suggest exercising in the new time zone at the same time of day when you would work out at home.

32. Is there an optimal time of day to exercise?

The best time to exercise is whenever you can fit it in. Scientifically, alas, the data are mixed. Some studies say morning is best, in part because you can do it before your day gets away from you. Others say late afternoon is best, perhaps because that's when body temperature peaks and perceived exertion (how hard you feel you are working) is lowest. This may be especially true for non-aerobic exercise.

33. Does exercise affect sleep?

Yes. Regular, aerobic exercise during the day can help relieve stress and in other ways help with sleep, though it may take four months for the benefits—including falling asleep more rapidly and staying asleep longer—to solidify. Interestingly, in the short run, a good night's sleep may have a stronger effect on exercising well the next day than the reverse, at least in people with diagnosed insomnia.

The mechanisms are not totally clear, but exercise does help keep circadian rhythms humming along nicely. And it temporarily increases body temperature, with the subsequent drop in temperature helping to promote sleep.

That said, research suggests avoiding exercise within three hours of bedtime, lest it rev you up and interfere with falling asleep. Among other things, the body needs to cool down in the late evening, which sets the stage for sleep. But a small study found that late-night exercise does not seem to disturb subjects' sleep quality, though it was linked to a faster heartbeat during the first three hours of sleep.

34. Is exercise addictive?

To some extent, in some people, but it's tough to tell exercise addicts from people who just like to exercise a lot. Exercise addiction is not recognized in the DSM-5, the *Diagnostic and Statistical Manual of Mental Disorders*, a handbook of psychiatric disorders.

Exercise may be viewed as addictive if you prioritize it above all else, potentially damaging your work and personal life—in other words, when exercise becomes life's organizing principle. Some researchers estimate the prevalence of exercise addiction to be about 3 percent of the general population.

The psychological effects of exercise, as we've seen earlier in this book, can be powerful—so powerful, in fact, that "exercise may be considered as a psychoactive drug," write Spanish researchers. This may pose a risk for extreme exercisers, such as ultra-marathoners, bodybuilders, and sports science students, they add. Exercise does trigger release of important biochemicals, including endorphins, dopamine, BDNF, and stress hormones. Exercise also boosts endocannabinoids, marijuana-like substances made in the body. (See Chapter 9.) Whether this triggers a genuine physical addiction is not fully clear. In addition, exercise may reduce anxiety by raising body temperature.

To qualify as a genuine "behavioral addiction," California psychologists argue that several features must be present.

These include the following: tolerance (you need more and more exercise to get the desired effect); withdrawal (skipping exercise triggers negative emotions like anxiety and irritability); lack of control (unsuccessful attempts to cut back on exercise); intention effects (inability to stick to your normal routine because exercise gets in the way); time (large amounts of time go toward exercising and planning and recovering from it); reduction in other activities (like family, work, or socializing); and continuance (keeping up exercise despite knowing it is contributing to physical or psychological problems).

On the plus side, it's possible that exercise may help combat drug addiction. A small 2010 study in rats showed that running on a little exercise wheel may help reduce relapses with cocaine addiction.

35. Is running the best exercise?

Maybe. Running is efficient, in the sense that you expend more calories per unit of time spent than walking, biking, or many other activities. Compared to non-runners, runners have a reduced risk of dying early from any cause by between 25 and 40 percent, regardless of drinking, smoking, or being overweight. An hour of running can increase life expectancy by about 7 hours, making it a better way to prolong life than walking, cycling, or swimming, although, as we've consistently noted, any exercise is far better than none. Running achieves this mainly by reducing the risks of heart disease and cancer.

36. Endurance versus resistance—Do you have to choose?

Yes, if you're an elite athlete dedicated to a specific event, such as weightlifting or marathon running. No, if you're just trying to stay as fit and strong as possible. In fact, except for truly elite athletes, the ideal path is a combination, to both ward off sarcopenia and maintain overall fitness.

Doing both makes sense, evolutionarily. After all, we evolved both to be fit enough to escape predators and hunt food, and to be strong enough to carry animal carcasses back to the fire.

On the other hand, you can't be great at both. It is "hardly surprising that simultaneously training for both endurance and strength results in a compromised adaptation compared with training for either exercise alone, a phenomenon known as the 'interference effect,'" writes Australian researcher John A. Hawley.

Then again, consider a 1980 study that compared strength and endurance training. Researchers divided participants into three groups: one did endurance training only, one did strength training only, and one did both. Only the folks whose workouts included endurance training showed increases in VO2max. Only the strength training group showed improvement in leg strength.

Research in rats seems to verify the idea that there is a "master switch" that, depending on the stimulus, sends a muscle along either the mitochondrial or the hypertrophy pathway (see Chapters 5 and 6). Whether such a master switch occurs in humans is not so clear.

In one 2006 study, researchers used highly trained endurance athletes and highly trained resistance athletes and had both groups do a tough bout of exercise in their own expertise. They then "crossed over" to the other type of exercise—and did just fine, suggesting considerable "response plasticity."

In his excellent 2011 book, *Which Comes First, Cardio or Weights?*, Canadian physicist and journalist Alex Hutchinson writes, "You can't fulfill your ultimate potential as both a weight lifter and a marathoner at the same time." But for most of us, he says, you can mix it up, that is, do both.

Bottom line? Unless you're an elite athlete, "[y]ou don't have to choose," says Mark Tarnopolsky, a mitochondrial disease specialist at McMaster University. "My conclusion is to combine the two, resistance and endurance, either on the same day or on alternate days."

37. **Does exercise offset the cancer and heart disease mortality risks of drinking?**

Yes, according to a study of more than 36,000 men and women aged 40 and over. So long as a person meets the recommended physical activity guidelines, exercise can offset *some* of the risks of cancer and all-cause mortality that are associated with drinking. But you can't rely on exercise to cancel out the effects of heavy drinking.

38. **If you do all this exercise, will you live forever?**

No, but you'll die buff!

CHAPTER 16
Dodging Bullets

WHAT WILL GET YOU WHEN

Like all other creatures on earth, we are dodging bullets all the time.

From the moment we are born until the last cancer cell, bacterium, heart spasm—or real bullet—does us in, we live in peril. In a very real sense, we're lucky if we live long enough to age at all.

But in case you're curious, here's what's likely to do you in. And when.

As a newborn American baby, the worst danger you face is being born with a congenital abnormality. By age one—and up until age 45—unintentional injury is the biggest risk of death, though starting in adolescence, homicide and suicide also begin to be big risks. In your mid-30s, cancer and heart disease begin to creep up as threats.

Once you hit 45, you've made it through a huge statistical mine-field. But it's also at midlife that your bad habits—smoking and Dante's deadliest sins (sloth and gluttony)—start to catch up with you. (Unless you're a Seventh Day Adventist. These religious folks don't smoke or drink, are physically active, eat their veggies, and have strong social ties. It pays off: Their life expectancy is 86 years for men, 89 for women.)

For the rest of us, the picture begins to change between 45 and 54. Cancer suddenly becomes the biggest killer, followed by heart disease. This pattern holds from age 55 to 64, with cancer the biggest danger, followed by heart disease, and diseases triggered mostly by ciga-rettes: chronic lower respiratory disease (COPD, or chronic obstructive pulmonary disease), chronic bronchitis, and emphysema.

Even so, once you make it to 65, your odds of making to 100 keep getting better. Dangers still lurk, with heart disease being the biggest, followed by cancer, chronic respiratory disease, strokes, Alzheimer's disease, diabetes, influenza, kidney failure, injury, and septicemia (blood poisoning).

By age 85 or 90, you're a statistical rocket. Your biggest risks now are heart disease, cancer, and Alzheimer's, in that order. But your chances of making it to 100 are terrific. (And if you're a woman who has been able to have a baby later in life without technical assistance, you've probably got the great genes for an exceptionally long life.)

This is remarkable. One hundred years ago, most people didn't make it past 50. Today, the average life expectancy at birth for Americans is 78.6 years, though this number has dipped slightly of late.

We're living longer today mostly because of better sanitation, cleaner drinking water, refrigeration, better diets, antibiotics, other medical advances, and, especially, childhood immunizations. (After all, if many children die in their early years, the pool of people with a fighting chance to make it to old age is greatly diminished.)

Growing numbers of us—55,000 at last count—are making it to 100 and beyond. Two decades ago, it was half that. And the odds are still improving, thanks to better treatment of high blood pressure, better surgical techniques, and better treatments of some cancers. These advances have made it possible for many Americans who otherwise would have died in mid-life to make it to old age.

And your chances for making it to 100? They get better the older you get.

Right now, for a newborn baby, the odds of making it to 100 are 1.939 percent. For a teenager (aged 15), they're slightly better, 1.944. For a 30-year-old, they're a bit better still, 1.965. If you make it to 45, your odds of reaching 100 improve again—to 2.012 percent.

By 60, things are looking even brighter—you have a 2.172 percent chance of making it to 100. By 75, you have a 2.277 percent chance. And once you make it to 90, luck—or the "hardy survivor" effect—is with you. Your chances of making it to 100 are 8.101 percent.

Until very late in life, your lifestyle choices—including exercise—control 75 percent of your health and longevity, with only 25 or 30 percent depending on your genes. In other words, until extreme old age, it's good behavior, not good genes, that determines successful aging. It's only at very old ages—100 or more—that good genes trump good behavior.

Thomas Perls, a Boston University gerontologist who studies centenarians, puts it this way: The older you are, the healthier you've been.

APPENDIX
Determining Your "Fitness Age"

Short of having a cardiac stress test on a treadmill at a medical institution, you can make some reasonable estimates with a few simple measurements at home. One way is to use the online methodology developed by researchers at the Norwegian University of Science and Technology. You can also follow the procedure on the Mayo Clinic website.

How fit are you, really? *World Fitness Level*. Retrieved from https://www.worldfitnesslevel.org/#/

The Fitness Calculator (2017). *Cardiac Exercise Research Group, NTNU*. Retrieved from https://www.ntnu.edu/cerg/vo2max

Reynolds, G. (2014, October 15). What's your fitness age? *New York Times, Well*. Retrieved from https://well.blogs.nytimes.com/2014/10/15/whats-your-fitness-age/

Mayo Clinic Staff (2017, March 14). How fit are you? See how you measure up. *Mayo Clinic*. Retrieved from http://www.mayoclinic.org/healthy-lifestyle/fitness/in-depth/fitness/art-20046433

REFERENCES

CHAPTER 1

Abrams, L. (2012, Oct. 24). The evolutionary importance of grandmothers. *The Atlantic*. Retrieved from https://www.theatlantic.com/health/archive/2012/10/the-evolutionary-importance-of-grandmothers/264039/

American Federation for Aging Research. (n.d.). *Theories of aging*. Retrieved from http://www.afar.org/docs/migrated/111121_INFOAGING_GUIDE_THEORIES_OF_AGINGFR.pdf

Andziak, B., O'Connor, T. P., Qi, W., DeWaal, E. M., Pierce, A., Chaudhuri, A. R., ... Buffenstein, R. (2006). High oxidative damage levels in the longest-living rodent, the naked mole-rat. *Aging Cell, 5*(6), 463–471.

Aronson, D., & Rayfield, E. J. (2002). How hyperglycemia promotes atherosclerosis: molecular mechanisms. *Cardiovascular Diabetology, 1*(1), 1.

Austad, S. N. (1997). *Why we age—what science is discovering about the body's journey through life*. New York, NY: John Wiley & Sons.

Baker, D. J., Childs, B. G., Durik, M., Wijers, M. E., Sieben, C. J., Zhong, J., ... van Deursen, J. M. (2016). Naturally occurring p16(Ink4a)-positive cells shorten healthy lifespan. *Nature, 530*, 184–189.

Bartlett, Z. (2014). The Hayflick limit. *The Embryo Project Encyclopedia at Arizona State University*. Retrieved from https://embryo.asu.edu/pages/hayflick-limit

Bock, E. (2016). Biological clock can help researchers understand aging process. *NIH Record, 68*(17). Retrieved from https://nihrecord.nih.gov/newsletters/2016/08_12_2016/story2.htm

Bodnar, A. G., & Coffman, J. A. (2016). Maintenance of somatic tissue regeneration with age in short- and long-lived species of sea urchins. *Aging Cell, 15*(4), 778–787.

Bratic, A., & Larsson, N.-G. (2013). The role of mitochondria in aging. *Journal of Clinical Investigation, 123*(3), 9511–9517.

Breitling, L. P., Saum, K.-U., Perna, L., Schöttker, B., Holleczek, B., & Brenner, H. (2016). Frailty is associated with the epigenetic clock but not with telomere length in a German cohort. *Clinical Epigenetics, 8*, 21.

Brodwin, E. (2016, Apr. 27). Everything you thought you knew about aging is wrong. *Business Insider*. Retrieved from http://www.businessinsider.com/forget-everything-you-know-about-aging-2016-4

Callaway, E. (2016, Feb. 3). Destroying worn-out cells makes mice live longer. *Nature/News*.

Chen, B. H., Marioni, R. E., Colicino, E., Peters, M. J., Ward-Caviness, C. K., Tsai, P.-C., ... Horvath, S. (2016). DNA methylation-based measures of biological age: meta-analysis predicting time to death. *Aging (Albany, NY), 8*(9), 1844–1859.

Christiansen, L., Lenart, A., Tan, Q., Vaupel, J. W., Aviv, A., McGue, M., & Christensen, K. (2016). DNA methylation age is associated with mortality in a longitudinal Danish twin study. *Aging Cell, 15*(1), 149–154.

Cohen, H. Y., Miller, C., Bitterman, K. J., Wall, N. R., Hekking, B., Kessler, B., . . . Sinclair, D. A. (2004). Calorie restriction promotes mammalian cell survival by inducing the SIRT1 deacetylase. *Science, 305*(5682), 390–392.

Cohen, J. (2015). Death-defying experiments. *Science, 350*(6265), 1186–1187.

Diamond, J. (2013, Nov.). *How societies can grow old better* [Lecture transcript]. *TED*. Retrieved from https://www.ted.com/talks/jared_diamond_how_societies_can_grow_old_better/transcript?language=en

Efeyan, A., Comb, W. C., & Sabatini, D. M. (2015). Nutrient sensing mechanisms and pathways. *Nature, 517*(7534), 302–310.

Erikson, G. A., Bodian, D. L., Rueda, M., Molparia, B., Scott, E. R., Scott-Van Zeeland, A. A., . . . Torkamani, A. (2016). Whole-genome sequencing of a healthy aging cohort. *Cell, 165*(4), 1002–1011.

Fishlock, V. (2011, Jun. 9). Why matriarchs matter in elephant society. *International Fund for Animal Welfare*. Retrieved from http://www.ifaw.org/united-states/node/2842

Fontana, L., Partridge, L., & Longo, V. D. (2010). Dietary restriction, growth factors and aging: from yeast to humans. *Science, 328*(5976), 321–326.

Foreman, J. (1993a, Jun. 7). CDC seeks further tests at reservation for clues to disease. *Boston Globe*. Retrieved from https://www.highbeam.com/doc/1P2-8231069.html

Foreman, J. (1993b, Jun. 14), Stalking a mystery illness. *Boston Globe*. Retrieved from https://www.highbeam.com/doc/1P2-8232177.html

Garatachea, N., Pareja-Galeano, H., Sanchis-Gomar, F., Santos-Lozano, A., Fiuza-Luces, C., Moran, M., . . . Lucia, A. (2015). Exercise attenuates the major hallmarks of aging. *Rejuvenation Research, 18*(1), 57–89.

Gibbs, W. W. (2014). Biomarkers and ageing: the clock-watcher. *Nature, 508*(7495), 168–170.

Goldman, D. P., Cutler, D., Rowe, J. W., Michaud, P. C., Sullivan, J., Peneva, D., . . . Olshansky, S. J. (2013). Substantial health and economic returns from delayed aging may warrant a new focus for medical research. *Health Affairs, 32*(10), 1698–1705.

Gredilla, R., Sanz, A., Lopez-Torres, M., & Barja, G. (2001). Caloric restriction decreases mitochondrial free radical generation at complex I and lowers oxidative damage to mitochondrial DNA in the rat heart. *FASEB Journal, 15*(9), 1589–1591.

Greenfieldboyce, N. (2016, Aug. 11). Talk about an ancient mariner! Greenland shark is at least 272 years old. *Shots NPR*. Retrieved from http://www.npr.org/sections/health-shots/2016/08/11/489229041/talk-about-an-ancient-mariner-greenland-shark-is-at-least-272-years-old

Grigorian-Shamagian, L., Liu, W., Fereydooni, S., Middleton, R. C., Valle, J., Cho, J. H., & Marban, E. (2017). Cardiac and systemic rejuvenation after cardiosphere-derived cell therapy in senescent rats. *European Heart Journal, 38*(39), 2957–2967.

Grimm, D. (2015). Why we outlive our pets. *Science (New York, NY), 350*(6265), 1182–1185.

Harmon, A. (2016, May 16). Dogs test drug aimed at humans' biggest killer: age. *New York Times*. Retrieved from https://www.nytimes.com/2016/05/17/us/aging-research-disease-dogs.html

He, C., Bassik, M. C., Moresi, V., Sun, K., Wei, Y., Zou, Z., . . . Levine, B. (2012). Exercise-induced BCL2-regulated autophagy is required for muscle glucose homeostasis. *Nature, 481*(7382), 511–515.

He, C., Sumpter, R., Jr., & Levine, B. (2012). Exercise induces autophagy in peripheral tissues and in the brain. *Autophagy, 8*(10), 1548–1551.

He, W., Goodkind, D., & Kowal, P. (2016, Mar.). An aging world: 2015, international population reports. *United States Census Bureau.* Retrieved from http://www.census.gov/content/dam/Census/library/publications/2016/demo/p95-16-1.pdf

Higashi, Y., Sukhanov, S., Anwar, A., Shai, S.-Y., & Delafontaine, P. (2012). Aging, atherosclerosis, and IGF-1. *Journals of Gerontology Series A: Biological Sciences and Medical Sciences, 67A*(6), 626–639.

Hood, D. A. (2009). Mechanisms of exercise-induced mitochondrial biogenesis in skeletal muscle. *Applied Physiology, Nutrition, and Metabolism, 34*(3), 465–472.

Horvath, S. (2013). DNA methylation age of human tissues and cell types. *Genome Biology, 14*(10), R115.

Horvath, S., Erhart, W., Brosch, M., Ammerpohl, O., von Schönfels, W., Ahrens, M., . . . Hampe, J. (2014). Obesity accelerates epigenetic aging of human liver. *Proceedings of the National Academy of Sciences of the United States of America, 111*(43), 15538–15543.

Horvath, S., Garagnani, P., Bacalini, M. G., Pirazzini, C., Salvioli, S., Gentilini, D., . . . Franceschi, C. (2015). Accelerated epigenetic aging in Down syndrome. *Aging Cell, 14*(3), 491–495.

Horvath, S., Gurven, M., Levine, M. E., Trumble, B. C., Kaplan, H., Allayee, H., . . . Assimes, T. L. (2016). An epigenetic clock analysis of race/ethnicity, sex, and coronary heart disease. *Genome Biology, 17*, 171.

Horvath, S., & Levine, A. J. (2015). HIV-1 infection accelerates age according to the epigenetic clock. *Journal of Infectious Diseases, 212*(10), 1563–1573.

Horvath, S., Mah, V., Lu, A. T., Woo, J. S., Choi, O.-W., Jasinska, A. J., . . . Coles, L. S. (2015). The cerebellum ages slowly according to the epigenetic clock. *Aging (Albany, NY), 7*(5), 294–306.

Horvath, S., Pirazzini, C., Bacalini, M. G., Gentilini, D., Di Blasio, A. M., Delledonne, M., . . . Franceschi, C. (2015). Decreased epigenetic age of PBMCs from Italian semi-supercentenarians and their offspring. *Aging (Albany, NY), 7*(12), 1159–1170.

Jin, K. (2010). Modern biological theories of aging. *Aging and Disease, 1*(2), 72–74.

Johnson, S. C., Rabinovitch, P. S., & Kaeberlein, M. (2013). mTOR is a key modulator of ageing and age-related disease. *Nature, 493*(7432), 338–345.

Jones, O. R., Scheuerlein, A., Salguero-Gómez, R., Camarda, C. G., Schaible, R., Casper, B. B., . . . Vaupel, J. W. (2014). Diversity of ageing across the tree of life. *Nature, 505*(7482), 169–173.

Kaeberlein, M. (2016, Oct. 8). Personal communication.

Kaeberlein, M., Rabinovitch, P. S., & Martin, G. M. (2015). Adapted from "Healthy aging: The ultimate preventative medicine," Box 1. Geroscience interventions with translational potential. *Science, 350*(6265), 1192.

Klass, P. (2017, Apr. 3). Good news for older mothers. *New York Times.*

Kochanek, K. D., Murphy, S. L., Xu, J. Q., & Arias, E. (2017, Dec.) Mortality in the United States, 2016. *NCHS Data Brief No. 293.* Hyattsville, MD: National Center for Health Statistics. Retrieved from https://www.cdc.gov/nchs/data/databriefs/db293.pdf

Kolata, G., & Chan, S. (2016, Oct. 3). Yoshinori Ohsumi of Japan wins Nobel Prize for study of "self-eating" cells. *New York Times.*

Leslie, M. (2016, Feb. 3). Suicide of aging cells prolongs life span in mice. *Science.* Retrieved from http://www.sciencemag.org/news/2016/02/suicide-aging-cells-prolongs-life-span-mice

Letzter, R. (2016, Aug. 12). Here's everything scientists know about how to avoid aging. *Business Insider*. Retrieved from http://www.businessinsider.com/best-ways-to-avoid-aging-2016-8

Lieberman, D. (2014). *The story of the human body*. New York, NY: Vintage Books.

Lieberman, D. E. (2015). Is exercise really medicine? An evolutionary perspective. *Current Sports Medicine Reports, 14*(4), 313–319.

Lindholm, M. E., Marabita, F., Gomez-Cabrero, D., Rundqvist, H., Ekstrom, T. J., & Sundberg, C. J. (2014). An integrative analysis reveals coordinated reprogramming of the epigenome and the transcriptome in human skeletal muscle after training. *Epigenetics, 9*(12), 1557–1569.

López-Otín, C., Blasco, M. A., Partridge, L., Serrano, M., & Kroemer, G. (2013). The hallmarks of aging. *Cell, 153*(6), 1194–1217.

López-Otín, C., Galluzzi, L., Freije, J. M. P., Madeo, F., & Kroemer, G. (2016). Metabolic control of longevity. *Cell, 166*(4), 802–821.

Lu, A. T., Salfati, E. L., Chen, B. H., Ferucci, L., Levy, D., Joehanes, R., . . . Horvath, S. (2018). GWAS of epigenetic aging rates in blood reveals a critical role for TERT. *Nature Communications, 9*(1), 387.

Ma, J., Ward, E. M., Siegel, R. L., & Jemal, A. (2015). Temporal trends in mortality in the United States, 1969–2013. *Journal of the American Medical Association, 314*(16), 1731–1739.

Madeo, F., Pietrocola, F., Eisenberg, T., & Kroemer, G. (2014). Caloric restriction mimetics: towards a molecular definition. *Nature Reviews Drug Discovery, 13*(10), 727–740.

Mannick, J. B., Del Giudice, G., Lattanzi, M., Valiante, N. M., Praestgaard, J., Huang, B., . . . Klickstein, L. B. (2014). mTOR inhibition improves immune function in the elderly. *Science Translational Medicine, 6*(268), 268ra179.

Marioni, R. E., Harris, S. E., Shah, S., McRae, A. F., von Zglinicki, T., Martin-Ruiz, C., . . . Deary, I. J. (2016). The epigenetic clock and telomere length are independently associated with chronological age and mortality. *International Journal of Epidemiology, 45*(2), 424–432.

Marioni, R. E., Shah, S., McRae, A. F., Chen, B. H., Colicino, E., Harris, S. E., . . . Deary, I. J. (2015). DNA methylation age of blood predicts all-cause mortality in later life. *Genome Biology, 16*(1), 25.

Mattson, M. P. (2008). Dietary factors, hormesis and health. *Ageing Research Reviews, 7*(1), 43–48.

Mistriotis, P., Bajpai, V. K., Wang, X., Rong, N., Shahini, A., Asmani, M., . . . Andreadis, S. T. (2017). NANOG reverses the myogenic differentiation potential of senescent stem cells by restoring ACTIN filamentous organization and SRF-dependent gene expression. *Stem Cells, 35*(1), 207–221.

Mitteldorf, J. (2017, Dec. 6). The varieties of aging in nature. Retrieved from https://josh-mitteldorf.scienceblog.com/2017/12/06/the-varieties-of-aging-in-nature/

National Institutes of Health. (2015, Sept. 1). NIH study finds calorie restriction lowers some risk factors for age-related diseases. Retrieved from https://www.nih.gov/news-events/news-releases/nih-study-finds-calorie-restriction-lowers-some-risk-factors-age-related-diseases

Nelson, P., & Masel, J. (2017). Intercellular competition and the inevitability of multicellular aging. *Proceedings of the National Academy of Sciences of the United States of America, 114*(49), 12982–12987.

New England Centenarian Study. (2017). *Boston University School of Medicine*. Retrieved from http://www.bumc.bu.edu/centenarian/

Nielsen, J., Hedeholm, R. B., Heinemeier, J., Bushnell, P. G., Christiansen, J. S., Olsen, J., . . . Steffensen, J. F. (2016). Eye lens radiocarbon reveals centuries of longevity in the Greenland shark (*Somniosus microcephalus*). *Science, 353*(6300), 702–704.

NIH VideoCast. (2016, May 10). *Demystifying medicine 2016: cholesterol: too much and too little are bad for your health.* [Video file]. Retrieved from https://www.youtube.com/watch?v=O8oBZ5639ds

Nobel Media AB. (2009, Oct. 5). *The 2009 Nobel Prize in Physiology or Medicine Elizabeth H. Blackburn, Carol W. Greider, Jack W. Szostak.* [Press release]. Retrieved from http://www.nobelprize.org/nobel_prizes/medicine/laureates/2009/press.html

Nóbrega-Pereira, S., Fernandez-Marcos, P. J., Brioche, T., Gomez-Cabrera, M. C., Salvador-Pascual, A., Flores, J. M., . . . Serrano, M. (2016). G6PD protects from oxidative damage and improves healthspan in mice. *Nature Communications, 7*, 10894.

Ogden, L. E. (2015, Jan. 26). The power of elephant matriarchs. *National Wildlife Federation.* Retrieved from https://www.nwf.org/News-and-Magazines/National-Wildlife/Animals/Archives/2015/Elephant-Family-Behavior.aspx

Olshansky, S. J., & Carnes, B. A. (2013). *A measured breath of life.* Retrieved from https://itunes.apple.com/us/book/a-measured-breath-of-life/id604410007?mt=11

Ortman, J. M., & Velkoff, V.A. (2014). An aging nation: the older population in the United States. *Population Estimates and Projections, Current Population Reports, US Department of Commerce, US Census Bureau.* Retrieved from https://www.census.gov/prod/2014pubs/p25-1140.pdf

Paterson, R., & Rose, M. R. (2011, Mar. 8). Thesis 14. [Web log post]. *Michael Rose's 55.* Retrieved from https://55theses.org/2011/03/18/thesis-14/

Patrick, A., Seluanov, M., Hwang, C., Tam, J., Khan, T., Morgenstern, A., . . . Gorbunova, V. (2016). Sensitivity of primary fibroblasts in culture to atmospheric oxygen does not correlate with species lifespan. *Aging, 8*(5), 841–847.

Perna, L., Zhang, Y., Mons, U., Holleczek, B., Saum, K.-U., & Brenner, H. (2016). Epigenetic age acceleration predicts cancer, cardiovascular, and all-cause mortality in a German case cohort. *Clinical Epigenetics, 8*, 64.

Quach, A., Levine, M. E., Tanaka, T., Lu, A. T., Chen, B. H., Ferrucci, L., . . . Horvath, S. (2017). Epigenetic clock analysis of diet, exercise, education, and lifestyle factors. *Aging (Albany, NY), 9*(2), 419–446.

Ravussin, E. (2015). A 2-year randomized controlled trial of human caloric restriction: feasibility and effects on predictors of health span and longevity. *Journal of Gerontology A, Biological Sciences and Medical Sciences, 70*(9), 1097–1104.

Reynolds, G. (2014, Dec. 17). How exercise changes our DNA. *New York Times.*

Robertson, S. (2015, Sep.17). What is DNA methylation? *News Medical, Life Sciences.* Retrieved from http://www.news-medical.net/life-sciences/What-is-DNA-Methylation.aspx

Rose, M., Flatt, T., Graves Jr., J., Greer, L. F., Martínez, D., Matos, M., . . . Shahrestani, P. (2012). What is aging? *Frontiers in Genetics, 3*, 134.

Roth, G. S., Ingram, D. K., & Lane, M. A. (2001). Caloric restriction in primates and relevance to humans. *Annals of the New York Academy of Sciences, 928*, 305–315.

Ruby, J. G., Smith, M., & Buffenstein, R. (2018, Jan. 24). Naked mole-rate mortality rates defy Gompertzian laws by not increasing with age. *eLIFE.* Retrieved from https://elifesciences.org/articles/31157

Schmidt, E. (2015, Feb. 18). Brains of people with Down syndrome age faster, UCLA study discovers. *UCLA Newsroom, Health + Behavior.* Retrieved from http://newsroom.ucla.edu/releases/brains-of-people-with-down-syndrome-age-faster-ucla-study-discovers

Schmidt, E. (2016, Aug. 16). Latinos age slower than other ethnicities, UCLA study shows. *UCLA Newsroom, Health + Behavior.* Retrieved from http://newsroom.ucla.edu/releases/latinos-age-slower-than-other-ethnicities-ucla-study-shows

Schmidt, E. (2016, Sep. 28). Epigenetic clock predicts life expectancy. *UCLA Newsroom, Health + Behavior.* Retrieved from http://newsroom.ucla.edu/releases/epigenetic-clock-predicts-life-expectancy-ucla-led-study-shows

Schulz, T. J., Zarse, K., Voigt, A., Urban, N., Birringer, M., & Ristow, M. (2007). Glucose restriction extends *Caenorhabditis elegans* life span by inducing mitochondrial respiration and increasing oxidative stress. *Cell Metabolism, 6*(4), 280–293.

Sebastiani, P., Bae, H., Sun, F. X., Anderson, S. L., Daw, E. W., & Malovini, A. (2013). Meta-analysis of genetic variants associated with human exceptional longevity. *Aging (Albany, NY), 5*(9), 653–661.

Sebastiani, P., Solovieff, N., DeWan, A. T., Walsh, K. M., Puca, A., Hartley, S. W., . . . Perls, T. T. (2012). Genetic signatures of exceptional longevity in humans. *PLoS ONE, 7*(1), e29848.

Sebastiani, P., Thyagarajan, B., Sun, F., Schupf, N., Newman, A. B., Montanao, M., & Perls, T. T. (2017). Biomarker signatures of aging. *Aging Cell, 16*(2), 329–338.

Stroustrup, N., Anthony, W. E., Nash, Z. M., Gowda, V., Gomez, A., López-Moyado, I. F., . . . Fontana, W. (2016). The temporal scaling of *Caenorhabditis elegans* ageing. *Nature, 530*(7588), 103–107.

Sun, F., Sebastiani, P., Schupf, N., Bae, H., Andersen, S. L., McIntosh, A., . . . Perls, T. T. (2015). Extended maternal age at birth of last child and women's longevity in the long life family study. *Menopause (New York, NY), 22*(1), 26–31.

Thanos, P. K., Hamilton, J., O'Rourke, J. R., Napoli, A., Febo, M., Volkow, N. D., . . . Gold, M. (2016). Dopamine D2 gene expression interacts with environmental enrichment to impact lifespan and behavior. *Oncotarget, 7*(15), 19111–19123.

Vermeij, W. P., Dollé, M. E. T., Reiling, E., Jaarsma, D., Payan-Gomez, C., Bombardieri, C. R., . . . Hoeijmakers, J. H. J. (2016). Diet restriction delays accelerated aging and genomic stress in DNA repair deficient mice. *Nature, 537*(7620), 427–431.

Wehner, M. (2018, Jan. 30). Naked mole rats are immune to aging. *New York Post.*

Willcox, B. J., Donlon, T. A., He, Q., Chen, R., Grove, J. S., Yano, K., . . . Curb, J. D. (2008). FOXO3A genotype is strongly associated with human longevity. *Proceedings of the National Academy of Sciences of the United States of America, 105*(37), 13987–13992.

Willcox, B. J., Tranah, G. J., Chen, R., Morris, B. J., Masaki, K. H., He, Q., . . . Donlon, T. A. (2016). The FoxO3 gene and cause-specific mortality. *Aging Cell, 15*(4), 617–624.

Wood, J. G., Jones, B. C., Jiang, N., Chang, C., Hosier, S., Wickremesinghe, P., . . . Helfand, S. L. (2016). Chromatin-modifying genetic interventions suppress age-associated transposable element activation and extend life span in *Drosophila. Proceedings of the National Academy of Sciences of the United States of America, 113*(40), 11277–11282.

Wrobel, S. (1995). Serendipity, science, and a new hantavirus. *FASEB Journal, 9*(13), 1247–1254.

Yong, E. (2015, Mar. 5). Why killer whales go through menopause but elephants don't. *Phenomena, National Geographic.* Retrieved from http://phenomena.nationalgeographic.com/2015/03/05/why-killer-whales-go-through-menopause-but-elephants-dont/

CHAPTER 2

Akesson, A., Larsson, S. C., Discacciati, A., & Wolk, A. (2014). Low-risk diet and lifestyle habits in the primary prevention of myocardial infarction in men: a population-based prospective cohort study. *Journal of the American College of Cardiology, 64*(13), 1299–1306.

American Heart Association. (2014). Statistical report tracks global figures for first time. Highest cardiovascular disease death rates [Data set]. Retrieved from http://news. heart.org/american-heart-association-statistical-report-tracks-global-figures-first-time/

Archer, E., Shook, R. P., Thomas, D. M., Katzmarzyk, P. T., McIver, K. L., . . . Blair, S. N. (2013). 45-year trends in women's use of time and household management energy expenditures. *PLoS ONE, 8*(2), 3566620.

Ardern, C. I., Katzmarzyk, P. T., Janssen, I., Leon, A. S., Wilmore, J. H., Skinner, J. S., . . . Bouchard, C. (2004). Race and sex similarities in exercise-induced changes in blood lipids and fatness. *Medicine and Science in Sports and Exercise, 36*(9), 1610–1615.

Arem, H., Moore, S. C., Patel, A., Hartge, P., de Gonzalez, B., Visnanathan, K., . . . Matthews, C. E. (2015). Leisure time physical activity and mortality: a detailed pooled analysis of the dose-response relationship. *JAMA Internal Medicine, 175*(6), 959–967.

Balady, G. J., Larson, M. G., Vasan, R. S., Leip, E. P., O'Donnell, C. J., & Levy, D. (2004). Usefulness of exercise testing in the prediction of coronary disease risk among asymptomatic persons as a function of the Framingham risk score. *Circulation, 110*(14), 1920–1925.

Ballantyne, C. (2009, Jan. 2). Does exercise really make you healthier? *Scientific American.* Retrieved from http://www.scientificamerican.com/article/does-exercise-really-make/

Baltimore Longitudinal Study of Aging. (n.d.). About BLSA. *National Institute on Aging.* Retrieved from https://www.blsa.nih.gov/about

Bassuk, S. S., Church, T. S., & Manson, J.-A. E. (2013). Why exercise works magic. *Scientific American, 509,* 74–79.

Blair, S. N., Kohl, H. W., Barlow, C. E., Paffenbarger, R. S., Gibbons, L. W., & Macera, C. A. (1995). Changes in physical fitness and all-cause mortality. A prospective study of healthy and unhealthy men. *Journal of the American Medical Association, 273*(14), 1093–1098.

Blair, S. N., Kohl, H. W., Paffenbarger, R. S., Clark, D. G., Cooper, K. H., & Gibbons, L. W. (1989). Physical fitness and all-cause mortality: a prospective study of healthy men and women. *Journal of the American Medical Association, 262*(17), 2395–2401.

Blair, S. N., & Powell, K.E. (2014). The evolution of the physical activity field. *Journal of Physical Education, Recreation and Dance, 85*(7), 9–12.

Bouchard, C., An, P., Rice, T., Skinner, J. S., Wilmore, J. H., Gagnon, J., . . . Rao, D. C. (1999). Familial aggregation of VO(2max) response to exercise training: results from the HERITAGE Family Study. *Journal of Applied Physiology (Bethesda, MD: 1985), 87*(3), 1003–1008.

Boule, N. G., Weisnagel, S. J., Tremblay, A., Bergman, R. N., Rankinen, T., Leon, A.S., . . . Bouchard, C. (2005). Effects of exercise training on glucose homeostasis: the HERITAGE Family Study. *Diabetes Care, 28*(1), 108–114.

Brown, D. (2016, Feb. 22). We all know exercise makes you live longer: but this will actually get you off the couch. *Washington Post.* Retrieved from https://www. washingtonpost.com/national/health-science/we-all-know-exercise-makes-you-live-longer-but-this-will-actually-get-you-off-the-couch/2016/02/22/833e0128-d0d5-11e5-88cd-753e80cd29ad_story.html?utm_term=.c438d3444088

Centers for Disease Control and Prevention. (2016). More than 1 in 4 US adults over 50 do not engage in regular physical activity. Retrieved from https://www.cdc.gov/media/releases/2016/p0915-physical-activity.html

Cooper Center Longitudinal Study. (2014). Overview. *The Cooper Institute.* Retrieved from https://www.cooperinstitute.org/ccls/

Fleg, J. L. (2016). Healthy lifestyle and risk of heart failure: an ounce of prevention well worth the effort. *Circulation Heart Failure, 9*(4), e003155.

Gebel, K., Ding, D., Chey, T., Stamatakis, E., Brown, W. J., & Bauman, A. E. (2015). Effect of moderate to vigorous physical activity on all-cause mortality in middle-aged and older Australians. *JAMA Internal Medicine, 175*(6), 970–977.

Glazer, N. L., Lyass, A., Esliger, D. W., Blease, S. J., Freedson, P. S., Massaro, J. M., . . . Vasan, R. S. (2013). Sustained and shorter bouts of physical activity are related to cardio-vascular health. *Medicine and Science in Sports and Exercise, 45*(1), 109–115.

Glynn, N. W., Santanasto, A. J., Simonsick, E. M., Boudreau, R. M., Beach, S. R., Schulz, R., & Newman, A. B. (2015). The Pittsburgh Fatigability Scale for Older Adults: development and validation. *Journal of the American Geriatrics Society, 63*(1), 130–135.

Gremeaux, V., Gayda, M., Lepers, R., Sosner, P., Juneau, M., & Nigam, A. (2012). Exercise and longevity. *Maturitas, 73*(4), 312–317.

Hakim, A. A., Curb, J. D., Petrovitch, H., Rodriguez, B. L., Yano, K., Ross, G. W., . . . Abbott, R. D. (1999). Effects of walking on coronary heart disease in elderly men: the Honolulu Heart Program. *Circulation, 100*(1), 9–13.

Hakim, A. A., Petrovitch, H., Burchfiel, C. M., Ross, G. W., Rodriguez, B. L., White, L. R., . . . Abbott, R. D. (1998). Effects of walking on mortality among nonsmoking retired men. *New England Journal of Medicine, 338*(2), 94–99.

Harvard Alumni Study. (2012). *University of Minnesota Twin Cities.* Retrieved from http://www.epi.umn.edu/cvdepi/study-synopsis/harvard-alumni-study

Health ABC. (n.d.). *Dynamics of Health, Aging and Body Composition.* Retrieved from National Institute of Aging https://www.nia.nih.gov/research/intramural-research-program/dynamics-health-aging-and-body-composition-health-abc

Heritage Family Study. (n.d.). HERITAGE—Genetics, Response to Exercise, Risk Factors. Retrieved from https://www.pbrc.edu/heritage/

History of the Framingham Heart Study. (2016). *Framingham Heart Study: A project of the National Heart, Lung and Blood Institute and Boston University.* Retrieved from https://www.framinghamheartstudy.org/about-fhs/history.php.

Hubert, H. B., Eaker, E. D., Garrison, R. J., & Castelli, W. P. (1987). Life-style correlates of risk factor change in young adults: an eight-year study of coronary heart disease risk factors in the Framingham offspring. *American Journal of Epidemiology, 125*(5), 812–831.

Hurford, M. (2017). This 69-year-old grandmother is still crushing the BMX race scene. *Bicycling.* Retrieved from https://www.bicycling.com/womens-cycling/this-69-year-old-grandmother-still-crushing-the-bmx-race-scene

Kannel, W. B., & Sorlie, P. (1979). Some health benefits of physical activity: the Framingham Study. *Archives of Internal Medicine, 139*(8), 857–861.

Katzmarzyk, P. T., Leon, A. S., Wilmore, J. H., Skinner, J. S., Rao, D. C., Rankinen, T., & Bouchard, C. (2003). Targeting the metabolic syndrome with exercise: evidence from the HERITAGE Family Study. *Medicine and Science in Sports and Exercise, 35*(10), 1703–1709.

Kiely, D. K., Wolf, P. A., Cupples, L. A., Beiser, A., & Kannel, W. B. (1994). Physical activity and stroke rise. *American Journal of Epidemiology, 140*(7), 608–620.

Kim, J. H., Malhotra, R., Chiampas, G., d'Hemecourt, P., Troyanos, C., Cianca, J., . . . Race Associated Cardiac Arrest Event Registry (RACER) Study Group. (2012). Cardiac arrest during long-distance running races. *New England Journal of Medicine, 366*(2), 130–140.

Kodama, S., Saito, K., Tanaka, S., Maki, M., Yachi, Y., Asumi, M., . . . Sone, H. (2009). Cardiorespiratory fitness as a quantitative predictor of all-cause mortality and cardiovascular events in healthy men and women: a meta-analysis. *Journal of the American Medical Association, 301*(19), 2024–2035.

Kolata, G. (2008, January 8). Does exercise really keep us healthy? *New York Times, Reporter's File.* Retrieved from http://www.nytimes.com/ref/health/healthguide/esn-exercise-ess.html

Kritchevsky, S. B., Nicklas, B. J., Visser, M., Simonsick, E. M., Newman, A. B., Harris, T. B., . . . Pahor, M. (2005). Angiotensin-converting enzyme insertion/deletion genotype, exercise and physical decline. *Journal of the American Medical Association, 294*(6), 691–698.

Kyu, H. H., Bachman, V. F., Alexander, L. T., Mumford, J. E., Afshin, A., Estep, K., . . . Forouzanfar, M. H. (2016). Physical activity and risk of breast cancer, colon cancer, diabetes, ischemic heart disease, and ischemic stroke events: systematic review and dose-response meta-analysis for the Global Burden of Disease Study 2013. *BMJ, 354,* i3857.

Lear, S. A., Hu, W., Rangarajan, S., Gasevic, D., Leong, D., & Iqbal, R. (2017). The effect of physical activity on mortality and cardiovascular disease in 130,000 people from 17 high-income, middle-income, and low-income countries: the PURE study. *Lancet, 390*(10113), 1643–1654.

Lee, D. C., Brellenthin, A. G., Thompson, P. D., Sui, X., Lee, I. M., & Lavie, C. J. (2017). Running as a key lifestyle medicine for longevity. *Progressive Cardiovascular Diseases, 60*(1), 45–55.

Lee, D., Pate, R. R., Lavie, C. J., Sui, X., Church, T. S., & Blair, S. N. (2014). Leisure-time running reduces all-cause and cardiovascular mortality risk. *Journal of the American College of Cardiology, 64*(5), 472–481.

Lee, D., Sui, X., Artero, E. G., Lee, I.-M., Church, T. S., McAuley, P. A., . . . Blair, S. N. (2011). Long-term effects of changes in cardiorespiratory fitness and body mass index on all-cause and cardiovascular disease mortality in men: the Aerobics Center Longitudinal Study. *Circulation, 124*(23), 2483–2490.

Leon, A. S., Gaskill, S. E., Rice, T., Bergeron, J., Gagnon, J., Rao, D.C., . . . Bouchard, C. (2002). Variability in the response of HDL cholesterol to exercise training in the HERITAGE Family Study. *International Journal of Sports Medicine, 23*(1), 1–9.

Leon, A. S., Rice, T., Mandel, S., Després, J. P., Bergeron, J., Gagnon, J., . . . Bouchard, C. (2000). Blood lipid response to 20 weeks of supervised exercise in a large biracial population: the HERITAGE Family Study. *Metabolism, 49*(4), 513–520.

Longman, J. (2016, Dec. 28). 85-year-old marathoner is so fast that even scientists marvel. *Sports, New York Times.* Retrieved from https://www.nytimes.com/2016/12/28/sports/ed-whitlock-marathon-running.html

Mineo, L. (2017, Apr. 11). Good genes are nice, but joy is better. *Harvard Gazette.*

Misu, H., Takayama, H., Saito, Y., Mita, Y., Kikichi, A., & Ishii, K.-A. (2017). Deficiency of the hepatokine selenoprotein P increases responsiveness to exercise in mice through upregulation of reactive oxygen species and AMP-activated protein kinase in muscle. *Nature Medicine, 23,* 508–516.

Moore, S. C., Lee, I.-M., Weiderpass, E., Campbell, P. T., Sampson, J. N., Kitahara, C. M., . . . Patel, A.V. (2016). Association of leisure-time physical activity with risk of 26 types of cancer in 1.44 million adults. *JAMA Internal Medicine, 176*(6), 816–825.

Moore, S. C., Patel, A. V., Matthews, C. E., Berrington de Gonzalez, A., Park, Y., Katki, H. A., . . . Lee, I. M. (2012). Leisure time physical activity of moderate to vigorous intensity and mortality: a large pooled cohort analysis. *PLoS Medicine, 9*(11), e1001335.

Morris, J. N. (1953). London Transport Workers Study, coronary heart disease and physical activity of work. *Lancet, 265,* 1053–1057. Retrieved from http://www.epi.umn.edu/cvdepi/study-synopsis/london-transport-workers-study

Morris, J. N., Clayton, D. G., Everitt, M. G., Semmence, A. M., & Burgess, E. H. (1990). Exercise in leisure time: coronary attack and death rates. *British Heart Journal, 63*(6), 325–334.

Morris, J. N., & Raffle, P. A. B. (1954). Coronary heart disease in transport workers: a progress report. *British Journal of Industrial Medicine, 11*(4), 260–264.

Murabito, J. M., Pedley, A., Massaro, J. M., Vasan, R. S., Esliger, D., Blease, S. J., . . . Fox, C. S. (2015). Moderate-to-vigorous physical activity with accelerometry is associated with visceral adipose tissue in adults. *Journal of the American Heart Association: Cardiovascular and Cerebrovascular Disease, 4*(3), e001379.

Murphy, J. (2017, Jan. 28). An ageless wonder of cross-country skiing. *Wall Street Journal.*

National Institute on Aging. (2010, July). *Healthy aging: lessons from the Baltimore Longitudinal Study of Aging* [Brochure]. Bethesda, MD: National Institute of Aging. Retrieved from https://www.nia.nih.gov/health/publication/healthy-aging-lessons-baltimore-longitudinal-study-aging/introduction

National Institutes of Health. (2015, Jun. 11). *NIH Common Fund launches physical activity research program.* [Press release]. Retrieved from https://www.nih.gov/news-events/news-releases/nih-common-fund-launches-physical-activity-research-program

Nocon, M., Hiemann, T., Muller-Riemenschneider, F., Thalau, F., Roll, S., & Willich, S. N. (2008). Association of physical activity with all-cause and cardiovascular morality: a systematic review and meta-analysis. *European Journal of Cardiovascular and Prevention and Rehabilitation, 15*(3), 239–246.

O'Donovan, G., Lee, I.-M., Hamer, M., & Stamatakis, E. (2017). Association of "weekend warrior" and other leisure time physical activity patterns with risk for all-cause, cardiovascular disease and cancer mortality, *JAMA Internal Medicine, 177*(3), 335–342.

O'Keefe, J. H., Patil, H. R., Lavie, C. J., Magalski, A., Vogel, R. A., & McCullough, P. A. (2012). Potential adverse cardiovascular effects from excessive endurance exercise. *Mayo Clinic Proceedings, 87*(6), 587–595.

Ortega, J. D., Beck, O. N., Roby, J. M., Turney, A. L., & Kram, R. (2014). Running for exercise mitigates age-related deterioration of walking economy. *PLoS ONE, 9*(11), e113471.

Paffenbarger, R. S., Blair, S. N., & Lee, I.-M. (2001). A history of physical activity, cardiovascular health and longevity: the scientific contributions of Jeremy N. Morris, DSc, DPH, FRCP. *International Journal of Epidemiology, 30*(5), 1184–1192.

Paffenbarger, R. S., & Hale, W. E. (1975). Work activity and coronary heart disease. *New England Journal of Medicine, 292*(11), 545–550.

Paffenbarger, R. S., Wing, A. L., & Hyde, R. T. (1978). Physical activity as an index of heart attack risk in college alumni. *American Journal of Epidemiology, 108*(3), 161–175.

Paganini-Hill, A., Kawas, C. H., & Corrada, M. M. (2011). Activities and mortality in the elderly: the Leisure World Cohort Study. *Journals of Gerontology Series A: Biological Sciences and Medical Sciences, 66A*(5), 559–567.

Pandey, A., Garg, S., Khunger, M., Darden, D., Ayers, C., Kumbhani, D. J., . . . Berry, J. D. (2015). Dose-response relationship between physical activity and risk of heart failure: a meta-analysis. *Circulation, 132*(19), 1786–1794.

Physical Activity Guidelines Advisory Committee. (2008). *Physical Activity Guidelines Advisory Committee Report, 2008.* Washington, DC: US Department of Health and

Services. Retrieved from https://health.gov/paguidelines/report/pdf/committeereport.pdf, A-3.

Pollock, R. D., Carter, S., Velloso, C. P., Duggal, N. A., Lord, J. M., Lazarus, N. R., ... Harridge, S. D. R. (2015). An investigation into the relationship between age and physiological function in highly active older adults. *Journal of Physiology, 593*(3), 657–680.

Predel, H.-G. (2014). Marathon run: cardiovascular adaptation and cardiovascular risk. *European Heart Journal, 35*(44), 3091–3098.

Reynolds, G. (2015, Apr. 15). The right dose of exercise. *New York Times.* Retrieved from http://well.blogs.nytimes.com/2015/04/15/the-right-dose-of-exercise-for-a-longer-life/

Reynolds, G. (2015a, Jan. 7). How exercise keeps us young. *New York Times.* Retrieved from http://well.blogs.nytimes.com/2015/01/07/how-exercise-keeps-us-young/

Reynolds, G. (2015b, July 1). Older athletes have a strikingly young fitness age. *New York Times.* Retrieved from http://well.blogs.nytimes.com/2015/07/01/older-athletes-have-a-strikingly-young-fitness-age/

Reynolds, R. (2017, Apr. 12). An hour of running may add 7 hours to your life. *New York Times.*

Research Milestones. (2016). *Framingham Heart Study: A Project of the National Heart, Lung and Blood Institute and Boston University.* Retrieved from https://www.framinghamheartstudy.org/about-fhs/research-milestones.php

Rodriguez, B. L., Curb, J. D., Burchfiel, C. M., Abbott, R. D., Petrovitch, H., Masaki, K., & Chiu, D. (1994). Physical activity and 23-year incidence of coronary heart disease morbidity and mortality among middle-aged men: the Honolulu Heart Program. *Circulation, 89*(6), 2540–2544.

Samitz, G., Egger, M., & Zwahlen, M. (2011). Domains of physical activity and all-cause mortality: systematic review and dose-response meta-analysis of cohort studies. *International Journal of Epidemiology, 40*(5), 1382–1400.

Sesso, H. D., Paffenbarger, R. S., & Lee, I. M. (2000). Physical activity and coronary heart disease in men: the Harvard Alumni Health Study. *Circulation, 102*(9), 975–980.

Simonsick, E. M., Schrack, J. A., Glynn, N. W., & Ferrucci, L. (2014). Assessing fatigability in mobility-intact older adults. *Journal of the American Geriatrics Society, 62*(2), 347–351.

Skinner, J. S., Wilmore, K. M., Krasnoff, J. B., Jaskólski, A., Jaskólska, A., Gagnon, J., ... Bouchard, C. (2000). Adaptation to a standardized training program and changes in fitness in a large, heterogeneous population: the HERITAGE Family Study. *Medicine and Science in Sports and Exercise, 32*(1), 157–161.

Snell, P. G., & Mitchell, J. H. (1999). Physical inactivity: an easily modified risk factor? *Circulation, 100*(1), 2–4.

Song, M., & Giovannucci, E. (2016). Preventable incidence and mortality of carcinoma associated with lifestyle factors among white adults in the United States. *JAMA Oncology, 2*(9), 1154–1161.

Stahl, L. (2014, May 4). Living to 90 and beyond. *CBS News.* Retrieved from http://www.cbsnews.com/news/living-to-90-and-beyond-60-minutes/

Stofan, J. R., DiPietro, L., Davis, D., Kohl, H. W., & Blair, S. N. (1998). Physical activity patterns associated with cardiorespiratory fitness and reduced mortality: the Aerobics Center Longitudinal Study. *American Journal of Public Health, 88*(12), 1807–1813.

Studenski, S., Perera, S., Patel, K., Rosano, C., Faulkner, K., Insitari, M., ... Guralnik, J. (2011). Gait speed and survival in older adults. *Journal of the American Medical Association, 305*(1), 50–58.

Sui, X., Li, H., Zhang, J., Chen, L., Zhu, L., & Blair, S. N. (2013). Percentage of deaths attributable to poor cardiovascular health lifestyle factors: findings from the Aerobics Center Longitudinal Study. *Epidemiology Research International.* https://doi.org/10.1155/2013/437465

Surrency, J. (2016). BMX racing keeps Des Moines grandmother young. *A Tribune Broadcasting Station.* Retrieved from http://whotv.com/2016/07/12/bmx-racing-keeps-des-moines-grandmother-young/

Talbot, L. A., Metter, E. J., & Fleg, J. L. (2000). Leisure-time physical activities and their relationship to cardiorespiratory fitness in healthy men and women 18–95 years old. *Medicine & Science in Sports & Exercise, 32*(2), 417–425.

Talbot, L. A., Morrell, C. H., Fleg, J. L., & Metter, E. J. (2007). Changes in leisure time physical activity and risk of all-cause mortality in men and women: the Baltimore Longitudinal Study of Aging. *Preventive Medicine, 45*(2–3), 169–176.

Talbot, L. A., Morrell, C. H., Metter, E. J., & Fleg, J. L. (2002). Comparison of cardio-respiratory fitness versus leisure time physical activity as predictors of coronary events in men aged < or = 65 years and >65 years. *American Journal of Cardiology, 89*(10), 1187–1192.

The 90+ Study, UCI Institute for Memory Impairments and Neurological Disorders. (n.d.). *The 90+ Study.* Retrieved from UCI MIND, http://www.mind.uci.edu/research-studies/90plus-study/

Wen, C. P., Wai, J. P. M., Tsai, M. K., & Chen, C. H. (2014). Minimal amount of exercise to prolong life: to walk, to run, or just mix it up? *Journal of the American College of Cardiology, 64*(5), 482–484.

Wen, C. P., Wai, J. P. M., Tsai, M. K., Yang, Y. C., Cheng, T. Y. D., Lee, M.-C., . . . Wu, X. (2011). Minimum amount of physical activity for reduced mortality and extended life expectancy: a prospective cohort study. *Lancet, 378*(9798), 1244–1253.

Wilhelm, M. (2014). Atrial fibrillation in endurance athletes. *European Journal of Preventive Cardiology, 21*(8), 1040–1048.

Wolfarth, B., Rankinen, T., Habgerg, J. M., Loos, R. J. F., Perusse, L., Roth, S. M., . . . Bouchard, C. (2014). Advances in exercise, fitness and performance gen-omics in 2013. *Medicine and Science in Sports and Exercise, 46*(5), 851–859.

World Fitness Level. (n.d.). Retrieved from https://www.worldfitnesslevel.org/#/

World Health Organization, Global Strategy on Diet, Physical Activity and Health. (n.d.). *Physical activity and adults.* Retrieved from http://www.who.int/dietphysicalactivity/factsheet_adults/en/

CHAPTER 3

AHA/ASA Newsroom. (2017). Risks for blood clots in a vein may rise with increased TV viewing. *American Heart Association Meeting Report Poster Presentation S5169, Session VA.APS.07.*

Althoff, T., Sosic, R., Hicks, J. L., King, A. C., Delp, S. L., & Leskovec, J. (2017). Large-scale physical inactivity data reveal worldwide activity inequality. *Nature, 547*(7663), 366–339.

Beddhu, S., Wei, G., Marcus, R. L., Chonchol, M., & Greene, T. (2015). Light-intensity physical activities and mortality in the United States general population and CKD subpopulation. *Clinical Journal of the American Society of Nephrology, 10*(7), 1145–1153.

Bergouignan, A., Latouche, C., Heywood, S., Grace, M. S., Reddy-Luthmoodoo, M., Natoli, A. K., . . . Kingwell, B. A. (2016). Frequent interruptions of sedentary time modulates contraction- and insulin-stimulated glucose uptake pathways in muscle: ancillary analysis from randomized clinical trials. *Scientific Reports, 6*, 32044.

Bey, L., & Hamilton, M. T. (2003). Suppression of skeletal muscle lipoprotein lipase activity during physical inactivity: a molecular reason to maintain daily low-intensity activity. *Journal of Physiology, 551*(Pt 2), 673–682.

Biswas, A., Oh, P. I., Faulkner, G. E., Bajaj, R. R., Silver, M. A., Mitchell, M. S., & Alter, D. A. (2015). Sedentary time and its association with risk for disease incidence, mortality, and hospitalization in adults: a systematic review and meta-analysis. *Annals of Internal Medicine, 162*(2), 123–132.

Blair, S. (2009). Physical inactivity: the biggest public health problem of the 21st century. *British Journal of Sports Medicine, 43*(1), 1–2.

Blotner, H. (1945). Effect of prolonged physical inactivity on tolerance of sugar. *Archives of Internal Medicine, 75*(1), 39–44.

Booth, F. W., Laye, M. J., & Roberts, M. D. (2011). Lifetime sedentary living accelerates some aspects of secondary aging. *Journal of Applied Physiology, 111*(5), 1497–1504.

Booth, F. W., Roberts, C. K., & Laye, M. J. (2012). Lack of exercise is a major cause of chronic diseases. *Comprehensive Physiology, 2*(2), 1143–1211.

Borodulin, K., Kärki, A., Laatikainen, T., Peltonen, M., & Luoto, R. (2015). Daily sedentary time and risk of cardiovascular disease: the National FINRISK 2002 Study. *Journal of Physical Activity & Health, 12*(7), 904–908.

Bouchard, C., Blair, S. N., & Katzmarzyk, P. T. (2015). Less sitting, more physical activity, or higher fitness? *Mayo Clinic Proceedings, 90*(11), 1533–1540.

Carlson, S. A., Fulton, J. E., Pratt, M., Yang, Z., & Adams, E. K. (2015). Inadequate physical activity and health care expenditures in the United States. *Progress in Cardiovascular Diseases, 57*(4), 315–323.

Centers for Disease Control and Prevention. (2017). New CDC report: more than 100 million Americans have diabetes or prediabetes. Retrieved from http://www.nbc12.com/story/35910974/new-cdc-report-more-than-100-million-americans-have-diabetes-or-prediabetes

Chau, J. Y., Grunseit, A. C., Chey, T., Stamatakis, E., Brown, W. J., Matthews, C. E., . . . van der Ploeg, H. P. (2013). Daily sitting time and all-cause mortality: a meta-analysis. *PLoS ONE, 8*(11), e80000.

Cherkas, L. F., Hunkin, J. L., Kato, B. S., Richards, J. B., Gardner, J. P., Surdulescu, G. L., . . . Aviv, A. (2008). The association between physical activity in leisure time and leukocyte telomere length. *Archives of Internal Medicine, 168*(2), 154–158.

Chomistek, A. K., Manson, J. E., Stefanick, M. L., Lu, B., Sands-Lincoln, M., Going, S. B., . . . Eaton, C. B. (2013). The relationship of sedentary behavior and physical activity to incident cardiovascular disease: results from the Women's Health Initiative. *Journal of the American College of Cardiology, 61*(23), 2346–2354.

Craft, L. L., Zderic, T. W., Gapstur, S. M., VanIterson, E. H., Thomas, D. M., Siddique, J., & Hamilton, M. T. (2012). Evidence that women meeting physical activity guidelines do not sit less: an observational inclinometry study. *International Journal of Behavioral Nutrition and Physical Activity, 9*, 122.

Das, P., & Horton, R. (2016). Physical activity: time to take it seriously and regularly. *Lancet, 388*(10051), 1254–1255.

Diaz, K. M., Howard, V. J., Hutto, B., Colabianchi, N., Vena, J. E., & Safford, M. M. (2017). Patterns of sedentary behavior and mortality in U.S. middle-aged and older adults: a national cohort study. *Annals of Internal Medicine, 167*(7), 465–475.

Ding, D., Lawson, K. D., Kolbe-Alexander, T. L., Finkelstein, E. A., Katzmarzyk, P. T., van Mechelen, W., . . . Lancet Physical Activity Series 2 Executive Committee.

(2016). The economic burden of physical inactivity: a global analysis of major non-communicable diseases. *Lancet, 388*(10051), 1311–1324.

Du, M., Prescott, J., Kraft, P., Han, J., Giovannucci, E., Hankinson, S. E., & De Vivo, I. (2012). Physical activity, sedentary behavior, and leukocyte telomere length in women. *American Journal of Epidemiology, 175*(5), 414–422.

Dunlop, D. D., Song, J., Arntson, E. K., Semanik, P. A., Lee, J., Chang, R. W., & Hootman, J. M. (2015). Sedentary time in U.S. older adults associated with disability in activities of daily living independent of physical activity. *Journal of Physical Activity & Health, 12*(1), 93–101.

Dunstan, D. W., Barr, E. L. M., Healy, G. N., Salmon, J., Shaw, J. E., Balkau, B., . . . Owen, N. (2010). Television viewing time and mortality: the Australian Diabetes, Obesity and Lifestyle Study (AusDiab). *Circulation, 121*(3), 384–391.

Duvivier, B. M. F. M., Schaper, N. C., Hesselink, C., van Kan, L., Stienen, N., & Winkens, B. (2017). Breaking sitting with light activities vs. structured exercise: a randomized crossover study demonstrating benefits for glycaemic control and insulin sensitivity in type 2 diabetes. *Diabetologia, 60*(3), 490–498.

Ekelund, U., Steene-Johannessen, J., Brown, W. J., Fagerland, M. W., Owen, N., Powell, K. E., . . . Lancet Sedentary Behaviour Working Group. (2016). Does physical activity attenuate, or even eliminate, the detrimental association of sitting time with mortality? A harmonised meta-analysis of data from more than 1 million men and women. *Lancet, 388*(10051), 1302–1310.

Figueiredo, P. A., Powers, S. K., Ferreira, R. M., Amado, F., Appell, H. J., & Duarte, J. A. (2009). Impact of lifelong sedentary behavior on mitochondrial function of mice skeletal muscle. *Journals of Gerontology Series A: Biological Sciences and Medical Sciences, 64*(9) 927–939.

Flegal, K. M., Kruszon-Moran, D., Carroll, M. D., Fryar, C. D., & Ogden, C. L. (2016). Trends in obesity among adults in the United States, 2005 to 2014. *Journal of the American Medical Association, 315*(21), 2284–2291.

Grøntved, A., & Hu, F. B. (2011). Television viewing and risk of type 2 diabetes, cardiovascular disease, and all-cause mortality: a meta-analysis. *Journal of the American Medical Association, 305*(23), 2448–2455.

Hamburg, N. M., McMackin, C. J., Huang, A. L., Shenouda, S. M., Widlansky, M. E., Schulz, E., . . . Vita, J. A. (2007). Physical inactivity rapidly induces insulin resistance and microvascular dysfunction in healthy volunteers. *Arteriosclerosis, Thrombosis, and Vascular Biology, 27*(12), 2650–2656.

Handschin, C., & Spiegelman, B. M. (2008). The role of exercise and PGC1a in inflammation and chronic disease. *Nature, 454*(7203), 463–469.

Harrington, J. L., Ayers, C., Berry, J. D., Omland, T., Pandey, A., & Seliger, S. L. (2017). Sedentary behavior and subclinical cardiac injury: results from the Dallas Heart Study. *Circulation, 136*(15), 1451–1453.

Healy, G. N., Dunstan, D. W., Salmon, J., Cerin, E., Shaw, J. E., Zimmet, P. Z., & Owen, N. (2007). Objectively measured light-intensity physical activity is independently associated with 2-h plasma glucose. *Diabetes Care, 30*(6), 1384–1389.

Healy, G. N., Dunstan, D. W., Salmon, J., Shaw, J. E., Zimmet, P. Z., & Owen, N. (2008). Television time and continuous metabolic risk in physically active adults. *Medicine and Science in Sports and Exercise, 40*(4), 639–645.

Healy, G. N., Matthews, C. E., Dunstan, D. W., Winkler, E. A. H., & Owen, N. (2011). Sedentary time and cardio-metabolic biomarkers in US adults: NHANES 2003–06. *European Heart Journal, 32*(5), 590–597.

Hein, H. O., Suadicani, P., & Gyntelberg, F. (1992). Physical fitness or physical activity as a predictor of ischaemic heart disease? A 17-year follow-up in the Copenhagen Male Study. *Journal of Internal Medicine, 232*(6), 471–479.

Hu, F. B., Li, T. Y., Colditz, G. A., Willett, W. C., & Manson, J. E. (2003). Television watching and other sedentary behaviors in relation to risk of obesity and type 2 diabetes mellitus in women. *Journal of the American Medical Association, 289*(14), 1785–1791.

Katzmarzyk, P. T. (2014). Standing and mortality in a prospective cohort of Canadian adults. *Medicine and Science in Sports and Exercise, 46*(5), 940–946.

Katzmarzyk, P. T., Church, T. S., Craig, C. L., & Bouchard, C. (2009). Sitting time and mortality from all causes, cardiovascular disease, and cancer. *Medicine and Science in Sports and Exercise, 41*(5), 998–1005.

Kim, Y., Wilkens, L. R., Park, S.-Y., Goodman, M. T., Monroe, K. R., & Kolonel, L. N. (2013). Association between various sedentary behaviours and all-cause, cardiovascular disease and cancer mortality: the Multiethnic Cohort Study. *International Journal of Epidemiology, 42*(4), 1040–1056.

LaMonte, M. J., Blair, S. N., & Church, T. S. (2005). Physical activity and diabetes prevention. *Journal of Applied Physiology, 99*(3), 1205–1213.

Lee, I.-M., Shiroma, E. J., Evenson, K. R., Kamada, M., LaCroix, A. Z., & Buring, J. E. (2018). Accelerometer-measured physical activity and sedentary behavior in relation to all-cause mortality. *Circulation, 137*, 203–205.

Lee, I. M., Shiroma, E. J., Lobelo, F., Puska, P., Blair, S. N., & Katzmarzyk, P. T. (2012). Effect of physical inactivity on major non-communicable diseases worldwide: an analysis of burden of disease and life expectancy. *Lancet, 380*(9838), 219–229.

Levine, J. (2014, Nov. 1). Killer chairs: how desk jobs ruin your health. *Scientific American.* Retrieved from https://www.scientificamerican.com/article/killer-chairs-how-desk-jobs-ruin-your-health/

Levine, J. A. (2015). Sick of sitting. *Diabetologia, 58*(8), 1751–1758.

Lieberman, D. (2014). *The story of the human body.* New York, NY: Vintage Books.

Loprinzi, P. D. (2015). Leisure-time screen-based sedentary behavior and leukocyte telomere length: implications for a new leisure-time screen-based sedentary behavior mechanism. *Mayo Clinic Proceedings, 90*(6), 786–790.

Lynch, B. M., & Owen, N. (2015). Too much sitting and chronic disease risk: steps to move the science forward. *Annals of Internal Medicine, 162*(2), 146–147.

Matthews, C. E., Chen, K. Y., Freedson, P. S., Buchowski, M. S., Beech, B. M., Pate, R. R., & Troiano, R. P. (2008). Amount of time spent in sedentary behaviors in the United States, 2003–2004. *American Journal of Epidemiology, 167*(7), 875–881.

Matthews, C. E., Cohen, S. S., Fowke, J. H., Han, X., Xiao, Q., Buchowski, M. S., . . . Blot, W. J. (2014). Physical activity, sedentary behavior, and cause-specific mortality in black and white adults in the Southern Community Cohort Study. *American Journal of Epidemiology, 180*(4), 394–405.

Matthews, C. E., George, S. M., Moore, S. C., Bowles, H. R., Blair, A., Park, Y., . . . Schatzkin, A. (2012). Amount of time spent in sedentary behaviors and cause-specific mortality in US adults. *American Journal of Clinical Nutrition, 95*(2), 437–445.

McGavock, J. M., Hastings, J. L., Snell, P. G., McGuire, D. K., Pacini, E. L., Levine, B. D., & Mitchell, J. H. (2009). A forty-year follow-up of the Dallas Bed Rest and Training Study: the effect of age on the cardiovascular response to exercise in men. *Journals of Gerontology Series A: Biological Sciences and Medical Sciences, 64A*(2), 293–299.

McGuire, D. K., Levine, B. D., Williamson, J. W., Snell, P. G., Blomqvist, C. G., Saltin, B., & Mitchell, J. H. (2001). A 30-year follow-up of the Dallas Bedrest and Training

Study: I. Effect of age on the cardiovascular response to exercise. *Circulation,* *104*(12), 1350–1357.

Measuring physical activity. (2016). *Harvard T. H. Chan School of Public Health.* Retrieved from https://www.hsph.harvard.edu/nutritionsource/mets-activity-table/

Messerli, F. H., Messerli, A. W., & Lüscher, T. F. (2005). Eisenhower's billion-dollar heart attack—50 years later. *New England Journal of Medicine, 353*(12), 1205–1207.

Ogden, C. L., Carroll, M. D., Lawman, H. G., Fryar, C. D., Kruszon-Moran, D., Kit, B. K., & Flegal, K. M. (2016). Trends in obesity prevalence among children and adolescents in the United States, 1988–1994 through 2013–2014. *Journal of the American Medical Association, 315*(21), 2292–2299.

O'Keefe, J. H., Vogel, R., Lavie, C. J., & Cordain, L. (2010). Achieving hunter-gatherer fitness in the 21st century: back to the future. *American Journal of Medicine, 123*(12), 1082–1086.

Pandey, A., Salahuddin, U., Garg, S., Ayers, C., Kulinski, J., Anand, V., . . . Berry, J. D. (2016). Continuous dose-response association between sedentary time and risk for cardiovascular disease: a meta-analysis. *JAMA Cardiology, 1*(5), 575–583.

Pate, R. R., O'Neill, J. R., & Lobelo, F. (2008). The evolving definition of "sedentary." *Exercise and Sport Sciences Reviews, 36*(4), 173–178.

Patel, A. V., Bernstein, L., Deka, A., Feigelson, H. S., Campbell, P. T., Gapstur, S. M., . . . Thun, M. J. (2010). Leisure time spent sitting in relation to total mortality in a prospective cohort of US adults. *American Journal of Epidemiology, 172*(4), 419–429.

Pavey, T. G., Peeters, G. G., & Brown, W. J. (2015). Sitting-time and 9-year all-cause mortality in older women. *British Journal of Sports Medicine, 49*(2), 95–99.

Pedersen, B. K., & Febbraio, M. A. (2012). Muscles, exercise and obesity: skeletal muscle as a secretory organ. *Nature Reviews Endocrinology, 8*(8), 457–465.

Petersen, C. B., Bauman, A., Grønbæk, M., Helge, J. W., Thygesen, L. C., & Tolstrup, J. S. (2014). Total sitting time and risk of myocardial infarction, coronary heart disease and all-cause mortality in a prospective cohort of Danish adults. *International Journal of Behavioral Nutrition and Physical Activity, 11*, 13.

Preidt, R. (2016, Aug. 16). Even if you exercise, too much sitting time is bad. *CBS News.* Retrieved from http://www.cbsnews.com/news/even-if-you-exercise-prolonged-sitting-time-is-bad-for-heart-health/

Proper, K. I., Singh, A. S., van Mechelen, W., & Chinapaw, M. J. M. (2011). Sedentary behaviors and health outcomes among adults: a systematic review of prospective studies. *American Journal of Preventive Medicine, 40*(2), 174–182.

Pulsford, R. M., Stamatakis, E., Britton, A. R., Brunner, E. J., & Hillsdon, M. (2015). Associations of sitting behaviours with all-cause mortality over a 16-year follow-up: the Whitehall II study. *International Journal of Epidemiology, 44*(6), 1909–1916.

Reis, R. S., Salvo, D., Ogilvie, D., Lambert, E. V., Goenka, S., Brownson, R. C., & Lancet Physical Activity Series 2 Executive Committee. (2016). Scaling up physical activity interventions across the globe: stepping up to larger and smarter approaches to get people moving. *Lancet, 388*(10051), 1337–1348.

Reynolds, G. (2014, Sept. 17). Sit less, live longer? *New York Times.* Retrieved from https://well.blogs.nytimes.com/2014/09/17/sit-less-live-longer/

Reynolds, G. (2015, May 13). A 2-minute walk may counter the harms of sitting. *New York Times.* Retrieved from https://well.blogs.nytimes.com/2015/05/13/a-2-minute-walk-may-counter-the-harms-of-sitting/

Rottensteiner, M., Leskinen, T., Niskanen, E., Aaltonen, S., Mutikainen, S., Wikgren, J., . . . Kujala, U. M. (2015). Physical activity, fitness, glucose homeostasis, and brain morphology in twins. *Medicine and Science in Sports and Exercise, 47*(3), 509–518.

Sallis, J. F., Bull, F., Guthold, R., Heath, G. W., Inoue, S., Kelly, P., . . . Hallal, P. C. (2016). Progress in physical activity over the Olympic quadrennium. *Lancet, 388*(10051), 1325–1336.

Schmid, D., & Leitzmann, M. F. (2014). Television viewing and time spent sedentary in relation to cancer risk: a meta-analysis. *Journal of the National Cancer Institute, 106*(7).

Seguin, R., Buchner, D. M., Liu, J., Allison, M., Manini, T., Wang, C.-Y., . . . LaCroix, A. Z. (2014). Sedentary behavior and mortality in older women: the Women's Health Initiative. *American Journal of Preventive Medicine, 46*(2), 122–135.

Shrestha, N., Kukkonen-Harula, K. T., Verbeek, J. H., Ijaz, S., Hermans, V., & Bhaumik, S. (2016, Mar. 17). Workplace interventions for reducing sitting time at work. *Cochrane Database of Systemic Reviews.* Retrieved from http://www.cochrane.org/CD010912/OCCHEALTH_workplace-interventions-reducing-sitting-time-work

Sjögren, P., Fisher, R., Kallings, L., Svenson, U., Roos, G., & Hellénius, M.-L. (2014). Stand up for health—avoiding sedentary behaviour might lengthen your telomeres: secondary outcomes from a physical activity RCT in older people. *British Journal of Sports Medicine, 48*(19), 1407–1409.

Stephens, B. R., Granados, K., Zderic, T. W., Hamilton, M. T., & Braun, B. (2011). Effects of 1 day of inactivity on insulin action in healthy men and women: interaction with energy intake. *Metabolism: Clinical and Experimental, 60*(7), 941–949.

Thorp, A. A., Owen, N., Neuhaus, M., & Dunstan, D. W. (2011). Sedentary behaviors and subsequent health outcomes in adults: a systematic review of longitudinal studies, 1996–2011. *American Journal of Preventive Medicine, 41*(2), 207–215.

Tremblay, M. S., Colley, R. C., Saunders, T. J., Healy, G. N., & Owen, N. (2010). Physiological and health implications of a sedentary lifestyle. *Applied Physiology, Nutrition, and Metabolism, 35*(6), 725–740.

van der Ploeg, H. P., Chey, T., Korda, R. J., Banks, E., & Bauman, A. (2012). Sitting time and all-cause mortality risk in 222 497 Australian adults. *Archives of Internal Medicine, 172*(6), 494–500.

Walsh, N. P., Gleeson, M., Shephard, R. J., Gleeson, M., Woods, J. A., Bishop, N. C., . . . Simon, P. (2011). Position statement. Part one: immune function and exercise. *Exercise Immunology Review, 17*, 33.

Wenner, M. (2009, Dec. 1). Does inflammation trigger insulin resistance and diabetes? *Scientific American.* Retrieved from https://www.scientificamerican.com/article/inflammatory-clues/

Wijndacle, K., Brage, S., Besson, H., Khaw, K.-T., Sharp, S. J., Luben, R., . . . Ekelund, U. (2011). Television viewing time independently predicts all-cause and cardiovascular mortality: the EPIC Norfolk Study. *International Journal of Epidemiology, 40*(1), 150–159.

Young, D. R., Hivert, M.-F., Alhassan, S., Camhi, S. M., Ferguson, J. F., . . . Yong, C. M. (2016). Sedentary behavior and cardiovascular morbidity and mortality: a science advisory from the American Heart Association, endorsed by the Obesity Society. *Circulation, 134*(13), e262–e279.

CHAPTER 4

Agha, G., Loucks, E. B., Tinker, L. F., Waring, M. E., Michaud, D. S., Foraker, R. E., . . . Eaton, C. B. (2014). Healthy lifestyle and risk of heart failure in the Women's Health Initiative Observational Study. *Journal of the American College of Cardiology, 64*(17), 1777–1785.

Akesson, A., Larsson, S. C., Discacciati, A., & Wolk, A. (2014). Low-risk diet and lifestyle habits in the primary prevention of myocardial infarction in men: a population-based prospective cohort study. *Journal of the American College of Cardiology, 64*(13), 1299–1306.

Albert, C. M., Mittleman, M. A., Chae, C. U., Lee, I. M., Hennekens, C. H., & Manson, J. E. (2000). Triggering of sudden death from cardiac causes by vigorous exertion. *New England Journal of Medicine, 343*(19), 1355–1361.

Al-Lamee, R., Thompson, D., Dehbi, H.-M., Sen, S., Tang, K., Davies, J., . . . ORBITA investigators. (2017). Percutaneous coronary intervention in stable angina (ORBITA): a double-blind, randomised controlled trial. *Lancet.* Retrieved from https://doi.org/10.1016/S0140-6736(17)32714-9

American College of Cardiology. (2017, Nov. 13). New ACC/AHA high blood pressure guidelines lower definition of hypertension. [Press release]. Retrieved from https://www.acc.org/latest-in-cardiology/articles/2017/11/08/11/47/mon-5pm-bp-guideline-aha-2017

American Diabetes Association, National Heart, Lung, and Blood Institute, Juvenile Diabetes Foundation International, National Institute of Diabetes and Digestive and Kidney Diseases, & American Heart Association. (1999). Diabetes mellitus: a major risk factor for cardiovascular disease. [Editorial]. *Circulation, 100*(10), 1132.

American Heart Association. (2015). Cardiovascular diseases & diabetes. Retrieved from http://www.heart.org/HEARTORG/Conditions/More/Diabetes/WhyDiabetesMatters/Cardiovascular-Disease-Diabetes_UCM_313865_Article.jsp/

American Heart Association. (2017, Sept. 27). What is heart failure? Retrieved from http://www.heart.org/HEARTORG/Conditions/HeartFailure/AboutHeartFailure/What-is-Heart-Failure_UCM_002044_Article.jsp#

American Heart Association. (2017, Nov. 12). Sexual activity rarely a heart-stopping activity. *AHA/ASA Newsroom.* Retrieved from https://newsroom.heart.org/news/sexual-activity-rarely-a-heart-stopping-activity

Anderson, L., Oldridge, N., Thompson, D. R., Zwisler, A. D., Rees, K., Martin, N., . . . Taylor, R. S. (2016). Exercise-based cardiac rehabilitation for coronary heart disease: Cochrane systematic review and meta-analysis. *Journal of the American College of Cardiology, 67*(1), 1–12.

Aoyagi, Y., & Shephard, R. J. (2010). Habitual physical activity and health in the elderly: the Nakanojo Study. *Geriatrics & Gerontology International, 10*(Suppl 1), S236–S243.

Apullan, F. J., Bourassa, M. G., Tardif, J.-C., Fortier, A., Gayda, M., & Nigam, A. (2008). Usefulness of self-reported leisure-time physical activity to predict long-term survival in patients with coronary heart disease. *American Journal of Cardiology, 102*(4), 375–379.

Arbab-Zadeh, A., Dijk, E., Prasad, A., Fu, Q., Torres, P., Zhang, R., . . . Levine, B. D. (2004). Effect of aging and physical activity on left ventricular compliance. *Circulation, 110*(13), 1799–1805.

Ardern, C. I., Katzmarzyk, P. T., Janssen, I., Leon, A. S., Wilmore, J. H., Skinner, J. S., . . . Bouchard, C. (2004). Race and sex similarities in exercise-induced changes in blood lipids and fatness. *Medicine and Science in Sports and Exercise, 36*(9), 1610–1615.

Arem, H., Moore, S. C., Patel, A., Hartge, P., de Gonzalez, A. B., Visvanathan, K., . . . Matthews, C. E. (2015). Leisure time physical activity and mortality: a detailed pooled analysis of the dose-response relationship. *JAMA Internal Medicine, 175*(6), 959–967.

Armstrong, M. E. G., Green, J., Reeves, G. K., Beral, V., Cairns, B. J., & Million Women Study Collaborators. (2015). Frequent physical activity may not reduce vascular disease risk as much as moderate activity: large prospective study of women in the United Kingdom. *Circulation, 131*(8), 721–729.

Autonomic nervous system. (n.d.). MedicineNet.com Retrieved from https://www.medicinenet.com/script/main/art.asp?articlekey=2403

Balady, G. J., Larson, M. G., Vasan, R. S., Leip, E. P., O'Donnell, C. J., & Levy, D. (2004). Usefulness of exercise testing in the prediction of coronary disease risk among asymptomatic persons as a function of the Framingham risk score. *Circulation, 110*(14), 1920–1925.

Ballantyne, C. (2009, Jan. 2). Does exercise really make you healthier? *Scientific American.* Retrieved from https://www.scientificamerican.com/article/does-exercise-really-make/

Beckerman, J. (2016, Sept. 14). Heart disease and C-reactive protein (CRP) testing. *WebMD.* Retrieved from https://www.webmd.com/heart-disease/guide/heart-disease-c-reactive-protein-crp-testing#1

Benjamin, E. J., Blaha, M. J., Chiuve, S. E., Cushman, M., Das, S. R., Deo, R., . . . Muntner, P. (2017). Heart disease and stroke statistics—2017 update: a report from the American Heart Association. *Circulation, 135*(10), e146–e603.

Bergouignan, A., Latouche, C., Heywood, S., Grace, M. S., Reddy-Luthmoodoo, M., Natoli, A. K., . . . Kingwell, B. A. (2016). Frequent interruptions of sedentary time modulates contraction- and insulin-stimulated glucose uptake pathways in muscle: ancillary analysis from randomized clinical trials. *Scientific Reports, 6*, 32044.

Bhella, P. S., Hastings, J. L., Fujimoto, N., Shibata, S., Carrick-Ranson, G., Adams-Huet, B., & Levine, B. D. (2014). Impact of lifelong exercise "dose" on left ventricular compliance and distensibility. *Journal of the American College of Cardiology, 64*(12), 1257–1266.

Blair, S. N. (2009). Physical inactivity: the biggest public health problem of the 21st century. *British Journal of Sports Medicine, 43*(1), 1–2.

Blair, S. N., Kohl, H. W., Paffenbarger, R. S., Clark, D. G., Cooper, K. H., & Gibbons, L. W. (1989). Physical fitness and all-cause mortality: a prospective study of healthy men and women. *Journal of the American Medical Association, 262*(17), 2395–2401.

Booth, F. W., Roberts, C. K., & Laye, M. J. (2012). Lack of exercise is a major cause of chronic diseases. *Comprehensive Physiology, 2*(2), 1143–1211.

Bouchard, C. (2012). Genomic predictors of trainability. *Experimental Physiology, 97*(3), 347–352.

Bouchard, C., An, P., Rice, T., Skinner, J. S., Wilmore, J. H., Gagnon, J., . . . Rao, D. C. (1999). Familial aggregation of VO(2max) response to exercise training: results from the HERITAGE Family Study. *Journal of Applied Physiology, 87*(3), 1003–1008.

Bouchard, C., Blair, S. N., Church, T. S., Earnest, C. P., Hagberg, J. M., Häkkinen, K., . . . Rankinen, T. (2012). Adverse metabolic response to regular exercise: is it a rare or common occurrence? *PLoS ONE, 7*(5), e37887.

Boulé, N. G., Weisnagel, S. J., Lakka, T. A., Tremblay, A., Bergman, R. N., Rankinen, T., . . . HERITAGE Family Study. (2005). Effects of exercise training on glucose homeostasis: the HERITAGE Family Study. *Diabetes Care, 28*(1), 108–114.

Braith, R. W., & Stewart, K. J. (2006). Resistance exercise training: its role in the prevention of cardiovascular disease. *Circulation, 113*(22), 2642–2650.

Broom, D. R., Batterham, R. L., King, J. A., & Stensel, D. J. (2009). Influence of resistance and aerobic exercise on hunger, circulating levels of acylated ghrelin, and peptide

YY in healthy males. *American Journal of Physiology. Regulatory, Integrative and Comparative Physiology, 296*(1), R29–35.

Burgomaster, K. A., Howarth, K. R., Phillips, S. M., Rakobowchuk, M., MacDonald, M. J., McGee, S. L., & Gibala, M. J. (2008). Similar metabolic adaptations during exercise after low-volume sprint interval and traditional endurance training in humans. *Journal of Physiology, 586*(Pt 1), 151–160.

Carrick-Ranson, G., Hastings, J. L., Bhella, P. S., Fujimoto, N., Shibata, S., Palmer, M. D., . . . Levine, B. D. (2014). The effect of lifelong exercise dose on cardiovascular function during exercise. *Journal of Applied Physiology, 116*(7), 736–745.

Carter, A. (2011, Apr. 11). Boston Marathon legend Johnny Kelley will always be "young at heart." *Newton Patch.* Retrieved from https://patch.com/massachusetts/newton/boston-marathon-legend-johnny-kelley-will-always-be-y8fc4a089a1

Centers for Disease Control and Prevention. (2016, June 16). Defining adult overweight & obesity. Retrieved from https://www.cdc.gov/obesity/adult/defining.html

Centers for Disease Control and Prevention. (2017, Jan. 20). Exercise or physical activity. National Center for Health Statistics. Retrieved from https://www.cdc.gov/nchs/fastats/exercise.htm

Centers for Disease Control and Prevention. (2017, Mar. 17). Leading causes of death. Retrieved from https://www.cdc.gov/nchs/fastats/leading-causes-of-death.htm

Centers for Disease Control and Prevention. (2017, May 3). Obesity and overweight. Retrieved from https://www.cdc.gov/nchs/fastats/obesity-overweight.htm

Chaudhary, S., Kang, M. K., & Sandhu, J. S. (2010). The effects of aerobic versus resistance training on cardiovascular fitness in obese sedentary females. *Asian Journal of Sports Medicine, 1*(4), 177–184.

Chomistek, A. K., Chasman, D. I., Cook, N. R., Rimm, E. B., & Lee, I.-M. (2013). Physical activity, genes for physical fitness, and risk of coronary heart disease. *Medicine and Science in Sports and Exercise, 45*(4), 691–697.

Ciolac, E. G., Bocchi, E. A., Bortolotto, L. A., Carvalho, V. O., Greve, J. M., & Guimarães, G. V. (2010). Effects of high-intensity aerobic interval training vs. moderate exercise on hemodynamic, metabolic and neuro-humoral abnormalities of young normotensive women at high familial risk for hypertension. *Hypertension Research, 33*(8), 836–843.

Competitor.com. (2013, Oct. 29). True inspiration from a 91-year-old runner. *Competitor Runner.* Retrieved from http://running.competitor.com/2013/10/news/true-inspiration-from-91-year-old-runner_87694

Cornelissen, V. A., Fagard, R. H., Coeckelberghs, E., & Vanhees, L. (2011). Impact of resistance training on blood pressure and other cardiovascular risk factors: a meta-analysis of randomized, controlled trials. *Hypertension, 58*(5), 950–958.

Curtis, B. M., & O'Keefe, J. H. (2002). Autonomic tone as a cardiovascular risk factor: the dangers of chronic fight or flight. *Mayo Clinic Proceedings, 77*(1), 45–54.

Del Gobbo, L. C., Kalantarian, S., Imamura, F., Lemaitre, R., Siscovick, D. S., Psaty, B. M., & Mozaffarian, D. (2015). Contribution of major lifestyle risk factors for incident heart failure in older adults: the Cardiovascular Health Study. *JACC Heart Failure, 3*(7), 520–528.

Dokken, B. B. (2008). The pathophysiology of cardiovascular disease and diabetes: beyond blood pressure and lipids. *Diabetes Spectrum, 21*(3), 160–165.

Dorn, J., Naughton, J., Imamura, D., & Trevisan, M. (1999). Results of a multicenter randomized clinical trial of exercise and long-term survival in myocardial infarction patients: the National Exercise and Heart Disease Project (NEHDP). *Circulation, 100*(17), 1764–1769.

Feldman, D. I., Al-Mallah, M. H., Keteyian, S. J., Brawner, C. A., Feldman, T., Blumenthal, R. S., & Blaha, M. J. (2015). No evidence of an upper threshold for mortality benefit at high levels of cardiorespiratory fitness. *Journal of the American College of Cardiology, 65*(6), 629–630.

Fleg, J. L. (2012). Aerobic exercise in the elderly: a key to successful aging. *Discovery Medicine, 13*(70), 223–228.

Fleg, J. L., Morrell, C. H., Bos, A. G., Brant, L. J., Talbot, L. A., Wright, J. G., & Lakatta, E. G. (2005). Accelerated longitudinal decline of aerobic capacity in healthy older adults. *Circulation, 112*(5), 674–682.

Fogoros, R. N. (2017, Sept. 28). Exercise and HDL cholesterol. Verywell. Retrieved from https://www.verywell.com/exercise-and-hdl-cholesterol-1745833

Foreman, J. (2004, Mar. 29). Blood, sweat and insulin. *Boston Globe.*

Froelicher, V. (2010). Exercise and health, PM&R program. Cardiology.org. Retrieved from http://www.cardiology.org/slides.html

Fujimoto, N., Hastings, J. L., Bhella, P. S., Shibata, S., Gandhi, N. K., Carrick-Ranson, G., . . . Levine, B. D. (2012). Effect of ageing on left ventricular compliance and distensibility in healthy sedentary humans. *Journal of Physiology, 590*(Pt 8), 1871–1880.

Fujimoto, N., Hastings, J. L., Carrick-Ranson, G., Shafer, K. M., Shibata, S., Bhella, P. S., . . . Levine, B. D. (2013). Cardiovascular effects of 1 year of alagebrium and endurance exercise training in healthy older individuals. *Circulation Heart Failure, 6*(6), 1155–1164.

Fujimoto, N., Prasad, A., Hastings, J. L., Arbab-Zadeh, A., Bhella, P. S., Shibata, S., . . . Levine, B. D. (2010). Cardiovascular effects of 1 year of progressive and vigorous exercise training in previously sedentary individuals older than 65 years of age. *Circulation, 122*(18), 1797–1805.

Gillen, J. B., Martin, B. J., MacInnis, M. J., Skelly, L. E., Tarnopolsky, M. A., & Gibala, M. J. (2016). Twelve weeks of sprint interval training improves indices of cardiometabolic health similar to traditional endurance training despite a five-fold lower exercise volume and time commitment. *PLoS ONE, 11*(4), e0154075.

Goraya, T. Y., Jacobsen, S. J., Pellikka, P. A., Miller, T. D., Khan, A., Weston, S. A., . . . Roger, V. L. (2000). Prognostic value of treadmill exercise testing in elderly persons. *Annals of Internal Medicine, 132*(11), 862–870.

Gore, J. M. (2017, Oct. 12). Physical activity benefits patients with stable coronary disease. *NEJM Journal Watch.* Retrieved from https://www.jwatch.org/na45167/2017/10/12/physical-activity-benefits-patients-with-stable-coronary

Gormley, S. E., Swain, D. P., High, R., Spina, R. J., Dowling, E. A., Kotipalli, U. S., & Gandrakota, R. (2008). Effect of intensity of aerobic training on VO2max. *Medicine and Science in Sports and Exercise, 40*(7), 1336–1343.

Greenberg, A. (2015, Jun. 1). This 92-year-old is the oldest woman to ever run (and finish) a marathon. *Time Health.* Retrieved from http://time.com/3902968/marathon-oldest-woman-harriette-thompson-cancer/

Gremeaux, V., Gayda, M., Lepers, R., Sosner, P., Juneau, M., & Nigam, A. (2012). Exercise and longevity. *Maturitas, 73*(4), 312–317.

Gulati, M., Black, H. R., Shaw, L. J., Arnsdorf, M. F., Merz, C. N. B., Lauer, M. S., . . . Thisted, R. A. (2005). The prognostic value of a nomogram for exercise capacity in women. *New England Journal of Medicine, 353*(5), 468–475.

Gulati, M., Pandey, D. K., Arnsdorf, M. F., Lauderdale, D. S., Thisted, R. A., Wicklund, R. H., . . . Black, H. R. (2003). Exercise capacity and the risk of death in women: the St. James Women Take Heart Project. *Circulation, 108*(13), 1554–1559.

Haapanen, N., Miilunpalo, S., Vuori, I., Oja, P., & Pasanen, M. (1996). Characteristics of leisure time physical activity associated with decreased risk of premature all-cause and cardiovascular disease mortality in middle-aged men. *American Journal of Epidemiology, 143*(9), 870–880.

Hambrecht, R., Adams, V., Erbs, S., Linke, A., Kränkel, N., Shu, Y., . . . Schuler, G. (2003). Regular physical activity improves endothelial function in patients with coronary artery disease by increasing phosphorylation of endothelial nitric oxide synthase. *Circulation, 107*(25), 3152–3158.

Hambrecht, R., Walther, C., Möbius-Winkler, S., Gielen, S., Linke, A., Conradi, K., . . . Schuler, G. (2004). Percutaneous coronary angioplasty compared with exercise training in patients with stable coronary artery disease: a randomized trial. *Circulation, 109*(11), 1371–1378.

Hambrecht, R., Wolf, A., Gielen, S., Linke, A., Hofer, J., Erbs, S., . . . Schuler, G. (2000). Effect of exercise on coronary endothelial function in patients with coronary artery disease. *New England Journal of Medicine, 342*(7), 454–460.

Harris, K. M., Creswell, L. L., Haas, T. S., Thomas, T., Tung, T., Isaacson, E., . . . Maron, B. J. (2017). Death and cardiac arrest in U.S. triathlon participants, 1985–2016: a case series. *Annals of Internal Medicine, 167*(8), 529–535.

Hastings, J. L., Krainski, F., Snell, P. G., Pacini, E. L., Jain, M., Bhella, P. S., . . . Levine, B. D. (2012). Effect of rowing ergometry and oral volume loading on cardiovascular structure and function during bed rest. *Journal of Applied Physiology, 112*(10), 1735–1743.

Hawley, J. A., Hargreaves, M., Joyner, M. J., & Zierath, J. R. (2014). Integrative biology of exercise. *Cell, 159*(4), 738–749.

Healy, G. N., Dunstan, D. W., Salmon, J., Cerin, E., Shaw, J. E., Zimmet, P. Z., & Owen, N. (2007). Objectively measured light-intensity physical activity is independently associated with 2-h plasma glucose. *Diabetes Care, 30*(6), 1384–1389.

Heber, S., & Volf, I. (2015). Effects of physical (in)activity on platelet function. *BioMed Research International.* Article ID 165078.

Helgerud, J., Høydal, K., Wang, E., Karlsen, T., Berg, P., Bjerkaas, M., . . . Hoff, J. (2007). Aerobic high-intensity intervals improve VO2max more than moderate training. *Medicine and Science in Sports and Exercise, 39*(4), 665–671.

Helliker, K. (2015, Nov. 4). The potential cardiac dangers of extreme exercise. *Wall Street Journal.* Retrieved from https://www.wsj.com/articles/ the-potential-cardiac-dangers-of-extreme-exercise-1446681536

Howden, E. J., Sarma, S., Lawley, J. S., Opondo, M., Cornwell, W., Stoller, D., . . . Levine, B. D. (2018). Reversing the cardiac effects of sedentary aging in middle age—a randomized controlled trial: implications for heart failure prevention. *Circulation, 137*(15), 1549–1560.

Jackson, A. S., Sui, X., Hébert, J. R., Church, T. S., & Blair, S. N. (2009). Role of lifestyle and aging on the longitudinal change in cardiorespiratory fitness. *Archives of Internal Medicine, 169*(19), 1781–1787.

Kavanagh, T., Mertens, D. J., Hamm, L. F., Beyene, J., Kennedy, J., Corey, P., & Shephard, R. J. (2003). Peak oxygen intake and cardiac mortality in women referred for cardiac rehabilitation. *Journal of the American College of Cardiology, 42*(12), 2139–2143.

Kawano, M., Shono, N., Yoshimura, T., Yamaguchi, M., Hirano, T., & Hisatomi, A. (2009). Improved cardio-respiratory fitness correlates with changes in the number and size of small dense LDL: randomized controlled trial with exercise training and dietary instruction. *Internal Medicine, 48*(1), 25–32.

Kelley, G. A., Kelley, K. S., & Tran, Z. V. (2005). Exercise, lipids, and lipoproteins in older adults: a meta-analysis. *Preventive Cardiology, 8*(4), 206–214.

Khera, A., Mitchell, J. H., & Levine, B. D. (2007). Preventative cardiology: the effects of exercise. In Willerson, J. T., Wellens, H. J. J., Cohn, J. N., & Holmes, D. R. (Ed.), *Cardiovascular medicine* (pp. 2631–2648). London: Springer.

Kim, J. H., Malhotra, R., Chiapas, G., d'Hemecourt, P., Troyanos, C., Cianca, J., ... Baggish, A. L. (2012). Cardiac arrest during long-distance running races. *New England Journal of Medicine, 366*, 130–140.

Kodama, S., Saito, K., Tanaka, S., Maki, M., Yachi, Y., Asumi, M., . . . Sone, H. (2009). Cardiorespiratory fitness as a quantitative predictor of all-cause mortality and cardiovascular events in healthy men and women: a meta-analysis. *Journal of the American Medical Association, 301*(19), 2024–2035.

Kodama, S., Tanaka, S., Saito, K., Shu, M., Sone, Y., Onitake, F., ... Sone, H. (2007). Effect of aerobic exercise training on serum levels of high-density lipoprotein cholesterol: a meta-analysis. *Archives of Internal Medicine, 167*(10), 999–1008.

Kokkinos, P., & Myers, J. (2010). Exercise and physical activity: clinical outcomes and applications. *Circulation, 122*(16), 1637–1648.

Kokkinos, P., Myers, J., Faselis, C., Panagiotakos, D. B., Doumas, M., Pittaras, A., ... Fletcher, R. (2010). Exercise capacity and mortality in older men: a 20-year follow-up study. *Circulation, 122*(8), 790–797.

Kokkinos, P., Myers, J., Kokkinos, J. P., Pittaras, A., Narayan, P., Manolis, A., . . . Singh, S. (2008). Exercise capacity and mortality in black and white men. *Circulation, 117*(5), 614–622.

Kravitz, L. (2014). High-intensity interval training [brochure]. American College of Sports Medicine. Retrieved from https://www.acsm.org/docs/brochures/high-intensity-interval-training.pdf

Kroeger, L. (2017, Sept. 10). Mike Fremont, 95, seeks world record at Sept. 16 marathon. SHARE. Retrieved from http://local.cincinnati.com/share/story/252264

Kulshreshtha, A., Vaccarino, V., Judd, S., Howard, V. J., McClellan, W., Muntner, P., ... Cushman, M. (2013). Life's simple 7 and risk of incident stroke: Reasons for Geographic And Racial Differences in Stroke (REGARDS) Study. *Stroke, 44*(7), 1904–1914.

LaMonte, M. J., Blair, S. N., & Church, T. S. (2005). Physical activity and diabetes prevention. *Journal of Applied Physiology, 99*(3), 1205–1213.

Landry, C. H., Allan, K. S., Connelly, K. A., Cunningham, K., Morrison, L. J., & Dorian, P. (2017). Sudden cardiac arrest during participation in competitive sports. *New England Journal of Medicine, 377*, 1943–1953.

Larsson, S. C., Tektonidis, T. G., Gigante, B., Åkesson, A., & Wolk, A. (2016). Healthy lifestyle and risk of heart failure: results from 2 prospective cohort studies. *Circulation Heart Failure, 9*(4), e002855.

Lear, S. A., Hu, W., Rangarajan, S., Gasevic, D., Leong, D., Iqbal, R., ... Yusuf, S. (2017). The effect of physical activity on mortality and cardiovascular disease in 130 000 people from 17 high-income, middle-income, and low-income countries: the PURE study. *Lancet.* Retrieved from https://doi.org/10.1016/S0140-6736(17)31634-3.

Lee, D., Artero, E. G., Sui, X., & Blair, S. N. (2010). Mortality trends in the general population: the importance of cardiorespiratory fitness. *Journal of Psychopharmacology, 24*(4 Suppl), 27–35.

Lee, D., Pate, R. R., Lavie, C. J., Sui, X., Church, T. S., & Blair, S. N. (2014). Leisure-time running reduces all-cause and cardiovascular mortality risk. *Journal of the American College of Cardiology, 64*(5), 472–481.

Lee, I.-M., Shiroma, E. J., Evenson, K. R., Kamada, M., LaCroix, A. Z., & Buring, J. E. (2018). Accelerometer-measured physical activity and sedentary behavior in relation to all-cause mortality: the Women's Health Study. *Circulation, 137,* 203–205.

Leon, A. S., & Bloor, C. M. (1968). Effects of exercise and its cessation on the heart and its blood supply. *Journal of Applied Physiology, 24*(4), 485–490.

Leon, A. S., & Bloor, C. M. (1976). The effect of complete and partial deconditioning on exercise-induced cardiovascular changes in the rat. *Advances in Cardiology, 18,* 81–92.

Leon, A. S., & Bronas, U. G. (2009). Pathophysiology of coronary heart disease and biological mechanisms for the cardioprotective effects of regular aerobic exercise. *American Journal of Lifestyle Medicine, 3*(5), 379–385.

Leon, A. S., Gaskill, S. E., Rice, T., Bergeron, J., Gagnon, J., Rao, D. C., . . . Bouchard, C. (2002). Variability in the response of HDL cholesterol to exercise training in the HERITAGE Family Study. *International Journal of Sports Medicine, 23*(1), 1–9.

Leon, A. S., Rice, T., Mandel, S., Després, J. P., Bergeron, J., Gagnon, J., . . . Bouchard, C. (2000). Blood lipid response to 20 weeks of supervised exercise in a large biracial population: the HERITAGE Family Study. *Metabolism: Clinical and Experimental, 49*(4), 513–520.

Levine, B. D. (2014). Can intensive exercise harm the heart? The benefits of competitive endurance training for cardiovascular structure and function. *Circulation, 130*(12), 987–991.

Levine, J. (2014, Nov. 1). Killer chairs: how desk jobs ruin your health. *Scientific American.* Retrieved from https://www.scientificamerican.com/article/killer-chairs-how-desk-jobs-ruin-your-health/

Levine, J. A. (2015). Sick of sitting. *Diabetologia, 58*(8), 1751–1758.

Lieberman, D. (2014). *The story of the human body.* New York, NY: Vintage Books.

Lin, X., Zhang, X., Guo, J., Roberts, C. K., McKenzie, S., Wu, W.-C., . . . Song, Y. (2015). Effects of exercise training on cardiorespiratory fitness and biomarkers of cardiometabolic health: a systematic review and meta-analysis of randomized controlled trials. *Journal of the American Heart Association, 4*(7), e002014.

Linke, A., Schoene, N., Gielen, S., Hofer, J., Erbs, S., Schuler, G., & Hambrecht, R. (2001). Endothelial dysfunction in patients with chronic heart failure: systemic effects of lower-limb exercise training. *Journal of the American College of Cardiology, 37*(2), 392–397.

Litsky, F. (2004, Oct. 8). John A. Kelley, marathoner, dies at 97. *New York Times.* Retrieved from http://www.nytimes.com/2004/10/08/sports/othersports/john-a-kelley-marathoner-dies-at-97.html

Löllgen, H., Böckenhoff, A., & Knapp, G. (2009). Physical activity and all-cause mortality: an updated meta-analysis with different intensity categories. *International Journal of Sports Medicine, 30*(3), 213–224.

Macias-Cervantes, M. H., Rodriguez-Soto, J. M., Uribarri, J., Diaz-Cisneros, F. J., Cai, W., Garay-Sevilla, M. E. (2015). Effect of an advanced glycation end product-restricting diet and exercise on metabolic parameters in adult overweight men. *Nutrition, 31*(3), 446–451.

McMaster University. (2017, Sept. 21). Being active saves lives whether a gym workout, walking to work or washing the floor. *ScienceDaily.* Retrieved from www.sciencedaily.com/releases/2017/09/170921185009.htm

Moake, J. L. (n.d.) How blood clots. *Merck Manual* (*Consumer Version*). Retrieved from https://www.merckmanuals.com/home/blood-disorders/blood-clotting-process/how-blood-clots

Möbius-Winkler, S., Walther, C., Linke, A., Erbs, S., Gielen, S., Lenk, K., . . . Schuler, G. C. (2007). Abstract 3713: five-year follow-up of thePCI vs. Exercise Training in Stable Coronary Artery Disease Pilot Trial (PET-PILOT). *Circulation, 116*(Suppl 16), II_844.

Moholdt, T. T., Amundsen, B. H., Rustad, L. A., Wahba, A., Løvø, K. T., Gullikstad, L. R., . . . Slørdahl, S. A. (2009). Aerobic interval training versus continuous moderate exercise after coronary artery bypass surgery: a randomized study of cardiovascular effects and quality of life. *American Heart Journal, 158*(6), 1031–1037.

Mons, U., Hahmann, H., & Brenner, H. (2014). A reverse J-shaped association of leisure time physical activity with prognosis in patients with stable coronary heart disease: evidence from a large cohort with repeated measurements. *Heart, 100*(13), 1043–1049.

Mora, S., Redberg, R. F., Cui, Y., Whiteman, M. K., Flaws, J. A., Sharrett, A. R., & Blumenthal, R. S. (2003). Ability of exercise testing to predict cardiovascular and all-cause death in asymptomatic women: a 20-year follow-up of the Lipid Research Clinics Prevalence Study. *Journal of the American Medical Association, 290*(12), 1600–1607.

Mousavi, N., Czarnecki, A., Kumar, K., Fallah-Rad, N., Lytwyn, M., Han, S.-Y., . . . Jassal, D. S. (2009). Relation of biomarkers and cardiac magnetic resonance imaging after marathon running. *American Journal of Cardiology, 103*(10), 1467–1472.

Myers, J., Kaykha, A., George, S., Abella, J., Zaheer, N., Lear, S., . . . Froelicher, V. (2004). Fitness versus physical activity patterns in predicting mortality in men. *American Journal of Medicine, 117*(12), 912–918.

Myers, J., McAuley, P., Lavie, C. J., Despres, J.-P., Arena, R., & Kokkinos, P. (2015). Physical activity and cardiorespiratory fitness as major markers of cardiovascular risk: their independent and interwoven importance to health status. *Progress in Cardiovascular Diseases, 57*(4), 306–314.

Myers, J., Prakash, M., Froelicher, V., Do, D., Partington, S., & Atwood, J. E. (2002). Exercise capacity and mortality among men referred for exercise testing. *New England Journal of Medicine, 346*(11), 793–801.

Naci, H., & Ioannidis, J. P. A. (2013). Comparative effectiveness of exercise and drug interventions on mortality outcomes: metaepidemiology study. *British Medical Journal, 347*, f5577.

Naoki, F., Prasad, A., Hastings, J. L., Bhella, P. S., Shibata, S., Palmer, D., & Levine, B. D. (2012). Cardiovascular effects of 1 year of progressive endurance exercise training in patients with heart failure with preserved ejection fraction. *American Heart Journal, 164*(6), 869–877.

National Health Service. (2017). Any type of physical exercise is good for the heart. *NHS Choices.* Retrieved from https://www.nhs.uk/news/lifestyle-and-exercise/any-type-physical-exercise-good-heart/

National Heart, Lung and Blood Institute, National Institutes of Health. (2016, June 22). What is atherosclerosis? Retrieved from https://www.nhlbi.nih.gov/health/health-topics/topics/atherosclerosis

National Heart, Lung and Blood Institute, National Institutes of Health. (n.d.). What is cholesterol? Retrieved from https://www.nhlbi.nih.gov/health/health-topics/topics/hbc/

National Institute of Diabetes and Digestive and Kidney Diseases, National Institutes of Health. (2014, Sept.). The A1C test & diabetes. Retrieved from https://www.niddk.nih.gov/health-information/diabetes/overview/tests-diagnosis/a1c-test

Nes, B. M., Vatten, L. J., Nauman, J., Janszky, I., & Wisløff, U. (2014). A simple nonexercise model of cardiorespiratory fitness predicts long-term mortality. *Medicine and Science in Sports and Exercise, 46*(6), 1159–1165.

Niebauer, J., & Cooke, J. P. (1996). Cardiovascular effects of exercise: role of endothelial shear stress. *Journal of the American College of Cardiology, 28*(7), 1652–1660.

Nocon, M., Hiemann, T., Müller-Riemenschneider, F., Thalau, F., Roll, S., & Willich, S. N. (2008). Association of physical activity with all-cause and cardiovascular mortality: a systematic review and meta-analysis. *European Journal of Cardiovascular Prevention and Rehabilitation, 15*(3), 239–246.

Norcross, D. (2017, Jun. 4). 94-year-old woman makes history in San Diego Half Marathon. *San Diego Union-Tribune.* Retrieved from http://www.sandiegouniontribune.com/sports/sd-sp-rock-roll-marathon-winners-20170604-story.html

Ogden, C. L., Carroll, M. D., Fryar, C. D., & Flegal, K. M. (2015). Prevalence of obesity among adults and youth: United States, 2011–2014. *NCHS Data Brief, 219.* Retrieved from https://www.cdc.gov/nchs/data/databriefs/db219.pdf

O'Keefe, J. H., Patil, H. R., Lavie, C. J., Magalski, A., Vogel, R. A., & McCullough, P. A. (2012). Potential adverse cardiovascular effects from excessive endurance exercise. *Mayo Clinic Proceedings, 87*(6), 587–595.

Ornish, D., Scherwitz, L. W., Billings, J. H., Brown, S. E., Gould, K. L., Merritt, T. A., . . . Brand, R. J. (1998). Intensive lifestyle changes for reversal of coronary heart disease. *Journal of the American Medical Association, 280*(23), 2001–2007.

Osborn, C. O., & Falck, S. (2017). Type 1 and type 2 diabetes: what's the difference? *Healthline.* Retrieved from https://www.healthline.com/health/difference-between-type-1-and-type-2-diabetes

Ouchi, N., Parker, J. L., Lugus, J. J., & Walsh, K. (2011). Adipokines in inflammation and metabolic disease. *Nature Reviews Immunology, 11*(2), 85–97.

Parmenter, B. J., Dieberg, G., Phipps, G., & Smart, N. A. (2015). Exercise training for health-related quality of life in peripheral artery disease: a systematic review and meta-analysis. *Vascular Medicine, 20*(1), 30–40.

Parmenter, B. J., Raymond, J., Dinnen, P., Lusby, R. J., & Fiatarone Singh, M. A. (2013). High-intensity progressive resistance training improves flat-ground walking in older adults with symptomatic peripheral arterial disease. *Journal of the American Geriatrics Society, 61*(11), 1964–1970.

Piña, I. L., Apstein, C. S., Balady, G. J., Belardinelli, R., Chaitman, B. R., Duscha, B. D., . . . American Heart Association Committee on Exercise, Rehabilitation, and Prevention. (2003). Exercise and heart failure: a statement from the American Heart Association Committee on exercise, rehabilitation, and prevention. *Circulation, 107*(8), 1210–1225.

Pollock, M. L., Franklin, B. A., Balady, G. J., Chaitman, B. L., Fleg, J. L., Fletcher, B., . . . Bazzarre, T. (2000). AHA Science Advisory. Resistance exercise in individuals with and without cardiovascular disease: benefits, rationale, safety, and prescription. *Circulation, 101*(7), 828–833.

Qiu, S., Cai, X., Schumann, U., Velders, M., Sun, Z., & Steinacker, J. M. (2014), Impact of walking on glycemic control and other cardiovascular risk factors in type 2 diabetes: a meta-analysis. *PLoS ONE, 9*(10), e109767.

Reference Health. How many steps burn 1000 calories? (n.d.). Retrieved from https://www.reference.com/health/many-steps-burn-1000-calories-cb780cf847073dbd#

Reynolds, G. (2011, Dec. 21). For older runners, good news and bad. *New York Times, Well.* Retrieved from https://well.blogs.nytimes.com/2011/12/21/for-older-runners-good-news-and-bad/

Reynolds, G. (2015, May 6). An unexpected death rattles the fitness community. *New York Times.* Retrieved from https://well.blogs.nytimes.com/2015/05/06/an-unexpected-death-rattles-the-fitness-community/

Ritti-Dias, R. M., Wolosker, N., de Moraes Forjaz, C. L., Carvalho, C. R. F., Cucato, G. G., Leão, P. P., & de Fátima Nunes Marucci, M. (2010). Strength training increases walking tolerance in intermittent claudication patients: randomized trial. *Journal of Vascular Surgery, 51*(1), 89–95.

Rosenbaum, L. (2014, July 15). Extreme exercise and the heart. *New Yorker.* Retrieved from https://www.newyorker.com/tech/elements/extreme-exercise-and-the-heart

Ross, R., Blair, S. N., Arena, R., Church, T. S., Després, J.-P., Franklin, B. A., . . . Wisløff, U. (2016). Importance of assessing cardiorespiratory fitness in clinical practice: a case for fitness as a clinical vital sign: a scientific statement from the American Heart Association. *Circulation, 134*(24), e653–e699.

Runners who dread slowing down can get faster even as they get older. (2013, Jun. 9). *The Columbian.* Retrieved from http://www.columbian.com/news/2013/jun/09/runners-who-dread-slowing-down-can-get-faster-even/

Sagar, V. A., Davies, E. J., Briscoe, S., Coats, A. J., Dalal, H. M., Lough, F., . . . Taylor, R. S. (2015). Exercise-based rehabilitation for heart failure: systematic review and meta-analysis. *Open Heart, 2*(1), e000163.

Samitz, G., Egger, M., & Zwahlen, M. (2011). Domains of physical activity and all-cause mortality: systematic review and dose-response meta-analysis of cohort studies. *International Journal of Epidemiology, 40*(5), 1382–1400.

Sanchis-Gomar, F., Lucia, A., & Levine, B. D. (2016). Editorial commentary: relationship between strenuous exercise and cardiac "morbimortality": benefits outweigh the potential risks. *Trends in Cardiovascular Medicine, 26*(3), 241–244.

Sattelmair, J., Pertman, J., Ding, E. L., Kohl, H. W., Haskell, W., & Lee, I.-M. (2011). Dose-response between physical activity and risk of coronary heart disease: a meta-analysis. *Circulation, 124*(7), 789–795.

Schnohr, P., Marott, J. L., Jensen, J. S., & Jensen, G. B. (2012). Intensity versus duration of cycling, impact on all-cause and coronary heart disease mortality: the Copenhagen City Heart Study. *European Journal of Preventive Cardiology, 19*(1), 73–80.

Schnohr, P., Marott, J. L., Lange, P., & Jensen, G. B. (2013). Longevity in male and female joggers: the Copenhagen City Heart Study. *American Journal of Epidemiology, 177*(7), 683–689.

Schnohr, P., O'Keefe, J. H., Marott, J. L., Lange, P., & Jensen, G. B. (2015). Dose of jogging and long-term mortality: the Copenhagen City Heart Study. *Journal of the American College of Cardiology, 65*(5), 411–419.

Shibata, S., & Levine, B. D. (2012). Effect of exercise training on biologic vascular age in healthy seniors. *American Journal of Physiology—Heart and Circulatory Physiology, 302*(6), H1340–H1346.

Simmons, R. K., Griffin, S. J., Steele, R., Wareham, N. J., & Ekelund, U., on behalf of the ProActive Research Team. (2008). Increasing overall physical activity and aerobic fitness is associated with improvements in metabolic risk: cohort analysis of the ProActive trial. *Diabetologia, 51*(5), 787–794.

Simon, H. B. (2015). Exercise and health: dose and response, considering both ends of the curve. *American Journal of Medicine, 128*(11), 1171–1177.

Skinner, J. S., Wilmore, K. M., Krasnoff, J. B., Jaskólski, A., Jaskólska, A., Gagnon, J., . . . Bouchard, C. (2000). Adaptation to a standardized training program and changes in fitness in a large, heterogeneous population: the HERITAGE Family Study. *Medicine and Science in Sports and Exercise, 32*(1), 157–161.

Slattery, M. L., Jacobs, D. R., & Nichaman, M. Z. (1989). Leisure time physical activity and coronary heart disease death: the US Railroad Study. *Circulation, 79*(2), 304–311.

Smyth, A., O'Donnell, M., Lamelas, P., Teo, K., Rangarajan, S., Yusuf, S., & INTERHEART Investigators. (2016). Physical activity and anger or emotional upset as triggers of acute myocardial infarction: the INTERHEART Study. *Circulation, 134*(15), 1059–1067.

Snedeker, J. G., & Gautieri, A. (2014). The role of collagen crosslinks in ageing and diabetes—the good, the bad, and the ugly. *Muscles, Ligaments and Tendons Journal, 4*(3), 303–308.

Stathokostas, L., Jacob-Johnson, S., Petrella, R. J., & Paterson, D. H. (2004). Longitudinal changes in aerobic power in older men and women. *Journal of Applied Physiology, 97*(2), 781–789.

Stephens, B. R., Granados, K., Zderic, T. W., Hamilton, M. T., & Braun, B. (2011). Effects of 1 day of inactivity on insulin action in healthy men and women: interaction with energy intake. *Metabolism: Clinical and Experimental, 60*(7), 941–949.

Sui, X., Jackson, A. S., Church, T. S., Lee, D.-C., O'Connor, D. P., Liu, J., & Blair, S. N. (2012). Effects of cardiorespiratory fitness on aging: glucose trajectory in a cohort of healthy men. *Annals of Epidemiology, 22*(9), 617–622.

Taylor, R. S., Brown, A., Ebrahim, S., Jolliffe, J., Noorani, H., Rees, K., . . . Oldridge, N. (2004). Exercise-based rehabilitation for patients with coronary heart disease: systematic review and meta-analysis of randomized controlled trials. *American Journal of Medicine, 116*(10), 682–692.

Thompson, P. D., Funk, E. J., Carleton, R. A., & Sturner, W. Q. (1982). Incidence of death during jogging in Rhode Island from 1975 through 1980. *Journal of the American Medical Association, 247*(18), 2535–2538.

Tjonna, A. E., Stolen, T. O., Bye, A., Volden, M., Slordahl, S. A., Odegard, R., . . . Wisloff, U. (2009). Aerobic interval training reduces cardiovascular risk factors more than a multi-treatment approach in overweight adolescents. *Clinical Science, 116*(4), 317–326.

Trappe, S. W., Costill, D. L., Vukovich, M. D., Jones, J., & Melham, T. (1996). Aging among elite distance runners: a 22-yr longitudinal study. *Journal of Applied Physiology, 80*(1), 285–290.

Trappe, S., Hayes, E., Galpin, A., Kaminsky, L., Jemiolo, B., Fink, W., . . . Tesch, P. (2013). New records in aerobic power among octogenarian lifelong endurance athletes. *Journal of Applied Physiology, 114*(1), 3–10.

Trivax, J. E., & McCullough, P. A. (2012). Phidippides cardiomyopathy: a review and case illustration. *Clinical Cardiology, 35*(2), 69–73.

US Department of Health and Human Services. (2008). Physical activity guidelines for Americans. Retrieved from https://health.gov/paguidelines/guidelines/summary. aspx

Wang, Y., Tuomilehto, J., Jousilahti, P., Antikainen, R., Mähönen, M., Katzmarzyk, P. T., & Hu, G. (2011). Lifestyle factors in relation to heart failure among finnish men and women. *Circulation Heart Failure, 4*(5), 607–612.

Warburton, D. E. R., McKenzie, D. C., Haykowsky, M. J., Taylor, A., Shoemaker, P., Ignaszewski, A. P., & Chan, S. Y. (2005). Effectiveness of high-intensity interval training for the rehabilitation of patients with coronary artery disease. *American Journal of Cardiology, 95*(9), 1080–1084.

Watson, K. B., Carlson, S. A., Gunn, J. P, Galuska, D. A., O'Connor, A., Greenlund, K. J., & Fulton, J. E. (2016). Physical inactivity among adults aged 50 years and older—United States, 2014. *Morbidity and Mortality Weekly Report, 65*(36), 954–958.

Wen, C. P., Wai, J. P. M., Tsai, M. K., Yang, Y. C., Cheng, T. Y. D., Lee, M.-C., . . . Wu, X. (2011). Minimum amount of physical activity for reduced mortality and extended life expectancy: a prospective cohort study. *Lancet, 378*(9798), 1244–1253.

Wienbergen, H., & Hambrecht, R. (2013). Physical exercise and its effects on coronary artery disease. *Current Opinion in Pharmacology, 13*(2), 218–225.

Wilmore, J. H., Green, J. S., Stanforth, P. R., Gagnon, J., Rankinen, T., Leon, A. S., . . . Bouchard, C. (2001). Relationship of changes in maximal and submaximal aerobic fitness to changes in cardiovascular disease and non-insulin-dependent diabetes mellitus risk factors with endurance training: the HERITAGE Family Study. *Metabolism: Clinical and Experimental, 50*(11), 1255–1263.

Wilmore, J. H., Stanforth, P. R., Gagnon, J., Rice, T., Mandel, S., Leon, A. S., . . . Bouchard, C. (2001). Heart rate and blood pressure changes with endurance training: the HERITAGE Family Study. *Medicine and Science in Sports and Exercise, 33*(1), 107–116.

Wilson, T. M., & Tanaka, H. (2000). Meta-analysis of the age-associated decline in maximal aerobic capacity in men: relation to training status. *American Journal of Physiology. Heart and Circulatory Physiology, 278*(3), H829–H834.

Wisløff, U., Støylen, A., Loennechen, J. P., Bruvold, M., Rognmo, Ø., Haram, P. M., . . . Skjaerpe, T. (2007). Superior cardiovascular effect of aerobic interval training versus moderate continuous training in heart failure patients: a randomized study. *Circulation, 115*(24), 3086–3094.

Wood, M. (2017, September 21). What is heart rate variability training? [Web log post]. Michael Wood Fitness. Retrieved from https://michaelwoodfitness.com/2017/09/21/what-is-heart-rate-variability-training/

CHAPTER 5

American Physiological Society. (2015). Could the bioenergetic health index become the next BMI?. *American Physiological Society Press Release*. Retrieved from http://www.the-aps.org/mm/hp/Audiences/Public-Press/2015-49.html

Austad, S. N. (1997). Why we age: what science is discovering about the body's journey through life. New York, NY: John Wiley & Sons, p. 126.

Bartlett, J. D., Close, G. L., Drust, B., & Morton, J. P. (2014). The emerging role of p53 in exercise metabolism. *Sports Medicine (Auckland, N.Z.), 44*(3), 303–309.

Bartlett, J. D., Close, G. L., MacLaren, D. P. M., Gregson, W., Drust, B., & Morton, J. P. (2011). High-intensity interval running is perceived to be more enjoyable than moderate-intensity continuous exercise: implications for exercise adherence. *Journal of Sports Sciences, 29*(6), 547–553.

Billat, V., Dhonneur, G., Mille-Hamard, L., Moyec, L. L., Momken, I., Launay, T., . . . Besse, S. (2017). Case studies in physiology: maximal oxygen consumption and performance in a centenarian cyclist. *Journal of Applied Physiology, 122*(3), 430–434.

Boutcher, S. H. (2011). High-intensity intermittent exercise and fat loss. *Journal of Obesity, 2011*, 868305. Retrieved from http://doi.org/10.1155/2011/868305

Bratic, A., & Larsson, N.-G. (2013). The role of mitochondria in aging. *Journal of Clinical Investigation, 123*(3), 951–957.

Bruno, N. E., Kelly, K. A., Hawkins, R., Bramah-Lawani, M., Amelio, A. L., Nwachukwu, J. C., . . . Conkright, M. D. (2014). Creb coactivators direct anabolic responses and enhance performance of skeletal muscle. *EMBO Journal, 33*(9), 1027–1043.

Burgomaster, K. A., Heigenhauser, G. J. F., & Gibala, M. J. (2006). Effect of short-term sprint interval training on human skeletal muscle carbohydrate metabolism during exercise and time-trial performance. *Journal of Applied Physiology, 100*(6), 2041–2047.

Burgomaster, K. A., Howarth, K. R., Phillips, S. M., Rakobowchuk, M., Macdonald, M. J., McGee, S. L., & Gibala, M. J. (2008). Similar metabolic adaptations during exercise after low-volume sprint interval and traditional endurance training in humans. *Journal of Physiology, 586*(1), 151–160.

Burgomaster, K. A., Hughes, S. C., Heigenhauser, G. J. F., Bradwell, S. N., & Gibala, M. J. (2005). Six sessions of sprint interval training increases muscle oxidative potential and cycle endurance capacity in humans. *Journal of Applied Physiology, 98*(6), 1985–1990.

Butler, S. L. (2018, Jan. 9). California woman qualifies for Olympic Marathon Trials at age 50. *Runner's World.*

Cann, R., Stoneking, M., & Wilson, A. C. (1987). Mitochondrial DNA and human evolution. *Nature, 325,* 31–36.

Centers for Disease Control and Prevention. (2015). How much physical activity do adults need? Retrieved from https://www.cdc.gov/physicalactivity/basics/adults/

Cheema, N., Herbst, A., McKenzie, D., & Aiken, J. M. (2015). Apoptosis and necrosis mediate skeletal muscle fiber loss in age-induced mitochondrial enzymatic abnormalities. *Aging Cell, 14*(6), 1085–1093.

Cobb, L. J., Lee, C., Xiao, J., Yen, K., Wong, R. G., Nakamura, H. K., . . . Cohen, P. (2016). Naturally occurring mitochondrial-derived peptides are age-dependent regulators of apoptosis, insulin sensitivity, and inflammatory markers. *Aging (Albany, NY), 8*(4), 796–808.

Crane, J. D., Devries, M. C., Safdar, A., Hamadeh, M. J., & Tarnopolsky, M. A. (2010). The effect of aging on human skeletal muscle mitochondrial and intramyocellular lipid ultrastructure. *Journals of Gerontology Series A: Biological Sciences and Medical Sciences, 65*(2), 119–128.

Crane, J. D., Ogborn, D. I., Cupido, C., Melov, S., Hubbard, A., Bourgeois, J. M., & Tarnopolsky, M. A. (2012). Massage therapy attenuates inflammatory signaling after exercise-induced muscle damage. *Science Translational Medicine, 4*(119), 119ra13.

DiCarlo, S. E., & Collins, H. L. (2001). Estimating ATP resynthesis during a marathon run: a method to introduce metabolism. *Advances in Physiology Education, 25*(2), 70–71.

Ding, W.-X., & Yin, X.-M. (2012). Mitophagy: mechanisms, pathophysiological roles, and analysis. *Biological Chemistry, 393*(7), 547–564.

Eaves, A. (2016, May 12). New study pits a 10-minute interval workout against 50 minutes of traditional cardio. *Men's Health.* Retrieved from http://www.menshealth.com/fitness/10-minute-sprint-interval-workout-benefits

Energy Production. (n.d.). *Wellcome Trust Centre for Mitochondrial Research Newcastle.* Retrieved from http://www.newcastle-mitochondria.com/patient-and-public-home-page/energy-production

Finsterer, J. (2007). Hematological manifestations of primary mitochondrial disorders. *Acta Haematologica, 118*(2), 88–98.

Fisher-Wellman, K. H., & Neufer, P. D. (2012). Linking mitochondrial bioenergetics to insulin resistance via redox biology. *Trends in Endocrinology and Metabolism, 23*(3), 142–153.

Gianni, P., Jan, K. J., Douglas, M. J., Stuart, P. M., & Tarnopolsky, M. A. (2004). Oxidative stress and the mitochondrial theory of aging in human skeletal muscle. *Experimental Gerontology, 39*(9), 1391–1400.

Gibala, M. (2017). *The one-minute workout: science shows a way to get fit that's smarter, faster, shorter*. New York, NY: Penguin Random House.

Gibala, M. J., & Jones, A. M. (2013). Physiological and performance adaptations to high-intensity interval training. *Nestle Nutrition Institute Workshop Series, 76*, 51–60.

Gibala, M. J., Little, J. P., Macdonald, M. J., & Hawley, J. A. (2012). Physiological adaptations to low-volume, high-intensity interval training in health and disease. *Journal of Physiology, 590*(5), 1077–1084.

Gibala, M. J., Little, J. P., van Essen, M., Wilkin, G. P., Burgomaster, K. A., Safdar, A., . . . Tarnopolsky, M. A. (2006). Short-term sprint interval versus traditional endurance training: similar initial adaptations in human skeletal muscle and exercise performance. *Journal of Physiology, 575*(Pt 3), 901–911.

Gillen, C. M. (2014). *The hidden mechanics of exercise: molecules that move us*. Cambridge, MA: The Belknap Press of Harvard University.

Gillen, J. B., Percival, M. E., Skelly, L. E., Martin, B. J., Tan, R. B., Tarnopolsky, M. A., & Gibala, M. J. (2014). Three minutes of all-out intermittent exercise per week increases skeletal muscle oxidative capacity and improves cardiometabolic health. *PLoS ONE, 9*(11), e111489.

Gliemann, L., Gunnarsson, T. P., Hellsten, Y., & Bangsbo, J. (2015). 10-20-30 training increases performance and lowers blood pressure and VEGF in runners. *Scandinavian Journal of Medicine & Science in Sports, 25*(5), e479–e489.

Gray, M. W. (2012). Mitochondrial evolution. *Cold Spring Harbor Perspectives in Biology, 4*(9), a011403.

Grierson, B. (2010, Nov. 25). The incredible flying nonagenarian. *New York Times*.

Hales, K. G. (2010). Mitochondrial fusion and division. *Nature Education, 3*(9), 12.

Hawley, J. A., Hargreaves, M., Joyner, M. J., & Zierath J. R. (2014). Integrative biology of exercise. *Cell, 159*(4), 738–749.

Heisz, J. J., Tejada, M. G. M., Paolucci, E. M., & Muir, C. (2016). Enjoyment for high-intensity interval exercise increases during the first six weeks of training: implications for promoting exercise adherence in sedentary adults. *PLoS ONE, 11*(12), e0168534.

Hepple, R. T. (2014). Mitochondrial involvement and impact in aging skeletal muscle. *Frontiers in Aging Neuroscience, 6*, 211.

Holloszy, J. O. (1967). Biochemical adaptations in muscle: effects of exercise on mitochondrial oxygen uptake and respiratory enzyme activity in skeletal muscle. *Journal of Biological Chemistry, 242*(9), 2278–2282.

Holloszy, J. O., & Coyle, E. F. (1984). Adaptations of skeletal muscle to endurance exercise and their metabolic consequences. *Journal of Applied Physiology: Respiratory, Environmental and Exercise Physiology, 56*(4), 831–838.

Hood, D. A. (2001). Invited review: contractile activity-induced mitochondrial biogenesis in skeletal muscle. *Journal of Applied Physiology (Bethesda, MD: 1985), 90*(3), 1137–1157.

Hood, D. A. (2009). Mechanisms of exercise-induced mitochondrial biogenesis in skeletal muscle. *Applied Physiology, Nutrition, and Metabolism, 34*(3), 465–472.

Hood, D. A., Irrcher, I., Ljubicic, V., & Joseph, A.-M. (2006). Coordination of metabolic plasticity in skeletal muscle. *Journal of Experimental Biology, 209*(12), 2265–2275.

Hood, D. A., Uguccioni, G., Vainshtein, A., & D'souza, D. (2011). Mechanisms of exercise-induced mitochondrial biogenesis in skeletal muscle: implications for health and disease. *Comprehensive Physiology, 1*(3), 1119–1134.

Hood, D. A., Zak, R., & Pette, D. (1989). Chronic stimulation of rat skeletal muscle induces coordinate increases in mitochondrial and nuclear mRNAs of cytochrome-c-oxidase subunits. *European Journal of Biochemistry, 179*(2), 275–280.

Karp, J. (2009, Feb.). The three metabolic energy systems. *IDEA Fitness Journal*. Retrieved from http://www.ideafit.com/fitness-library/the-three-metabolic-energy-systems

Karstoft, K., Winding, K., Knudsen, S. H., Nielsen, J. S., Thomsen, C., Pedersen, B. K., & Solomon, T. P. J. (2013). The effects of free-living interval-walking training on glycemic control, body composition, and physical fitness in type 2 diabetic patients: a randomized, controlled trial. *Diabetes Care, 36*(2), 228–236.

Khan Academy. (n.d.). Oxidative phosphorylation. Retrieved from https://www.khanacademy.org/science/biology/cellular-respiration-and-fermentation/oxidative-phosphorylation/a/oxidative-phosphorylation-etc

Kohl, T., Weninger, G., Zalk, R., Eaton, P., & Lehnart, S. E. (2015). Intensity matters: ryanodine receptor regulation during exercise. *Proceedings of the National Academy of Sciences of the United States of America, 112*(50), 15271–15272.

Laursen, P. B. (2010). Training for intense exercise performance: high-intensity or high-volume training? *Scandinavian Journal of Medicine & Science in Sports, 20*(Suppl 2), 1–10.

Lazarou, M. (2015). Keeping the immune system in check: a role for mitophagy. *Immunology and Cell Biology, 93*(1), 3–10.

Lee, D., Pate, R. R., Lavie, C. J., Sui, X., Church, T. S., & Blair, S. N. (2014). Leisure-time running reduces all-cause and cardiovascular mortality risk. *Journal of the American College of Cardiology, 64*(5), 472.

Lin, J., Handschin, C., & Spiegelman, B. M. (2005). Metabolic control through the PGC-1 family of transcription coactivators. *Cell Metabolism, 1*(6), 361–370.

Lindholm, M., & Appel, S. W. (2012). On your bike: how muscles respond to exercise. *Science in School* (23). Retrieved from http://www.scienceinschool.org/2012/issue23/exercise

López-Otín, C., Blasco, M. A., Partridge, L., Serrano, M., & Kroemer, G. (2013). The hallmarks of aging. *Cell, 153*(6), 1194–1217.

Lunt, H., Draper, N., Marshall, H. C., Logan, F. J., Hamlin, M. J., Shearman, J. P., . . . Frampton, C. M. A. (2014). High intensity interval training in a real world setting: a randomized controlled feasibility study in overweight inactive adults, measuring change in maximal oxygen uptake. *PLoS ONE, 9*(1), e83256.

MacInnis, M. J., & Gibala, M. J. (2016). Physiological adaptations to interval training and the role of exercise intensity. *Journal of Physiology*. Retrieved from http://dx.doi.org/10.1113/JP273196

MacInnis, M. J., Zacharewicz, E., Martin, B. J., Haikalis, M. E., Skelly, L. E., Tarnopolsky, M. A., . . . Gibala, M. J. (2017). Superior mitochondrial adaptations in human skeletal muscle after interval compared to continuous single-leg cycling matched for total work. *Journal of Physiology, 595*(1), 2955–2968.

Martin, W. F, & Mentel M. (2010). The origin of mitochondria, *Nature Education, 3*(9), 58.

Menshikova, E. V., Ritov, V. B., Fairfull, L., Ferrell, R. E., Kelley, D. E., & Goodpaster, B. H. (2006). Effects of exercise on mitochondrial content and function in aging human skeletal muscle. *Journals of Gerontology Series A: Biological Sciences and Medical Sciences, 61*(6), 534–540.

Mitochondria. (n.d.). *Scitable by Nature Education*. Retrieved from http://www.nature.com/scitable/topicpage/mitochondria-14053590

Moholdt, T. T., Amundsen, B. H., Rustad, L. A., Wahba, A., Løvø, K. T., Gullikstad, L. R., . . . Slørdahl, S. A. (2009). Aerobic interval training versus continuous moderate exercise after coronary artery bypass surgery: a randomized study of cardiovascular effects and quality of life. *American Heart Journal, 158*(6), 1031–1037.

National Science Foundation. (n.d.). The President's National Medal of Science: recipient details, Lynn Margulis. Retrieved from https://www.nsf.gov/od/nms/recip_details.jsp?recip_id=228

Ní Chéilleachair, N. J., Harrison, A. J., & Warrington, G. D. (2017). HIIT enhances endurance performance and aerobic characteristics more than high-volume training in trained rowers. *Journal of Sports Sciences, 35*(11), 1052–1058.

Olga Kotelko. (2018). *Wikipedia.* Retrieved from https://en.wikipedia.org/wiki/Olga_Kotelko

Olga Kotelko, track and field notable, dies at 95 amid book fame. (2014, Jun. 25). *Times of San Diego.*

Parikh, S., Goldstein, A., Koenig, M. K., Scaglia, F., Enns, G. M., Saneto, R., . . . DiMauro, S. (2015). Diagnosis and management of mitochondrial disease: a consensus statement from the Mitochondrial Medicine Society. *Genetics in Medicine: Official Journal of the American College of Medical Genetics, 17*(9), 689–701.

Place, N., Ivarsson, N., Venckunas, T., Neyroud, D., Brazaitis, M., Cheng, A. J., . . . Westerblad, H. (2015). Ryanodine receptor fragmentation and sarcoplasmic reticulum Ca2+ leak after one session of high-intensity interval exercise. *Proceedings of the National Academy of Sciences of the United States of America, 112*(50), 15492–15497

Polley, K. R., Jenkins, N., O'Connor, P., & McCully, K. (2015). Influence of exercise training with resveratrol supplementation on skeletal muscle mitochondrial capacity. *Applied Physiology, Nutrition, and Metabolism, 41*(1), 26–32.

Psilander, N. (2014). The effect of different exercise regiments on mitochondrial biogenesis and performance. *Karolinska Institutet.* Retrieved from http://gih.diva-portal.org/smash/get/diva2:766681/FULLTEXT01.pdf

Psilander, N., Niklas, P., Wang, L., Li, W., Westergren, J., Jens, W., . . . Kent, S. (2010). Mitochondrial gene expression in elite cyclists: effects of high-intensity interval exercise. *European Journal of Applied Physiology, 110*(3), 597–606.

Puigserver, P., Wu, Z., Park, C. W., Graves, R., Wright, M., & Spiegelman, B. M. (1998). A cold-inducible coactivator of nuclear receptors linked to adaptive thermogenesis. *Cell, 92*(6), 829–839.

Reynolds, G. (2011). Overestimating how hard we exercise. *New York Times.* Retrieved from https://well.blogs.nytimes.com/2014/06/11/judging-badly-how-hard-we-exercise/?_r=0

Reynolds, G. (2013). *The first 20 minutes: surprising science reveals how we can exercise better, train smarter, live longer.* New York, NY: Penguin.

Reynolds, G. (2017, Feb. 8). Lessons on aging well, from a 105-year-old cyclist. *New York Times.* Retrieved from https://www.nytimes.com/2017/02/08/well/move/lessons-on-aging-well-from-a-105-year-old-cyclist.html

Ristow, M., Zarse, K., Oberbach, A., Klöting, N., Birringer, M., Kiehntopf, M., . . . Blüher, M. (2009). Antioxidants prevent health-promoting effects of physical exercise in humans. *Proceedings of the National Academy of Sciences of the United States of America, 106*(21), 8665–8670.

Robinson, M. M., Dasari, S., Konopka, A. R., Johnson, M. L., Manjuanatha, S., & Esponda, R. R. (2017). Enhanced protein translation underlies improved metabolic and physical adaptations to different exercise training modes in young and old humans. *Cell Metabolism, 25*(3), 581–592.

Safdar, A., Bourgeois, J. M., Ogborn, D. I., Little, J. P., Hettinga, B. P., Akhar, M., . . . Tarnopolsky, M. A. (2011). Endurance exercise rescues progeroid aging and induces systemic mitochondrial rejuvenation in mtDNA mutator mice. *Proceedings* of the *National Academy of Sciences of the United States of America*, 108(10), 4135–4140.

Safdar, A., Little, J. P., Stokl, A. J., Hettinga, B. P., Akhtar, M., & Tarnopolsky, M. A. (2011). Exercise increases mitochondrial PGC-1alpha content and promotes nuclear-mitochondrial cross-talk to coordinate mitochondrial biogenesis. *Journal of Biological Chemistry*, 286(12), 10605–10617.

Taivassalo, T., & Haller, R. G. (2005). Exercise and training in mitochondrial myopathies. *Medicine and Science in Sports and Exercise*, 37(12), 2094–2101.

Terjung, R. L. (1995). Muscle adaptations to aerobic training. *Sports Science Exchange*, 54(8). Retrieved from http://www.gssiweb.org/Article/sse-54-muscle- adaptations-to-aerobic-training

Tjønna, A. E., Stølen, T. O., Bye, A., Volden, M., Slørdahl, S. A., Odegård, R., . . . Wisløff, U. (2009). Aerobic interval training reduces cardiovascular risk factors more than a multitreatment approach in overweight adolescents. *Clinical Science (London, England: 1979)*, 116(4), 317–326.

Treadwell, B.V., (2014). Endurance exercise: keeping the mitochondria furnaces burning. *Juvenon* 7(10). Retrieved from http://www.juvenon.com/endurance-exercise-keeping-the-mitochondria-furnaces-burning-1008/

Valero, T. (2014). Mitochondrial biogenesis: pharmacological approaches. *Current Pharmaceutical Design*, 20(35), 5507–5509.

Warburton, D. E. R., McKenzie, D. C., Haykowsky, M. J., Taylor, A., Shoemaker, P., Ignaszewski, A. P., & Chan, S. Y. (2005). Effectiveness of high-intensity interval training for the rehabilitation of patients with coronary artery disease. *American Journal of Cardiology*, 95(9), 1080–1084.

Whitaker, R. M., Corum, D., Beeson, C. C., & Schnellmann, R. G. (2016). Mitochondrial biogenesis as a pharmacological target: a new approach to acute and chronic diseases. *Annual Review of Pharmacology and Toxicology*, 56, 229–249.

Wisløff, U., Støylen, A., Loennechen, J. P., Bruvold, M., Rognmo, Ø., Haram, P. M., . . . Skjaerpe, T. (2007). Superior cardiovascular effect of aerobic interval training versus moderate continuous training in heart failure patients: a randomized study. *Circulation*, 115(24), 3086–3094.

Wu, Z., Puigserver, P., Andersson, U., Zhang, C., Adelmant, G., Mootha, V., . . . Spiegelman, B. M. (1999). Mechanisms controlling mitochondrial biogenesis and respiration through the thermogenic coactivator PGC-1. *Cell*, 98(1), 115–124.

Youle, R. J., & Narendra, D. P. (2011). Mechanisms of mitophagy. *Nature Reviews Molecular Cell Biology*, 12(1), 9–14.

Zhang, Y., Uguccioni, G., Ljubicic, V., Irrcher, I., Iqbal, S., Singh, K., . . . Hood, D. A. (2014). Multiple signaling pathways regulate contractile activity-mediated PGC-1a gene expression and activity in skeletal muscle cells. *Physiological Reports*, 2(5), e12008.

Zhang, Z.-W., Cheng, J., Xu, F., Chen, Y.-E., Du, J.-B., Yuan, M., . . . Yuan, S. (2011). Red blood cell extrudes nucleus and mitochondria against oxidative stress. *IUBMB Life*, 63(7), 560–565.

Zong, W.-X., Rabinowitz, J. D., & White, E. (2016). Mitochondria and cancer. *Molecular Cell*, 61(5), 667–676.

CHAPTER 6

Adams, G. R. (2002). Invited review: autocrine/paracrine IGF-I and skeletal muscle adaptation. *Journal of Applied Physiology (Bethesda, MD: 1985)*, 93(3), 1159–1167.

Ahima, R. S., & Park, H. K. (2015). Connecting myokines and metabolism. *Endocrinology and Metabolism (Seoul, Korea)*, 30(3), 235–245.

Andrews, M. A. W. (2003). How does exercise make your muscles stronger? *Scientific American*. Retrieved from https://www.scientificamerican.com/article/how-does-exercise-make-yo/

Aragon, A. A., & Schoenfeld, B. J. (2013). Nutrient timing revisited: is there a post-exercise anabolic window? *Journal of the International Society of Sports Nutrition, 10*(1), 5.

Associated Press. (2007, May 30). Rare condition gives toddler super strength. *CTV News*. Retrieved from http://www.ctvnews.ca/rare-condition-gives-toddler-super-strength-1.243163

Balakrishnan, V. S., Rao, M., Menon, V., Gordon, P. L., Pilichowska, M., Castaneda, F., & Castaneda-Sceppa, C. (2010). Resistance training increases muscle mitochondrial biogenesis in patients with chronic kidney disease. *Clinical Journal of the American Society of Nephrology, 5*(6), 996–1002.

Bassel-Duby, R., & Olson, E. N. (2006). Signaling pathways in skeletal muscle remodeling. *Annual Review of Biochemistry, 75*, 19–37.

Bazgir, B., Fathi, R., Rezazadeh Valojerdi, M., Mozdziak, P., & Asgari, A. (2016). Satellite cells contribution to exercise mediated muscle hypertrophy and repair. *Cell Journal (Yakhteh), 18*(4), 473–484.

BBC Science & Nature. (2014). Human body and mind—muscles layer. Retrieved from http://www.bbc.co.uk/science/humanbody/body/factfiles/workinpairs/biceps_animation.shtml

Bell, K. E., Snijders, T., Zulyniak, M., Kumbhare, D., Parie, G., Chabowski, A., . . . Phillips, S. M. (2017). A whey protein-based multi-ingredient nutritional supplement stimulates gains in lean body mass and strength in healthy older men: a randomized controlled study. *PLoS ONE, 12*(7), e0181387.

Benatti, F. B., & Pedersen, B. K. (2015). Exercise as an anti-inflammatory therapy for rheumatic diseases-myokine regulation. *Nature Reviews Rheumatology, 11*(2), 86–97.

Bischoff, R. (1986). A satellite cell mitogen from crushed adult muscle. *Developmental Biology, 115*(1), 140–147.

Bischoff, R. (1989). Analysis of muscle regeneration using single myofibers in culture. *Medicine and Science in Sports and Exercise, 21*(5 Suppl), S164–S172.

Boström, P., Wu, J., Jedrychowski, M. P., Korde, A., Ye, L., Lo, J. C., . . . Spiegelman, B. M. (2012). A PGC1-α-dependent myokine that drives brown-fat-like development of white fat and thermogenesis. *Nature, 481*(7382), 463–468. Retrieved from https://doi.org/10.1038/nature10777

Bouchard, C., Rankinen, T., & Timmons, J. A. (2011). Genomics and genetics in the biology of adaptation to exercise. *Comprehensive Physiology, 1*(3), 1603–1648.

Braith, R. W., & Stewart, K. J. (2006). Resistance exercise training: its role in the prevention of cardiovascular disease. *Circulation, 113*(22), 2642–2650.

Brose, A., Parise, G., & Tarnopolsky, M. A. (2003). Creatine supplementation enhances isometric strength and body composition improvements following strength exercise training in older adults. *Journals of Gerontology Series A: Biological Sciences and Medical Sciences, 58*(1), 11–19.

Candow, D. G., Chilibeck, P. D., Weisgarber, K., Vogt, E., & Baxter-Jones, A. D. G. (2013). Ingestion of low-dose ibuprofen following resistance exercise in postmenopausal women. *Journal of Cachexia, Sarcopenia and Muscle, 4*(1), 41–46.

Castaneda, C., Gordon, P. L., Uhlin, K. L., Levey, A. S., Kehayias, J. J., Dwyer, J. T., . . . Singh, M. F. (2001). Resistance training to counteract the catabolism of a low-protein diet in patients with chronic renal insufficiency. A randomized, controlled trial. *Annals of Internal Medicine, 135*(11), 965–976.

Castaneda, C., Layne, J. E., Munoz-Orians, L., Gordon, P. L., Walsmith, J., Foldvari, M., . . . Nelson, M. E. (2002). A randomized controlled trial of resistance exercise training to improve glycemic control in older adults with type 2 diabetes. *Diabetes Care, 25*(12), 2335–2341.

Chargé, S. B. P., & Rudnicki, M. A. (2004). Cellular and molecular regulation of muscle regeneration. *Physiological Reviews, 84*(1), 209–238.

Cheema, B. (2016, May 31). Research presented at the American College of Sports Medicine Conference, Boston, MA.

Cheema, B., Abas, H., Smith, B., O'Sullivan, A., Chan, M., Patwardhan, A., . . . Singh, M. F. (2007). Progressive exercise for anabolism in kidney disease (PEAK): a randomized, controlled trial of resistance training during hemodialysis. *Journal of the American Society of Nephrology, 18*(5), 1594–1601.

Cheema, B. S., Kilbreath, S. L., Fahey, P. P., Delaney, G. P., & Atlantis, E. (2014). Safety and efficacy of progressive resistance training in breast cancer: a systematic review and meta-analysis. *Breast Cancer Research and Treatment, 148*(2), 249–268.

Cheema, B. S. B., O'Sullivan, A. J., Chan, M., Patwardhan, A., Kelly, J., Gillin, A., & Fiatarone Singh, M. A. (2006). Progressive resistance training during hemodialysis: rationale and method of a randomized-controlled trial. *Hemodialysis International International Symposium on Home Hemodialysis, 10*(3), 303–310.

Christov, C., Chrétien, F., Abou-Khalil, R., Bassez, G., Vallet, G., Authier, F.-J., . . . Gherardi, R. K. (2007). Muscle satellite cells and endothelial cells: close neighbors and privileged partners. *Molecular Biology of the Cell, 18*(4), 1397–1409.

Churchward-Venne, T. A., Burd, N. A., & Phillips, S. M. (2012). Nutritional regulation of muscle protein synthesis with resistance exercise: strategies to enhance anabolism. *Nutrition & Metabolism, 9*(1), 40.

Coffey, V. G., & Hawley, J. A. (2007). The molecular bases of training adaptation. *Sports Medicine (Auckland, NZ), 37*(9), 737–763.

Colaianni, G., Cuscito, C., Mongelli, T., Pignataro, P., Buccoliero, C., Liu, P., . . . Grano, M. (2015). The myokine irisin increases cortical bone mass. *Proceedings of the National Academy of Sciences of the United States of America, 112*(39), 12157–12162.

Colker, C. (n.d.). Myostatin inhibition. *Flex.* Retrieved from http://www.flexonline.com/nutrition/myostatin-inhibition

Curtis, H. (1983). *Biology.* New York, NY: Worth.

Damas, F., Phillips, S. M., Libardi, C. A., Vechin, F. C., Lixandrão, M. E., Jannig, P. R., . . . Ugrinowitsch, C. (2016). Resistance training-induced changes in integrated myofibrillar protein synthesis are related to hypertrophy only after attenuation of muscle damage. *Journal of Physiology, 594*(18), 5209–5222.

Dana Farber Cancer Institute. (2012). Researchers discover regulator linking exercise to bigger, stronger muscles. Retrieved from http://www.dana-farber.org/Newsroom/News-Releases/researchers-discover-regulator-linking-exercise-to-bigger-stronger-muscles.aspx

Doyne, E. J., Ossip-Klein, D. J., Bowman, E. D., Osborn, K. M., McDougall-Wilson, I. B., & Neimeyer, R. A. (1987). Running versus weight lifting in the treatment of depression. *Journal of Consulting and Clinical Psychology, 55*(5), 748–754.

Drummond, M. J., Dreyer, H. C., Fry, C. S., Glynn, E. L., & Rasmussen, B. B. (2009). Nutritional and contractile regulation of human skeletal muscle protein synthesis and mTORC1 signaling. *Journal of Applied Physiology (Bethesda, MD: 1985), 106*(4), 1374–1384.

Fiatarone Singh, M. A., Gates, N., Saigal, N., Wilson, G. C., Meiklejohn, J., Brodaty, H., . . . Valenzuela, M. (2014). The Study of Mental and Resistance Training

(SMART) study—resistance training and/or cognitive training in mild cognitive impairment: a randomized, double-blind, double-sham controlled trial. *Journal of the American Medical Directors Association, 15*(12), 873–880.

Gianoudis, J., Bailey, C. A., Ebeling, P. R., Nowson, C. A., Sanders, K. M., Hill, K., & Daly, R. M. (2014). Effects of a targeted multimodal exercise program incorporating high-speed power training on falls and fracture risk factors in older adults: a community-based randomized controlled trial. *Journal of Bone and Mineral Research: The Official Journal of the American Society for Bone and Mineral Research, 29*(1), 182–191.

Gregory, S. M., Spiering, B. A., Alemany, J. A., Tuckow, A. P., Rarick, K. R., Staab, J. S., ██████ C. (2013). Exercise-induced insulin-like growth factor I system concentrations after training in women. *Medicine and Science in Sports and Exercise, 45*(3), 420–428.

Gremeaux, V., Gayda, M., Lepers, R., Sosner, P., Juneau, M., & Nigam, A. (2012). Exercise and longevity. *Maturitas, 73*(4), 312–317.

Hamrick, M. W. (2011). A role for myokines in muscle-bone interactions. *Exercise and Sport Sciences Reviews, 39*(1), 43–47.

Hardee, J. P., Porter, R. R., Sui, X., Archer, E., Lee, I.-M., Lavie, C. J., & Blair, S. N. (2014). The role of resistance exercise on all-cause mortality in cancer survivors. *Mayo Clinic Proceedings, 89*(8), 1108–1115.

Hawley, J. A., Hargreaves, M., Joyner, M. J., & Zierath, J. R. (2014). Integrative biology of exercise. *Cell, 159*(4), 738–749.

Henwood, T. R., Riek, S., & Taaffe, D. R. (2008). Strength versus muscle power-specific resistance training in community-dwelling older adults. *Journals of Gerontology Series A: Biological Sciences and Medical Sciences, 63*(1), 83–91.

Hoier, B., & Hellsten, Y. (2014). Exercise-induced capillary growth in human skeletal muscle and the dynamics of VEGF. *Microcirculation (New York, NY: 1994), 21*(4), 301–314.

Ibanez, J., Izquierdo, M., Arguelles, I., Forga, L., Larrion, J.l., Garcia-Unciti, M., . . . Gorostiaga, E. M. (2005). Twice-weekly progressive resistance training decreases abdominal fat and improves insulin sensitivity in older men with type 2 diabetes. *Diabetes Care, 28*(3), 662–667.

Jedrychowski, M. P., Wrann, C. D., Paulo, J. A., Gerber, K. K., Szpyt, J., Robinson, M. M., . . . Spiegelman, B. M. (2015). Detection and quantitation of circulating human irisin by tandem mass spectrometry. *Cell Metabolism, 22*(4), 734–740.

Joanisse, S., Nederveen, J. P., Baker, J. M., Snijders, T., Iacono, C., & Parise, G. (2016). Exercise conditioning in old mice improves skeletal muscle regeneration. *FASEB Journal, 30*(9), 3256–3268.

Kadi, F., Charifi, N., Denis, C., Lexell, J., Andersen, J. L., Schjerling, P., . . . Kjaer, M. (2005). The behaviour of satellite cells in response to exercise: what have we learned from human studies? *Pflugers Archiv: European Journal of Physiology, 451*(2), 319–327.

Khan Academy. (n.d.). Role of the sarcoplasmic reticulum in muscle cells. Retrieved from https://www.khanacademy.org/science/biology/human-biology/muscles/v/role-of-the-sarcoplasmic-reticulum-in-muscle-cells

Krentz, J. R., Quest, B., Farthing, J. P., Quest, D. W., & Chilibeck, P. D. (2008). The effects of ibuprofen on muscle hypertrophy, strength, and soreness during resistance training. *Applied Physiology, Nutrition, and Metabolism = Physiologie Appliquee, Nutrition et Metabolisme, 33*(3), 470–475.

Ledin, E. (2014). The protein interview: an interview with Dr. Stuart Phillips. *Lean Bodies Consulting.* Retrieved from https://www.leanbodiesconsulting.com/articles/the-protein-interview-an-interview-with-dr-stuart-phillips/

Lincoln, A. K., Shepherd, A., Johnson, P. L., & Castaneda-Sceppa, C. (2011). The impact of resistance exercise training on the mental health of older Puerto Rican adults with type 2 diabetes. *Journals of Gerontology Series B: Psychological Sciences and Social Sciences, 66B*(5), 567–570.

Liu, C.-J., & Latham, N. K. (2009). Progressive resistance strength training for improving physical function in older adults. *Cochrane Database of Systematic Reviews,* (3), CD002759.

Lo, M. S., Lin, L. L. C., Yao, W.-J., & Ma, M.-C. (2011). Training and detraining effects of the resistance vs. endurance program on body composition, body size, and physical performance in young men. *Journal of Strength and Conditioning Research, 25*(8), 2246–2254.

Marcell, T. J., Hawkins, S. A., & Wiswell, R. A. (2014). Leg strength declines with advancing age despite habitual endurance exercise in active older adults. *Journal of Strength and Conditioning Research, 28*(2), 504–513.

Mauro, A. (1961). Satellite cell of skeletal muscle fibers. *Journal of Biophysical and Biochemical Cytology, 9,* 493–495.

McPherron, A. C., Lawler, A. M., & Lee, S. J. (1997). Regulation of skeletal muscle mass in mice by a new TGF-beta superfamily member. *Nature, 387*(6628), 83–90.

Mekary, R. A., Grøntved, A., Despres, J.-P., De Moura, L. P., Asgarzadeh, M., Willett, W. C., . . . Hu, F. B. (2015). Weight training, aerobic physical activities, and long-term waist circumference change in men. *Obesity (Silver Spring, MD), 23*(2), 461–467.

Melov, S., Tarnopolsky, M. A., Beckman, K., Felkey, K., & Hubbard, A. (2007). Resistance exercise reverses aging in human skeletal muscle. *PLoS ONE, 2*(5), e465.

Moon, H. Y., Becke, A., Berron, D., Becker, B., Sah, N., Benoni, G., . . . van Praag, H. (2016). Running-induced systemic cathepsin B secretion is associated with memory function. *Cell Metabolism, 24*(2), 332–340.

Moreno, M., Moreno-Navarrete, J. M., Serrano, M., Ortega, F., Delgado, E., Sanchez-Ragnarsson, C., . . . Fernández-Real, J. M. (2015). Circulating irisin levels are positively associated with metabolic risk factors in sedentary subjects. *PLoS ONE, 10*(4), e0124100.

Morton, R. W., Oikawa, S. Y., Wavell, C. G., Mazara, N., McGlory, C., Quadrilatero, J., . . . Phillips, S. M. (2016). Neither load nor systemic hormones determine resistance training-mediated hypertrophy or strength gains in resistance-trained young men. *Journal of Applied Physiology (Bethesda, MD: 1985), 121*(1), 129–138.

Narkar, V. A., Downes, M., Yu, R. T., Embler, E., Wang, Y.-W., Banayo, E., . . . Evans, R. M. (2008). AMPK and PPAR delta agonists are exercise mimetics. *Cell, 134*(3), 405–415.

Pedersen, B. K. (2011). Muscles and their myokines. *Journal of Experimental Biology, 214*(Pt 2), 337–346.

Pedersen, B. K., Akerström, T. C. A., Nielsen, A. R., & Fischer, C. P. (2007). Role of myokines in exercise and metabolism. *Journal of Applied Physiology (Bethesda, MD: 1985), 103*(3), 1093–1098.

Pedersen, B. K., & Febbraio, M. A. (2012). Muscles, exercise and obesity: skeletal muscle as a secretory organ. *Nature Reviews Endocrinology, 8*(8), 457–465.

Pedersen, B. K., & Fischer, C. P. (2007). Beneficial health effects of exercise: the role of IL-6 as a myokine. *Trends in Pharmacological Sciences, 28*(4), 152–156.

Pedersen, B. K., Steensberg, A., Fischer, C., Keller, C., Keller, P., Plomgaard, P., . . . Saltin, B. (2003). Searching for the exercise factor: is IL-6 a candidate? *Journal of Muscle Research and Cell Motility, 24*(2–3), 113–119.

Petersen, A. M. W., & Pedersen, B. K. (2005). The anti-inflammatory effect of exercise. *Journal of Applied Physiology (Bethesda, MD: 1985), 98*(4), 1154–1162.

Peterson, M. D., & Gordon, P. M. (2011). Resistance exercise for the aging adult: clinical implications and prescription guidelines. *American Journal of Medicine, 124*(3), 194–198.

Peterson, M. D., Sen, A., & Gordon, P. M. (2011). Influence of resistance exercise on lean body mass in aging adults: a meta-analysis. *Medicine and Science in Sports and Exercise, 43*(2), 249–258.

Petrella, J. K., Kim, J., Cross, J. M., Kosek, D. J., & Bamman, M. M. (2006). Efficacy of myonuclear addition may explain differential myofiber growth among resistance-trained young and older men and women. *American Journal of Physiology, Endocrinology and Metabolism, 291*(5), E937–E946.

Petrella, J. K., Kim, J.-S., Mayhew, D. L., Cross, J. M., & Bamman, M. M. (2008). Potent myofiber hypertrophy during resistance training in humans is associated with satellite cell-mediated myonuclear addition: a cluster analysis. *Journal of Applied Physiology (Bethesda, MD: 1985), 104*(6), 1736–1742.

Phillips, S. M. (2014). A brief review of critical processes in exercise-induced muscular hypertrophy. *Sports Medicine (Auckland, NZ), 44*(Suppl 1), 71–77.

Phillips, S. M., & Van Loon, L. J. C. (2011). Dietary protein for athletes: from requirements to optimum adaptation. *Journal of Sports Sciences, 29*(Suppl 1), S29–38.

Philp, A., Hamilton, D. L., & Baar, K. (2011). Signals mediating skeletal muscle remodeling by resistance exercise: PI3-kinase independent activation of mTORC1. *Journal of Applied Physiology (Bethesda, MD: 1985), 110*(2), 561–568.

Physiological Society. (2016, Mar. 23). *Manipulating muscle protein turnover to maximize exercise adaptations, Stuart Phillips* [Video file]. Retrieved from https://www.youtube.com/watch?v=yvx7EhK6ixM

Pollock, R. D., O'Brien, K. A., Daniels, L. J., Nielsen, K. B., Rowlerson, A., & Duggal, N. A. (2018). Properties of the vastus lateralis muscle in relation to age and physiological function in master cyclists aged 55–79. *Aging Cell, 17*(2).

Power, G. A., Allen, M. D., Gilmore, K. J., Stashuk, D. W., Doherty, T. J., Hepple, R. T., . . . Rice, C. L. (2016). Motor unit number and transmission stability in octogenarian world class athletes: can age-related deficits be outrun? *Journal of Applied Physiology (Bethesda, MD: 1985), 121*(4), 1013–1020.

Power, G. A., Dalton, B. H., Behm, D. G., Vandervoort, A. A., Doherty, T. J., & Rice, C. L. (2010). Motor unit number estimates in masters runners: use it or lose it? *Medicine and Science in Sports and Exercise, 42*(9), 1644–1650.

Qiao, X., Nie, Y., Ma, Y., Chen, Y., Cheng, R., Yin, W., . . . Xu, L. (2016). Corrigendum: irisin promotes osteoblast proliferation and differentiation via activating the MAP kinase signaling pathways. *Scientific Reports, 6*, 21053.

Reynolds, G. (2015). Ask Well: why do muscles ache a day or two after exercise? *New York Times.* Retrieved from https://well.blogs.nytimes.com/2015/11/02/ask-well-why-do-muscles-ache-a-day-or-two-after-exercise/

Reynolds, G. (2016, Oct. 12). How exercise may turn white fat into brown. *New York Times.* Retrieved from https://www.nytimes.com/2016/10/12/well/move/how-exercise-may-fight-obesity-by-turning-white-fat-into-brown.html

Ruas, J. L., White, J. P., Rao, R. R., Kleiner, S., Brannan, K. T., Harrison, B. C., . . . Spiegelman, B. M. (2012). A PGC-1α isoform induced by resistance training regulates skeletal muscle hypertrophy. *Cell, 151*(6), 1319–1331.

Sarnataro, B. R. (n.d.). Delayed onset muscle soreness. *WebMD.* Retrieved from http://www.webmd.com/fitness-exercise/features/sore-muscles-dont-stop-exercising

Schnyder, S., & Handschin, C. (2015). Skeletal muscle as an endocrine organ: PGC-1α, myokines and exercise. *Bone, 80,* 115–125.

Schreckinger, B. (2017). I did Ruth Bader Ginsburg's workout. It nearly broke me. *Politico.* Retrieved from http://www.politico.com/magazine/story/2017/02/rbg-ruth-bader-ginsburg-workout-personal-trainer-elena-kagan-stephen-breyer-214821

Siegel, A. L., Kuhlmann, P. K., & Cornelison, D. D. W. (2011). Muscle satellite cell proliferation and association: new insights from myofiber time-lapse imaging. *Skeletal Muscle, 1*(1), 7.

Silvennoinen, M., Ahtiainen, J. P., Hulmi, J. J., Pekkala, S., Taipale, R. S., Nindl, B. C., . . . Kainulainen, H. (2015). PGC-1 isoforms and their target genes are expressed differently in human skeletal muscle following resistance and endurance exercise. *Physiological Reports, 3*(10).

Singh, N. A., Clements, K. M., & Fiatarone, M. A. (1997). A randomized controlled trial of progressive resistance training in depressed elders. *Journals of Gerontology Series A: Biological Sciences and Medical Sciences, 52*(1), M27–35.

Smith, G. I., Julliand, S., Reeds, D. N., Sinacore, D. R., Klein, S., & Mittendorfer, B. (2015). Fish oil-derived omega-3 PUFA therapy increases muscle mass and function in healthy older adults. *American Journal of Clinical Nutrition, 102*(1), 115–122.

Thevis, M., Schänzer, W., & Walpurgis, K. (2016). Analysis of antibody-based myostatin inhibitors. *World Anti-Doping Agency.* Retrieved from https://www.wada-ama.org/en/resources/analysis-of-antibody-based-myostatin-inhibitors

Trappe, T. A., Carroll, C. C., Dickinson, J. M., LeMoine, J. K., Haus, J. M., Sullivan, B. E., . . . Hollon, C. J. (2011). Influence of acetaminophen and ibuprofen on skeletal muscle adaptations to resistance exercise in older adults. *American Journal of Physiology: Regulatory, Integrative and Comparative Physiology, 300*(3), R655–662.

Trappe, S., Godard, M., Gallagher, P., Carroll, C., Rowden, G., & Porter, D. (2001). Resistance training improves single muscle fiber contractile function in older women. *American Journal of Physiology: Cell Physiology, 281*(2), C398–C406.

Trappe, S., Williamson, D., & Godard, M. (2002). Maintenance of whole muscle strength and size following resistance training in older men. *Journals of Gerontology Series A: Biological Sciences and Medical Sciences, 57*(4), B138–143.

Tsai, C.-L., Wang, C.-H., Pan, C.-Y., & Chen, F.-C. (2015). The effects of long-term resistance exercise on the relationship between neurocognitive performance and GH, IGF-1, and homocysteine levels in the elderly. *Frontiers in Behavioral Neuroscience, 9,* 23.

Walker, K. S., Kambadur, R., Sharma, M., & Smith, H. K. (2004). Resistance training alters plasma myostatin but not IGF-1 in healthy men. *Medicine and Science in Sports and Exercise, 36*(5), 7887–7793.

Wozniak, A. C., Kong, J., Bock, E., Pilipowicz, O., & Anderson, J. E. (2005). Signaling satellite-cell activation in skeletal muscle: markers, models, stretch, and potential alternate pathways. *Muscle & Nerve, 31*(3), 283–300.

Wroblewski, A. P., Amati, F., Smiley, M. A., Goodpaster, B., & Wright, V. (2011). Chronic exercise preserves lean muscle mass in masters athletes. *Physician and Sportsmedicine, 39*(3), 172–178.

Yablonka-Reuveni, Z. (2011). The skeletal muscle satellite cell: still young and fascinating at 50. *Journal of Histochemistry and Cytochemistry, 59*(12), 1041–1059.

Yablonka-Reuveni, Z., Seger, R., & Rivera, A. J. (1999). Fibroblast growth factor promotes recruitment of skeletal muscle satellite cells in young and old rats. *Journal of Histochemistry and Cytochemistry: Official Journal of the Histochemistry Society, 47*(1), 23–42.

Yin, H., Price, F., & Rudnicki, M. A. (2013). Satellite cells and the muscle stem cell niche. *Physiological Reviews, 93*(1), 23–67.

CHAPTER 7

American Society for Bone and Mineral Research. (2017). ICER Cost effectiveness report on treatments for osteoporosis, a "wake-up call" to address current crisis of under-treatment. *American Society for Bone and Mineral Research statement,* May 4.

Basaraba, S. (2017). How dangerous is a broken hip when you're older? Healthy Aging, Prevention. *Verywell.* Retrieved from https://www.verywell.com/healthy-aging-prevention-4014164

Bennett, D. (2016, Sept. 30). Exercise releases hormone that helps shed, prevent fat. *Science & Wellness, University of Florida* [Press release]. Retrieved from http://news.ufl.edu/articles/2016/09/exercise-releases-hormone-that-helps-shed-prevent-fat.php

Bergland, C. (2016, Oct. 5). Irisin: the "exercise hormone" is a fat-fighting phenomenon. *Psychology Today.* Retrieved from https://www.psychologytoday.com/blog/the-athletes-way/201610/irisin-the-exercise-hormone-is-a-fat-fighting-phenomenon

Black, D. M., Delmas, P. D., Eastell, R., Reid, I. R., Boonen, S., Cauley, J. A., . . . Cummings, S. R. (2007). Once-yearly zolendronic acid for treatment of postmenopausal osteoporosis. *New England Journal of Medicine, 356,* 1809–1822.

Black, D. M., & Rosen, C. J. (2016). Postmenopausal osteoporosis. *New England Journal of Medicine, 374,* 254–262.

Bonewald, L. D. (n.d.) The osteocyte: conductor of the bone cell orchestra. *Department of Oral and Craniofacial Sciences, School of Dentistry, University of Missouri-Kansas City.* Retrieved from http://www.nmbonecare.com/foundation/PDF/8%20-Bonewald.pdf

Bonewald, L. (2011). The amazing osteocyte. *Journal of Bone and Mineral Research, 26*(2), 229–238.

Bonewald, L. (2017). The role of the osteoclast in bone and nonbone disease. *Endocrinology & Metabolism Clinics, 46*(1), 1–18.

Bonnet, N., & Ferrari, S. L. (2010). Exercise and the skeleton: how it works and what it really does. *IBMS BoneKEy, 7,* 235–248.

Booth, F. W., Ruegsegger, G. N., & Olver, T. D. (2016). Exercise has a bone to pick with skeletal muscle. *Cell Metabolism, 23*(6), 961–962.

Bostrom, P., Wu, J., Jedrychowski, M. P., Korde, A., Ye, L., Lo, J. C., . . . Spiegelman, B. M. (2012). A PGC1-alpha-dependent myokine that drives brown-fat-like development of white fat and thermogenesis. *Nature, 481,* 463–468.

Brooks, M. (2017). FDA clears abaloparatide for high-risk osteoporosis patients. *News & Perspectives, Medscape Medical News, FDA Approvals.* Retrieved from http://www.medscape.com/viewarticle/879284

Centers for Disease Control and Prevention. (n.d.). Falls among older adults: an overview. Retrieved from http://www.arizonaafo.com/default/assets/File/CDC%20Fact%20Sheet.pdf

Centers for Disease Control and Prevention. (2016). Hip fractures among older adults. Retrieved from https://www.cdc.gov/homeandrecreationalsafety/falls/adulthipfx.html

Chubak, J., Ulrich, C. M., Tworoger, S. S., Sorensen, B., Yasui, Y., Irwin, M. L., . . . McTiernan, A. (2006). Effect of exercise on bone mineral density and lean mass in postmenopausal women. *Medicine and Science in Sports and Exercise, 38*(7), 1236–1244.

Colaianni, G., Cuscito, C., Mongelli, T., Pignataro, P., Buccoliero, C., Liu, P., . . . Grano, M. (2015). The myokine irisin increases cortical bone mass. *Proceedings of the National Academy of Sciences of the United States of America, 112*(39), 12157–12162.

Colaianni, G., Mongelli, T., Cuscito, C., Pignataro, P., Lippo, L., Spiro, G., . . . Grano, M. (2017). Irisin prevents and restores bone loss and muscle atrophy in hind-limb suspended mice. *Science Reports, 7*(1), 2811.

Dallas, S. L., Prideaux, M., & Bonewald, L. (2013). The osteocyte: an endocrine cell . . . and more. *Endocrine Review, 34*(5), 658–690.

Ducher, G., & Bass, S. L. (2007). Exercise during growth: compelling evidence for the primary prevention of osteoporosis?, *BoneKEy-Osteovision, 4*, 171–180.

Evans, R. K., Negus, C. H, Centi, A. J., Spiering, B. A., Kraemer, W. J., & Nindl, B. C. (2012). Peripheral QCT sector analysis reveals early exercise-induced increases in tibial bone mineral density. *Journal of Musculoskeletal and Neuronal Interactactions, 12*(3), 155–164.

Farr, J. N., Xu, M., Weivoda, M. M., Monroe, D. G., Fraser, D. G., Onken, J. L., . . . Khosla, S. (2017). Targeting cellular senescence prevents age-related bone loss in mice. *Nature Medicine, 23*(9), 1072–1079.

Feskanich, D., Willett, W., & Colditz, G. (2002). Walking and leisure-time activity and risk of hip fracture in postmenopausal women. *Journal of the American Medical Association, 288*(18), 2300–2306.

Foreman, J. (2001, Apr. 24). A "cure" for osteoporosis may be near. *Boston Globe.*

Gardinier, J. D., Mohamed, F., & Kohn, D. H. (2015). PTH signaling during exercise contributes to bone adaptation. *Journal of Bone and Mineral Research, 30*(6), 1053–1063.

Gremeaux, V., Gayda, M., Lepers, R., Sosner, P., Juneau, M., & Nigam, A. (2012). Exercise and longevity. *Maturitas, 73*, 312–317.

Guadelupe-Grau, A., Fuentes, T. Guerra, B., & Calbet, J. A. (2009). Exercise and bone mass in adults. *Sports Medicine, 39*(6), 439–468.

Haentjens, P., Magaziner, J., Colon-Emeric, C. S., Vanderschueren, D., Milisen, K., Velkeniers, B., & Boonen, S. (2010). Meta-analysis: excess mortality after hip fracture among older women and men. *Annals of Internal Medicine, 152*(6), 380–390.

Hamrick, M. W. (2011). A role for myokines in muscle-bone interactions. *Exercise and Sport Science Reviews, 39*(1), 43–47.

Hamrick, M. (2015, August 25). ASBMR webinar: exercise in muscle & bone. *ASMBR.* Retrieved from http://www.asbmr.org/education-detail?cid=8dcf2213-381e-4ec0-8652-ef8a80bdf6bf#.WYCl0BiZPvE

Harvard Women's Health Watch. (2008). What's the story with Fosamax? *Harvard Health Publications.* Retrieved from http://www.health.harvard.edu/diseases-and-conditions/whats_the_story_with_fosamax

Heinonen, A., Kannus, P., Sievanen, H., Oja, P., Pasanen, M., Rinne, M., . . . Vuori, I. (1996). Randomized controlled trial of effect of high-impact exercise on selected risk factors for osteoporotic fractures. *Lancet, 348*(9038), 1343–1347.

Hinton, P. S., Nigh, P., & Thyfault, J. (2015). Effectiveness of resistance training or jumping-exercise to increase bone mineral density in men with low bone mass: a 12-month randomized, controlled trial. *Bone, 79*, 203–212.

Jarvinen, T. L. N., Michaelsson, K., Aspenberg, P., & Sievanen, H. (2015). Osteoporosis: the emperor has no clothes. *Journal of Internal Medicine, 277*(6), 662–673.

Jedrychowski, M. P., Wrann, C. D., Paulo, J. A., Gerber, K. K., Szpyt, J., Robinson, M. M., . . . Spiegelman, B. M. (2015). Detection and quantitation of circulating human irisin by tandem mass spectrometry. *Cell Metabolism, 22*(4), 734–740.

Kawai, M., & Rosen, C. J. (2012). The insulin-like growth factor system in bone, basic and clinical implications. *Endocrinology and Metabolism Clinics of North America, 41*(2), 323–33

Kennel, K. A. (2015). Osteoporosis drugs: risk of bone problems in jaw, thigh? *MayoClinic*. Retrieved from http://www.mayoclinic.org/diseases-conditions/osteoporosis/expert-answers/osteoporosis-drug-risks/faq-20058121

Khan Academy. (n.d.). Cellular structure of bone. Retrieved from https://www.khanacademy.org/science/health-and-medicine/human-anatomy-and-physiology/skeletal-system/v/cellular-structure-of-bone

Khan Academy. (n.d.). Microscopic structure of bone: the Haversian system. Retrieved from https://www.khanacademy.org/science/health-and-medicine/human-anatomy-and-physiology/skeletal-system/v/microscopic-structure-of-bone-haversian-system

Kolata, G. (2016a, Apr. 1). Exercise is not the path to strong bones. *New York Times*.

Kolata, G. (2016b, Apr. 22). A second look at a "misconception" on exercise and bones. *New York Times*.

Lai, C. L., Tseng, S. Y., Chen, C. N., Liao, W. C., Wang, C. H., Lee, M. C., & Hsu, P. S. (2013). Effect of 6 months of whole body vibration on lumbar spine bone density in postmenopausal women: a randomized controlled trial. *Clinical Interventions in Aging, 8*, 1603–1609.

Landefeld, C. S. (2011). Goals of care for hip fracture. Invited commentary. *Archives of Internal Medicine, 171*(20), 1837–1838.

LeBlanc, E. S., Hillier, T. A., Pedula, K. L., Rizzo, J. H., Cawthon, P. M., Fink, H. A., . . . Browner, W. S. (2011). Hip fracture and increased short-term but not long-term mortality in healthy older women. *Archives of Internal Medicine, 171*(20), 1831–1837.

Lomas-Vega, R., Obrero-Gaitlan, E., Molina-Orega, F. J., & Del-Pino-Casado, R. (2017). Tai chi for risk of falls: a meta-analysis. *Journal of the American Geriatrics Society, 65*(9), 2017–2043.

Lorentzon, M., & Cummings, S. R. (2015). Osteoporosis: the evolution of a diagnosis. *Journal of Internal Medicine, 277*(6), 650–661.

Macias, B. R., Swift, J. M., Nilsson, M. I., Hogan, H. A., Bouse, S. D., & Bloomfield, S. A. (2012). Simulated resistance training, but not alendronate, increases cortical bone formation and suppressed sclerostin during disuse. *Journal of Applied Physiology, 112*(5), 918–925.

Manolagas, S. C. (2000). Birth and death of bone cells: basic regulatory mechanisms and implications for the pathogenesis and treatment of osteoporosis. *Endocrine Reviews, 21*(2), 115–137.

MedicineNet. (2002). Bones, how many and what do they do? Retrieved from http://www.medicalgeek.com/anatomy/21978-how-many-bones-human-body.html

Mera, P., Laue, K., Ferron, M., Confavreux, C., Wei, J., Galan-Diez, M., . . . Karsenty, G. (2016). Osteocalcin signaling in myofibers is necessary and sufficient for optimum adaptation to exercise. *Cell Metabolism, 23*(6), 1078–1092.

Michaelsson, K., Olofsson, H., Jenseevik, K., Larsson, S., Mallmin, H., Berglund, L., . . . Melhus, H. (2007). Leisure physical activity and the risk of fracture in men. *PLoS Medicine, 4*(6), e199.

Miller, P., Hattersley, G., Rils, B. J., Williams, G. C., Lau, E., Russo, L. A., . . . Christiansen, C. (2016). Effect of abaloparatide vs placebo on new vertebral fractures in postmenopausal women with osteoporosis. *Journal of the American Medical Association, 316*(7), 722–733.

Miller, M., Sturmer, T., Azrael, D., Levin, R., & Solomon, D. H. (2011). Opioid analgesics and the risk of fractures among older adults with arthritis. *Journal of the American Geriatrics Society, 59*(3), 430–438.

National Institute of Arthritis and Musculoskeletal and Skin Diseases. (2015). Preventing falls and related fractures. Retrieved from https://www.niams.nih.gov/Health_Info/Bone/Osteoporosis/Fracture/prevent_falls.asp

National Institute on Aging. (2017). Falls and fractures. *Age Page.* Retrieved from https://www.nia.nih.gov/health/publication/falls-and-fractures

National Institutes of Health. (2000). Osteoporosis prevention, diagnosis, and therapy. *National Institutes of Health Consensus Development Conference Statement, March 27–29, 17*(1), 1–36.

National Osteoporosis Foundation. (n.d.). What is osteoporosis and what causes it? Retrieved from https://www.nof.org/patients/what-is-osteoporosis/

Nelson, M. E., Fiatarone, M. A., & Morganti, C. M. (1994). Effects of high-intensity strength training on multiple risk factors for osteoporotic fractures: a randomized controlled trial. *Journal of the American Medical Association, 272*(24), 1909–1914.

Novotny, S. A., Warren, G. L., & Hamrick, M. W. (2015). Aging and the muscle–bone relationship. *Physiology (Bethesda, MD), 30*(1), 8–16.

Paiva-Fonseca, F., Santos-Silva, A. R., Della-Coletta, R., Vargas, P. A., & Lopes, M. A. (2013). Alendronate-associated osteonecrosis of the jaws: a review of the main topics. *Medicina Oral Patologia Oral y Cirugia Bucal, 19*(2), e106–e111.

Radiological Society of North America, Inc. (2017). Bone densitometry (DEXA). *RadiologyInfo.org.* Retrieved from https://www.radiologyinfo.org/en/info.cfm?pg=dexa

Russo, C. R. (2009). The effects of exercise on bone: basic concepts and implications for the prevention of fractures. *Clinical Cases in Mineral and Bone Metabolism, 6*(3), 223–228.

Sanudo, B., de Hoyo, M., Del Pozo-Cruz, J., Carrasco, L., Del Pozo-Cruz, B., Tejero, S., & Firth, E. (2017). A systematic review of the exercise effect on bone health: the importance of assessing mechanical loading in perimenopausal and postmenopausal women. *Menopause, 24*(10), 1208–1216.

Schiller, J. S., Kramarow, E. A., & Dey, A. N. (2007, Sept. 21). Fall injury episodes among noninstitutionalized older adults: United States, 2001–2003. *Advance data, from Vital and Health Statistics, Centers for Disease Control and Prevention, No. 392.*

Slovik, D. (2005). Osteoporosis. Chapter 15, *Exercise in rehabilitation medicine, human kinetics.* Retrieved from http://www.humankinetics.com/home

Stiles, V. H., Metcalf, B. S., Knapp, K. M., & Rowlands, A. V. (2017). A small amount of precisely measured high-intensity habitual physical activity predicts bone health in pre- and post-menopausal women in UK Biobank. *International Journal of Epidemiology, 46*(6), 1847–1856.

Taylor, R. B. (2009). Male osteoporosis: bone mass matters. *WebMD.* Retrieved from https://www.google.com/#q=Male+osteoporosis:+Bone+Mass+Matters

Thomas, G. A., Cartmel, B., Harrigan, M., Fiellin, M., Capozza, S., Zhou, Y., . . . Irwin, M. L. (2017). The effect of exercise on body composition and bone mineral density in breast cancer survivors taking aromatase inhibitors. *Obesity (Silver Spring), 25*(2), 346–351.

Trail blazer: Dr. Lynda Bonewald on new muscle-bone research models and breakthroughs. (2013, April 2). *Aging in Motion, American Society for Bone and Mineral Research.* Retrieved from http://www.asbmr.org/publications/news/newsdetail.aspx?cid=94319459-9028-4434-a39e-860f8b8e0d09#.WXYuPhiZOfc

Tucker, L. A., Strong, J. E., Le Cheminant, J. D., & Bailey, B. W. (2015). Effect of two jumping programs in hip bone mineral density in premenopausal women: a randomized controlled trial. *American Journal of Health Promotion, 29*(3), 158–164.

Wei, J., & Karsenty, G. (2015). An overview of the metabolic functions of osteocalcin. *Reviews in Endocrine and Metabolic Disorders, 16*(2), 93–98.

Wijenayaka, A. R, Kogawa, M., Lim, H. P., Bonewald, L. F., Findlay, D. M., & Atkins, G. J. (2011). Sclerostin stimulates osteocyte support of osteoclast activity by a RANKL-dependent pathway. *PLoS ONE, 6*(10), 325900.

Winters-Stone, K. M., & Snow, C. M. (2006). Site-specific response of bone to exercise in premenopausal women. *Bone, 39*(6), 1203–1209.

Wrann, C. D., White, J. P., Salogiannis, J., Laznik-Bogoslavski, D., Wu, J., Ma, D., . . . Spiegelman, B. M. (2013). Exercise induces hippocampal BDNF through a PGC-1 alpha/FNDC5 pathway. *Cell Metabolism, 18*(5), 649–659.

Zernicke, R., MacKay, C., & Lorincz, C. (2006). Mechanisms of bone remodeling during weight-bearing exercise. *Applied Physiology, Nutrition and Metabolism, 31*(6), 655–660.

Zhang, J., Valverde, P., Zhu, X., Murray, D., Wu, Y., Yu, L., . . . Chen, J. (2017). Exercise-induced irisin in bone and systemic irisin administration reveal new regulatory mechanisms of bone metabolism. *Bone Research, 5,* 16056.

Zhang, Y., Xie, C., Wang, H., Foss, R. M., Clare, M., George, E. V., . . . Yang, L. J. (2016). Irisin exerts dual effects on browning and adipogenesis of human white adipocytes. *American Journal of Physiology, 311*(2), E530–E541.

Zhao, R., Zhang, M., & Zhang, Q. (2017). The effectiveness of combined exercise interventions for preventing postmenopausal bone loss: a systematic review and meta-analysis. *Journal of Orthopaedic & Sports Physical Therapy, 47*(4), 225–295.

CHAPTER 8

Adlard, P. A., Perreau, V. M., Pop, V., & Cotman, C. W. (2005). Voluntary exercise decreases amyloid load in a transgenic model of Alzheimer's disease. *Journal of Neuroscience: The Official Journal of the Society for Neuroscience, 25*(17), 4217–4221.

Ahlskog, J. E., Geda, Y. E., Graff-Radford, N. R., & Petersen, R. C. (2011). Physical exercise as a preventive or disease-modifying treatment of dementia and brain aging. *Mayo Clinic Proceedings, 86*(9), 876–884.

Aichberger, M. C., Busch, M. A., Reischies, F. M., Ströhle, A., Heinz, A., & Rapp, M. A. (2010). Effect of physical inactivity on cognitive performance after 2.5 years of follow-up. *GeroPsych, 23*(1), 7–15.

Akst, J. (2016, Nov. 14). Probing exercise's effects on cognitive function. *The Scientist.* Retrieved from http://www.the-scientist.com/?articles.view/articleNo/47506/title/Probing-Exercise-s-Effects-on-Cognitive-Function

Albert, M. S., Jones, K., Savage, C. R., Berkman, L., Seeman, T., Blazer, D., & Rowe, J. W. (1995). Predictors of cognitive change in older persons: MacArthur studies of successful aging. *Psychology and Aging, 10*(4), 578–589.

Albinet, C. T., Boucard, G., Bouquet, C. A., & Audiffren, M. (2010). Increased heart rate variability and executive performance after aerobic training in the elderly. *European Journal of Applied Physiology, 109*(4), 617–624.

Alfini, A. J., Weiss, L. R., Leitner, B. P., Smith, T. J., Hagberg, J. M., & Smith, J. C. (2016). Hippocampal and cerebral blood flow after exercise cessation in master athletes. *Frontiers in Aging Neuroscience, 8,* 184.

Alzheimer's Association. (n.d.). Mild cognitive impairment. Retrieved from http://www.alz.org/dementia/mild-cognitive-impairment-mci.asp

Alzheimer's Association. (n.d.). What is Alzheimer's? Retrieved from http://www.alz. org/alzheimers_disease_what_is_alzheimers.asp

Alzheimer's Association. (2015, July 23). Going beyond risk reduction: physical exercise may be an effective treatment for Alzheimer's disease and vascular dementia. [Press release]. Retrieved from https://www.alz.org/aaic/_downloads/thurs-1130am-exercise.pdf

Angevaren, M., Aufdemkampe, G., Verhaar, H. J. J., Aleman, A., & Vanhees, L. (2008). Physical activity and enhanced fitness to improve cognitive function in older people without known cognitive impairment. *Cochrane Database of Systematic Reviews*, (3), CD005381.

Arden, C. I., & Rotondi, M. (2013). Knowledge synthesis report: the role of physical activity in the prevention and management of Alzheimer's disease—implications for Ontario. Ontario Brain Institute. Retrieved from http://www.alzheimer.ca/~/media/Files/on/Media%20Releases/2013/OBI%20Report%20March%208%20 2013.pdf

Azevedo, F. A. C., Carvalho, L. R. B., Grinberg, L. T., Farfel, J. M., Ferretti, R. E. L., Leite, R. E. P., ... Herculano-Houzel, S. (2009). Equal numbers of neuronal and nonneuronal cells make the human brain an isometrically scaled-up primate brain. *Journal of Comparative Neurology, 513*(5), 532–541.

Baker, L. D., Frank, L. L., Foster-Schubert, K., Green, P. S., Wilkinson, C. W., McTiernan, A., ... Craft, S. (2010). Effects of aerobic exercise on mild cognitive impairment: a controlled trial. *Archives of Neurology, 67*(1), 71–79.

Baker, L. D., Skinner, J. S., Craft, S., Sink, K. M., Montine, T., Hansen, A., ... Callaghan, M. (2015). Aerobic exercise reduces phosphorylated tau protein in cerebrospinal fluid in older adults with mild cognitive impairment. *Alzheimer's & Dementia: The Journal of the Alzheimer's Association, 11*(7), 324.

Barnes, D. E., & Yaffe, K. (2011). The projected impact of risk factor reduction on Alzheimer's disease prevalence. *Lancet Neurology, 10*(9), 819–828.

Barnes, D. E., Yaffe, K., Satariano, W. A., & Tager, I. B. (2003). A longitudinal study of cardiorespiratory fitness and cognitive function in healthy older adults. *Journal of the American Geriatrics Society, 51*(4), 459–465.

Begley, S. (2018, Mar. 7). Controversial study challenges scientific consensus that adult brains make new neurons. *STAT*.

Berchtold, N. C., Castello, N., & Cotman, C. W. (2010). Exercise and time-dependent benefits to learning and memory. *Neuroscience, 167*(3), 588–597.

Berchtold, N. C., Chinn, G., Chou, M., Kesslak, J. P., & Cotman, C. W. (2005). Exercise primes a molecular memory for brain-derived neurotrophic factor protein induction in the rat hippocampus. *Neuroscience, 133*(3), 853–861.

Berchtold, N. C., Kesslak, J. P., Pike, C. J., Adlard, P. A., & Cotman, C. W. (2001). Estrogen and exercise interact to regulate brain-derived neurotrophic factor mRNA and protein expression in the hippocampus. *European Journal of Neuroscience, 14*(12), 1992–2002.

Bherer, L., Erickson, K. I., & Liu-Ambrose, T. (2013a). A review of the effects of physical activity and exercise on cognitive and brain functions in older adults. *Journal of Aging Research, 2013,* 657508.

Bherer, L., Erickson, K. I., & Liu-Ambrose, T. (2013b). Physical exercise and brain functions in older adults. *Journal of Aging Research, 2013,* 197326.

Binder, D. K., & Scharfman, H. E. (2004). Brain-derived neurotrophic factor. *Growth Factors (Chur, Switzerland), 22*(3), 123–131.

Blumenthal, J. A., Emery, C. F., Madden, D. J., Schniebolk, S., Walsh-Riddle, M., George, L. K., . . . Coleman, R. E. (1991). Long-term effects of exercise on psychological functioning in older men and women. *Journal of Gerontology, 46*(6), 352–361.

Bolandzadeh, N., Tam, R., Handy, T. C., Nagamatsu, L. S., Hsu, C. L., Davis, J. C., . . . Liu-Ambrose, T. (2015). Resistance training and white matter lesion progression in older women: exploratory analysis of a 12-month randomized controlled trial. *Journal of the American Geriatrics Society, 63*(10), 2052–2060.

Boldrini, M., Fulmore, C. A., Tartt, A. N., Simeon, L. R., Pavlova, I., Poposka, V., . . . Hen, R. (2018). Human hippocampal neurogenesis persists throughout aging. *Cell Stem Cell, 22,* 589–599.

Buchman, A. S., Yu, L., Boyle, P. A., Schneider, J. A., De Jager, P. L., & Bennett, D. A. (2016). Higher brain BDNF gene expression is associated with slower cognitive decline in older adults. *Neurology, 86*(8), 735–741.

Burdette, J. H., Laurienti, P. J., Espeland, M. A., Morgan, A., Telesford, Q., Vechlekar, C. D., . . . Rejeski, W. J. (2010). Using network science to evaluate exercise-associated brain changes in older adults. *Frontiers in Aging Neuroscience, 2,* 23.

Burzynska, A. Z., Wong, C. N., Chaddock-Heyman, L., Olson, E. A., Gothe, N. P., Knecht, A., . . . Kramer, A. F. (2016). White matter integrity, hippocampal volume, and cognitive performance of a world-famous nonagenarian track-and-field athlete. *Neurocase, 22*(2), 135–144.

Cardona-Gómez, G. P., Mendez, P., DonCarlos, L. L., Azcoitia, I., & Garcia-Segura, L. M. (2001). Interactions of estrogens and insulin-like growth factor-I in the brain: implications for neuroprotection. *Brain Research Reviews, 37*(1–3), 320–334.

Carro, E., Trejo, J. L., Busiguina, S., & Torres-Aleman, I. (2001). Circulating insulin-like growth factor I mediates the protective effects of physical exercise against brain insults of different etiology and anatomy. *Journal of Neuroscience, 21*(15), 5678–5684.

Carvalho, A., Rea, I. M., Parimon, T., & Cusack, B. J. (2014). Physical activity and cognitive function in individuals over 60 years of age: a systematic review. *Clinical Interventions in Aging, 9,* 661–682.

Cassilhas, R. C., Viana, V. A. R., Grassmann, V., Santos, R. T., Santos, R. F., Tufik, S., & Mello, M. T. (2007). The impact of resistance exercise on the cognitive function of the elderly. *Medicine and Science in Sports and Exercise, 39*(8), 1401–1407.

Centers for Disease Control and Prevention. (2016, Jan. 26). The Healthy Brain Initiative: a national public health road map to maintaining cognitive health. Retrieved from https://www.cdc.gov/aging/healthybrain/roadmap.htm

Chang, M., Jonsson, P. V., Snaedal, J., Bjornsson, S., Saczynski, J. S., Aspelund, T., . . . Launer, L. J. (2010). The effect of midlife physical activity on cognitive function among older adults: AGES—Reykjavik Study. *Journals of Gerontology Series A: Biological Sciences and Medical Sciences, 65A*(12), 1369–1374.

Colcombe, S. J., Erickson, K. I., Raz, N., Webb, A. G., Cohen, N. J., McAuley, E., & Kramer, A. F. (2003). Aerobic fitness reduces brain tissue loss in aging humans. *Journals of Gerontology Series A: Biological Sciences and Medical Sciences, 58*(2), 176–180.

Colcombe, S. J., Erickson, K. I., Scalf, P. E., Kim, J. S., Prakash, R., McAuley, E., . . . Kramer, A. F. (2006). Aerobic exercise training increases brain volume in aging humans. *Journals of Gerontology Series A: Biological Sciences and Medical Sciences, 61*(11), 1166–1170.

Colcombe, S., & Kramer, A. F. (2003). Fitness effects on the cognitive function of older adults: a meta-analytic study. *Psychological Science, 14*(2), 125–130.

Colcombe, S. J., Kramer, A. F., Erickson, K. I., Scalf, P., McAuley, E., Cohen, N. J., . . . Elavsky, S. (2004). Cardiovascular fitness, cortical plasticity, and aging. *Proceedings of the National Academy of Sciences of the United States of America, 101*(9), 3316–3321.

Colcombe, S. J., Kramer, A. F., McAuley, E., Erickson, K. I., & Scalf, P. (2004). Neurocognitive aging and cardiovascular fitness: recent findings and future directions. *Journal of Molecular Neuroscience, 24*(1), 9–14.

Cotman, C. (2005). Exercise induces BDNF, improves learning and reduces B-amyloid. [PowerPoint slides]. Retrieved from https://www.alz.washington.edu/NONMEMBER/FALL05/cotman.pdf

Cotman, C. (2017, Feb. 22). Personal communication.

Cotman, C. W., & Berchtold, N. C. (2002). Exercise: a behavioral intervention to enhance brain health and plasticity. *Trends in Neurosciences, 25*(6), 295–301.

Cotman, C. W., Berchtold, N. C., & Christie, L.-A. (2007). Exercise builds brain health: key roles of growth factor cascades and inflammation. *Trends in Neurosciences, 30*(9), 464–472.

Dai, W., Lopez, O. L., Carmichael, O. T., Becker, J. T., Kuller, L. H., & Gach, H. M. (2009). Mild cognitive impairment and Alzheimer disease: patterns of altered cerebral blood flow at MR imaging. *Radiology, 250*(3), 856–866.

Daviglus, M. L., Bell, C. C., Berrettini, W., Bowen, P. E., Connolly, E. S., Cox, N. J., . . . Trevisan, M. (2010). NIH state-of-the-science conference statement: preventing Alzheimer's disease and cognitive decline. *NIH Consensus and State-of-the-Science Statements, 27*(4), 1–30.

Dennis, C. V., Suh, L. S., Rodriguez, M. L., Kril, J. J., & Sutherland, G. T. (2016). Human adult neurogenesis across the ages: an immunohistochemical study. *Neuropathology and Applied Neurobiology, 42*, 621–638.

Dik, M., Deeg, D. J. H., Visser, M., & Jonker, C. (2003). Early life physical activity and cognition at old age. *Journal of Clinical and Experimental Neuropsychology, 25*(5), 643–653.

Ding, Q., Vaynman, S., Akhavan, M., Ying, Z., & Gomez-Pinilla, F. (2006). Insulin-like growth factor I interfaces with brain-derived neurotrophic factor-mediated synaptic plasticity to modulate aspects of exercise-induced cognitive function. *Neuroscience, 140*(3), 823–833.

Don Carlos, L. L., Azcoitia, I., & Garcia-Segura, L. M. (2009). Neuroprotective actions of selective estrogen receptor modulators. *Psychoneuroendocrinology, 34*(S1), S113–S122.

Dustman, R. E., Ruhling, R. O., Russell, E. M., Shearer, D. E., Bonekat, H. W., Shigeoka, J. W., . . . Bradford, D. C. (1984). Aerobic exercise training and improved neuropsychological function of older individuals. *Neurobiology of Aging, 5*(1), 35–42.

Erickson, K. I., Colcombe, S. J., Elavsky, S., McAuley, E., Korol, D. L., Scalf, P. E., & Kramer, A. F. (2007). Interactive effects of fitness and hormone treatment on brain health in postmenopausal women. *Neurobiology of Aging, 28*(2), 179–185.

Erickson, K. I., Hillman, C. H., & Kramer, A. F. (2015). Physical activity, brain, and cognition. *Current Opinion in Behavioral Sciences, 4*, 27–32.

Erickson, K. I., Leckie, R. L., & Weinstein, A. M. (2014). Physical activity, fitness, and gray matter volume. *Neurobiology of Aging, 35*(Suppl 2), S20–S28.

Erickson, K. I., Miller, D. L., & Roecklein, K. A. (2012). The aging hippocampus: interactions between exercise, depression, and BDNF. *The Neuroscientist : A Review Journal Bringing Neurobiology, Neurology and Psychiatry, 18*(1), 82–97.

Erickson, K. I., Prakash, R. S., Voss, M. W., Chaddock, L., Heo, S., McLaren, M., . . . Kramer, A. F. (2010). BDNF is associated with age-related decline in hippocampal volume.

Journal of Neuroscience: The Official Journal of the Society for Neuroscience, 30(15), 5368–5375.

Erickson, K. I., Prakash, R. S., Voss, M. W., Chaddock, L., Hu, L., Morris, K. S., . . . Kramer, A. F. (2009). Aerobic fitness is associated with hippocampal volume in elderly humans. Hippocampus, 19(10), 1030–1039.

Erickson, K. I., Raji, C. A., Lopez, O. L., Becker, J. T., Rosano, C., Newman, A. B., . . . Kuller, L. H. (2010). Physical activity predicts gray matter volume in late adulthood: the Cardiovascular Health Study. Neurology, 75(16), 1415–1422.

Erickson, K. I., Voss, M. W., Prakash, R. S., Basak, C., Szabo, A., Chaddock, L., . . . Kramer, A. F. (2011). Exercise training increases size of hippocampus and improves memory. Proceedings of the National Academy of Sciences of the United States of America, 108(7), 3017–3022.

Eriksson, P. S., Perfilieva, E., Bjork-Eriksson, T., Alborn, A. M., Nordborg, C., Peterson, D. A., & Gage, F. H. (1998). Neurogenesis in the adult human hippocampus. Nature Medicine, 4, 1313–1317.

Etnier, J. L., Nowell, P. M., Landers, D. M., & Sibley, B. A. (2006). A meta-regression to examine the relationship between aerobic fitness and cognitive performance. Brain Research Reviews, 52(1), 119–130.

Fabel, K., Fabel, K., Tam, B., Kaufer, D., Baiker, A., Simmons, N., . . . Palmer, T. D. (2003). VEGF is necessary for exercise-induced adult hippocampal neurogenesis. European Journal of Neuroscience, 18(10), 2803–2812.

Fiatarone Singh, M. A., Gates, N., Saigal, N., Wilson, G. C., Meiklejohn, J., Brodaty, H., . . . Valenzuela, M. (2014). The Study of Mental and Resistance Training (SMART) study—resistance training and/or cognitive training in mild cognitive impairment: a randomized, double-blind, double-sham controlled trial. Journal of the American Medical Directors Association, 15(12), 873–880.

Firth, J., Stubbs, B., Rosenbaum, S., Vancampfort, D., Malchow, B., Schuch, F., . . . Yung, A. R. (2017). Aerobic exercise improves cognitive functioning in people with schizophrenia: a systematic review and meta-analysis. Schizophrenia Bulletin, 43(3), 546–556.

Firth, J., Stubbs, B., Vancampfort, D., Schuch, F., Lagopoulos, J., Rosenbaum, S., . . . Ward, P. B. (2018). Effect of aerobic exercise on hippocampal volume in humans: a systematic review and meta-analysis. NeuroImage, 166, 230–238.

Foster, A. C., & Kemp, J. A. (2006). Glutamate- and GABA-based CNS therapeutics. Current Opinion in Pharmacology, 6(1), 7–17.

Friedman, R. A. (2015, Oct. 23). Can you get smarter? New York Times. Retrieved from https://www.nytimes.com/2015/10/25/opinion/sunday/can-you-get-smarter.html

Gajewski, P. D., & Falkenstein, M. (2016). Physical activity and neurocognitive functioning in aging: a condensed updated review. European Review of Aging and Physical Activity, 13, 1.

Gant, J. C., Blalock, E. M., Chen, K.-C., Kadish, I., Thibault, O., Porter, N. M., & Landfield, P. W. (2018). FK506-binding protein 12.6/1b, a negative regulator of [Ca2+], rescues memory and restores genomic regulation in the hippocampus of aging rats. Journal of Neuroscience, 38(4),1030–1041.

Garcia-Segura, L. M., Cardona-Gómez, G. P., Chowen, J. A., & Azcoitia, I. (2000). Insulin-like growth factor-I receptors and estrogen receptors interact in the promotion of neuronal survival and neuroprotection. Journal of Neurocytology, 29(5–6), 425–437.

Gardener, H., Wright, C. B., Dong, C., Cheung, K., DeRosa, J., Nannery, M., . . . Sacco, R. L. (2016). Ideal cardiovascular health and cognitive aging in the Northern Manhattan Study. Journal of the American Heart Association, 5(3), e002731.

Geda, Y. E., Roberts, R. O., Knopman, D. S., Christianson, T. J. H., Pankratz, V. S., Ivnik, R. J., . . . Rocca, W. A. (2010). Physical exercise and mild cognitive impairment: a population-based study. *Archives of Neurology, 67*(1), 80–86.

Gitler, A. D. (2011). Neuroscience: another reason to exercise. *Science (New York, NY), 334*(6056), 606–607.

Gomez-Pinilla, F., & Hillman, C. (2013). The influence of exercise on cognitive abilities. *Comprehensive Physiology, 3*(1), 403–428.

Griffin, E. W., Mullally, S., Foley, C., Warmington, S. A., O'Mara, S. M., & Kelly, A. M. (2011). Aerobic exercise improves hippocampal function and increases BDNF in the serum of young adult males. *Physiology and Behavior, 104*(5), 934–941.

Guiney, H., & Machado, L. (2013). Benefits of regular aerobic exercise for executive functioning in healthy populations. *Psychonomic Bulletin & Review, 20*(1), 73–86.

Hamer, M., & Chida, Y. (2009). Physical activity and risk of neurodegenerative disease: a systematic review of prospective evidence. *Psychological Medicine, 39*(1), 3–11.

Hamilton, J. (2018, Mar. 7). Sorry, adults, no new neurons for your aging brains. NPR. Retrieved from https://www.npr.org/sections/health-shots/2018/03/07/591305604/sorry-adults-no-new-neurons-for-your-aging-brains

He, C., Sumpter, R., & Levine, B. (2012). Exercise induces autophagy in peripheral tissues and in the brain. *Autophagy, 8*(10), 1548–1551.

Henry Ford Quotes. (n.d.). BrainyQuote. Retrieved from https://www.brainyquote.com/quotes/quotes/h/henryford141720.html

Heyn, P., Abreu, B. C., & Ottenbacher, K. J. (2004). The effects of exercise training on elderly persons with cognitive impairment and dementia: a meta-analysis. *Archives of Physical Medicine and Rehabilitation, 85*(10), 1694–1704.

Horowitz, A. M., & Villeda, S. A. (2017). Therapeutic potential of systemic brain rejuvenation strategies for neurodegenerative disease. *F1000Res, 6*, 1291.

Horsburgh, K. (2015). Long-term reduction in blood flow: a cause of vascular dementia and Alzheimer's disease? Alzheimer's Society. Retrieved from https://www.alzheimers.org.uk/info/20053/research_projects/649/long-term_reduction_in_blood_flow_-_a_cause_of_vascular_dementia_and_alzheimers_disease

Hsu, C. L., Best, J. R., Davis, J. C., Nagamatsu, L. W., Wang, S., Boyd, L. A., . . . Liu-Ambrose, T. (2018). Aerobic exercise promotes executive functions and impacts functional neuronal activity among older adults with vascular impairment. *British Journal of Sports Medicine, 52*(3), 184–191.

Hyodo, K., Dan, I., Kyutoku, Y., Suwabe, K., Byun, K., Ochi, G., . . . Soya, H. (2016). The association between aerobic fitness and cognitive function in older men mediated by frontal lateralization. *NeuroImage, 125*, 291–300.

Jackson, P. A., Pialoux, V., Corbett, D., Drogos, L., Erickson, K. I., Eskes, G. A., & Poulin, M. J. (2016). Promoting brain health through exercise and diet in older adults: a physiological perspective. *Journal of Physiology, 594*(16), 4490.

Jedrziewski, M. K., Ewbank, D. C., Wang, H., & Trojanowski, J. Q. (2010). Exercise and cognition: results from the National Long Term Care Survey. *Alzheimer's & Dementia: The Journal of the Alzheimer's Association, 6*(6), 448–455.

Johnson, N. F., Gold, B. T., Bailey, A. L., Clasey, J. L., Hakun, J. G., White, M., . . . Powell, D. K. (2016). Cardiorespiratory fitness modifies the relationship between myocardial function and cerebral blood flow in older adults. *NeuroImage, 131*, 126–132.

Kirk-Sanchez, N. J., & McGough, E. L. (2014). Physical exercise and cognitive performance in the elderly: current perspectives. *Clinical Interventions in Aging, 9*, 51–62.

Kobilo, T., Liu, Q.-R., Gandhi, K., Mughal, M., Shaham, Y., & van Praag, H. (2011). Running is the neurogenic and neurotrophic stimulus in environmental enrichment. *Learning & Memory, 18*(9), 605–609.

Kramer, A. F., Bherer, L., Colcombe, S. J., Dong, W., & Greenough, W. T. (2004). Environmental influences on cognitive and brain plasticity during aging. *Journals of Gerontology Series A: Biological Sciences and Medical Sciences, 59*(9), M940–957.

Kramer, A. F., Erickson, K. I., & Colcombe, S. J. (2006). Exercise, cognition, and the aging brain. *Journal of Applied Physiology (Bethesda, MD: 1985), 101*(4), 1237–1242.

Kramer, A. F., Hahn, S., Cohen, N. J., Banich, M. T., McAuley, E., Harrison, C. R., . . . Colcombe, A. (1999). Ageing, fitness and neurocognitive function. *Nature, 400*(6743), 418–419.

Knoth, R., Singec, I., Ditter, M., Pantazis, G., Capetian, P., Meyer, R. P., . . . Kempermann, G. (2010). Murine features of neurogenesis in the human hippocampus across the lifespan from 0 to 100 years. *PLoS ONE, 5*, e8809.

Larson, E. B., Wang, L., Bowen, J. D., McCormick, W. C., Teri, L., Crane, P., & Kukull, W. (2006). Exercise is associated with reduced risk for incident dementia among persons 65 years of age and older. *Annals of Internal Medicine, 144*(2), 73–81.

Laurin, D., Verreault, R., Lindsay, J., MacPherson, K., & Rockwood, K. (2001). Physical activity and risk of cognitive impairment and dementia in elderly persons. *Archives of Neurology, 58*(3), 498–504.

Lautenschlager, N. T., Cox, K., & Cyarto, E. V. (2012). The influence of exercise on brain aging and dementia. *Biochimica et Biophysica Acta, 1822*(3), 474–481.

Lautenschlager, N. T., Cox, K. L., Flicker, L., Foster, J. K., van Bockxmeer, F. M., Xiao, J., . . . Almeida, O. P. (2008). Effect of physical activity on cognitive function in older adults at risk for Alzheimer disease: a randomized trial. *Journal of the American Medical Association, 300*(9), 1027–1037.

Li, M.-Y., Huang, M.-M., Li, S.-Z., Tao, J., Zheng, G.-H., & Chen, L.-D. (2017). The effects of aerobic exercise on the structure and function of DMN-related brain regions: a systematic review. *International Journal of Neuroscience, 127*(7), 634–649.

Lewis, T. (2016, Mar. 25). Human brain: facts, functions & anatomy. LiveScience. Retrieved from http://www.livescience.com/29365-human-brain.html

Liang, K. Y., Mintun, M. A., Fagan, A. M., Goate, A. M., Bugg, J. M., Holtzman, D. M., . . . Head, D. (2010). Exercise and Alzheimer's disease biomarkers in cognitively normal older adults. *Annals of Neurology, 68*(3), 311–318.

Liu-Ambrose, T., Donaldson, M. G., Ahamed, Y., Graf, P., Cook, W. L., Close, J., . . . Khan, K. M. (2008). Otago home-based strength and balance retraining improves executive functioning in older fallers: a randomized controlled trial. *Journal of the American Geriatrics Society, 56*(10), 1821–1830.

Liu-Ambrose, T., Nagamatsu, L. S., Graf, P., Beattie, B. L., Ashe, M. C., & Handy, T. C. (2010). Resistance training and executive functions: a 12-month randomised controlled trial. *Archives of Internal Medicine, 170*(2), 170–178.

Maddock, R. J., Casazza, G. A., Fernandez, D. H., & Maddock, M. I. (2016). Acute modulation of cortical glutamate and GABA content by physical activity. *Journal of Neuroscience: The Official Journal of the Society for Neuroscience, 36*(8), 2449–2457.

Marlatt, M. W., Potter, M. C., Lucassen, P. J., & van Praag, H. (2012). Running throughout middle-age improves memory function, hippocampal neurogenesis and BDNF levels in female C57Bl/6J mice. *Developmental Neurobiology, 72*(6), 943–952.

Matura, S., Fleckenstein, J., Deichmann, R., Engeroff, T., Fyzeki, E., Hattingen, E., . . . Pantel, J. (2017). Effects of aerobic exercise on brain metabolism and grey matter volume in older adults: results of the randomized controlled SMART trial. *Translational Psychiatry, 7*, e1172.

Mazza, M., Marano, G., Traversi, G., Bria, P., & Mazza, S. (2011). Primary cerebral blood flow deficiency and Alzheimer's disease: shadows and lights. *Journal of Alzheimer's Disease, 23*(3), 375–389.

McEwen, S. C., Hardy, A., Ellingson, B. M., Jarrahi, B., Sandu, N., Subotnik, K. L., . . . Nuechterlein, K. H. (2015). Prefrontal and hippocampal brain volume deficits: the role of low physical activity on brain plasticity in first-episode schizophrenia patients. *Journal of the International Neuropsychological Society, 21*(10), 868–879.

McMorris, T., & Hale, B. J. (2012). Differential effects of differing intensities of acute exercise on speed and accuracy of cognition: a meta-analytical investigation. *Brain and Cognition, 80*(3), 338–351.

Meeusen, R. (2014). Exercise, nutrition and the brain. *Sports Medicine (Auckland, NZ), 44*(Suppl 1), 47–56.

Michalski, B., Corrada, M., Kawas, C., & Fahnestock, M. (2015). Brain-derived neurotrophic factor and TrkB expression in the "oldest-old," the 90+ Study: correlation with cognitive status and levels of soluble amyloid-beta. *Neurobiology of Aging, 36*(12), 3130–3139.

Miller, D. I., Taler, V., Davidson, P. S. R., & Messier, C. (2012). Measuring the impact of exercise on cognitive aging: methodological issues. *Neurobiology of Aging, 33*(3), 622.e29–43.

Mischel, N. A., Llewellyn-Smith, I. J., & Mueller, P. J. (2014). Physical (in)activity-dependent structural plasticity in bulbospinal catecholaminergic neurons of rat rostral ventrolateral medulla. *Journal of Comparative Neurology, 522*(3), 499–513.

Moon, H. Y., Becke, A., Berron, D., Becker, B., Sah, N., Benoni, G., . . . van Praag, H. (2016). Running-induced systemic cathepsin B secretion is associated with memory function. *Cell Metabolism, 24*(2), 332–340.

Morris, J. K., Vidoni, E. D., Johnson, D. K., Van Sciver, A., Mahnken, J. D., Honea, R. A., . . . Burns, J. M. (2017). Aerobic exercise for Alzheimer's disease: a randomized controlled pilot trial. *PLoS ONE, 12*(2). Retrieved from https://doi.org/10.1371/journal.pone.0170547

Nagamatsu, L. S., Chan, A., Davis, J. C., Beattie, B. L., Graf, P., Voss, M. W., . . . Liu-Ambrose, T. (2013). Physical activity improves verbal and spatial memory in older adults with probable mild cognitive impairment: a 6-month randomized controlled trial. *Journal of Aging Research, 2013*, 861893.

Neeper, S. A., Gómez-Pinilla, F., Choi, J., & Cotman, C. (1995). Exercise and brain neurotrophins. *Nature, 373*(6510), 109.

Ngandu, T., Lehtisalo, J., Solomon, A., Levälahti, E., Ahtiluoto, S., Antikainen, R., . . . Kivipelto, M. (2015). A 2-year multidomain intervention of diet, exercise, cognitive training, and vascular risk monitoring versus control to prevent cognitive decline in at-risk elderly people (FINGER): a randomised controlled trial. *Lancet, 385*(9984), 2255–2263.

Nokia, M. S., Lensu, S., Ahtiainen, J. P., Johansson, P. P., Koch, L. G., Britton, S. L., & Kainulainen, H. (2016). Physical exercise increases adult hippocampal neurogenesis in male rats provided it is aerobic and sustained. *Journal of Physiology, 594*(7), 1855–1873.

Northey, J. M., Cherbuin, K. L., Smee, D. J., & Rattray, B. (2018). Exercise interventions for cognitive function in adults older than 50: a systematic review with meta-analysis. *British Journal of Sports Medicine, 52*(3), 154–160.

O'Toole, G. (2012, Jan. 13). I take my only exercise acting as a pallbearer to my friends who exercise [Web log post]. Quote Investigator. Retrieved from http://quoteinvestigator.com/2012/01/13/exercise-as-pallbearer/

Owen, A. M., Hampshire, A., Grahn, J. A., Stenton, R., Dajani, S., Burns, A. S., ... Ballard, C. G. (2010). Putting brain training to the test. *Nature, 465*(7299), 775–778.

Pereira, A. C., Huddleston, D. E., Brickman, A. M., Sosunov, A. A., Hen, R., McKhann, G. M., ... Small, S. A. (2007). An in vivo correlate of exercise-induced neurogenesis in the adult dentate gyrus. *Proceedings of the National Academy of Sciences of the United States of America, 104*(13), 5638–5643.

Radiological Society of North America. (2016, Nov. 30). Aerobic exercise preserves brain volume and improves cognitive function. [Press release]. Retrieved from https://press.rsna.org/timssnet/Media/pressreleases/14_pr_target.cfm?id=1921

Raichlen, D. A., Bharadwaj, P. K., Fitzhugh, M. C., Haws, K. A., Torre, G.-A., Trouard, T. P., & Alexander, G. E. (2016). Differences in resting state functional connectivity between young adult endurance athletes and healthy controls. *Frontiers in Human Neuroscience, 10*, 610.

Ratey, J. J., & Hagerman, E. (2008). *Spark: the revolutionary new science of exercise and the brain*. New York, NY: Little, Brown.

Reynolds, G. (2014, Jan. 21). How inactivity changes the brain. *New York Times*. Retrieved from https://well.blogs.nytimes.com/2014/01/22/how-inactivity-changes-the-brain/

Reynolds, G. (2014, July 2). Can exercise reduce Alzheimer's risk? *New York Times*. Retrieved from https://well.blogs.nytimes.com/2014/07/02/can-exercise-reduce-alzheimers-risk/

Reynolds, G. (2015, June 17). Does exercise help keep our bodies young? *New York Times*. Retrieved from https://well.blogs.nytimes.com/2015/12/09/does-exercise-help-keep-our-brains-young/

Reynolds, G. (2015, Sept. 2). Does exercise change your brain? *New York Times*. Retrieved from https://well.blogs.nytimes.com/2015/09/02/physed-4/

Rogers, R. L., Meyer, J. S., & Mortel, K. F. (1990). After reaching retirement age physical activity sustains cerebral perfusion and cognition. *Journal of the American Geriatrics Society, 38*(2), 123–128.

Roher, A. E., Debbins, J. P., Malek-Ahmadi, M., Chen, K., Pipe, J. G., Maze, S., ... Beach, T. G. (2012). Cerebral blood flow in Alzheimer's disease. *Vascular Health and Risk Management, 8*, 599–611.

Rolland, Y., Abellan van Kan, G., & Vellas, B. (2010). Healthy brain aging: role of exercise and physical activity. *Clinics in Geriatric Medicine, 26*(1), 75–87.

Rovio, S., Kåreholt, I., Helkala, E.-L., Viitanen, M., Winblad, B., Tuomilehto, J., ... Kivipelto, M. (2005). Leisure-time physical activity at midlife and the risk of dementia and Alzheimer's disease. *Lancet Neurology, 4*(11), 705–711.

Scarmeas, N., Luchsinger, J. A., Brickman, A. M., Cosentino, S., Schupf, N., Xin-Tang, M., ... Stern, Y. (2011). Physical activity and Alzheimer's disease course. *American Journal of Geriatric Psychiatry: Official Journal of the American Association for Geriatric Psychiatry, 19*(5), 471–481.

Schuit, A. J., Feskens, E. J., Launer, L. J., & Kromhout, D. (2001). Physical activity and cognitive decline, the role of the apolipoprotein e4 allele. *Medicine and Science in Sports and Exercise, 33*(5), 772–777.

Singh-Manoux, A., Hillsdon, M., Brunner, E., & Marmot, M. (2005). Effects of physical activity on cognitive functioning in middle age: evidence from the Whitehall II Prospective Cohort Study. *American Journal of Public Health, 95*(12), 2252–2258.

Sink, K. M., Espeland, M. A., Castro, C. M., Church, T., Cohen, R., Dodson, J. A., . . . Williamson, J. D. (2015). Effect of a 24-month physical activity intervention compared to health education on cognitive outcomes in sedentary older adults: the LIFE Randomized Trial. *Journal of the American Medical Association, 314*(8), 781–790.

Sleiman, S. F., Henry, J., Al-Haddad, R., El Hayek, L., Abou Haidar, E., Stringer, T., . . . Chao, M. V. (2016). Exercise promotes the expression of brain derived neurotrophic factor (BDNF) through the action of the ketone body β-hydroxybutyrate. *eLife, 5,* e15092.

Smiley-Oyen, A. L., Lowry, K. A., Francois, S. J., Kohut, M. L., & Ekkekakis, P. (2008). Exercise, fitness, and neurocognitive function in older adults: the "selective improvement" and "cardiovascular fitness" hypotheses. *Annals of Behavioral Medicine: A Publication of the Society of Behavioral Medicine, 36*(3), 280–291.

Smith, J. C., Nielson, K. A., Woodard, J. L., Seidenberg, M., Durgerian, S., Hazlett, K. E., . . . Rao, S. M. (2014). Physical activity reduces hippocampal atrophy in elders at genetic risk for Alzheimer's disease. *Frontiers in Aging Neuroscience, 6,* 61.

Smith, J. K. (2001). Exercise and atherogenesis. *Exercise and Sport Sciences Reviews, 29*(2), 49–53.

Smith, P. J., Blumenthal, J. A., Hoffman, B. M., Cooper, H., Strauman, T. A., Welsh-Bohmer, K., . . . Sherwood, A. (2010). Aerobic exercise and neurocognitive performance: a meta-analytic review of randomized controlled trials. *Psychosomatic Medicine, 72*(3), 239–252.

Snyder, J. S. (2018, Mar. 7). Questioning human neurogenesis. *Nature, New and Views.*

Sofi, F., Valecchi, D., Bacci, D., Abbate, R., Gensini, G. F., Casini, A., & Macchi, C. (2011). Physical activity and risk of cognitive decline: a meta-analysis of prospective studies. *Journal of Internal Medicine, 269*(1), 107–117.

Sorrells, S. F., Paredes, M. F., Cebrian-Sila, A., Sandoval, K., Qi, D., Keley, K. W., . . . Alvarez-Buylla, A. (2018). Human hippocampal neurogenesis drops sharply in children to undetectable levels in adults. *Nature, 555,* 377–381.

Soto, I., Graham, L. C., Richter, H. J., Simeone, S. N., Radell, J. E., Grabowska, W., . . . Howell, G. R. (2015). APOE stabilization by exercise prevents aging neurovascular dysfunction and complement induction. *PLoS Biology, 13*(10), e1002279.

Spalding, K. L., Bergmann, O., Alkass, K., Bernard, S., Salehpour, M., Huttner, H. B., . . . Frisen, J. (2013). Dynamics of hippocampal neurogenesis. *Cell, 153,* 1219–1227.

Spartano, N. L., Himali, J. J., Beiser, A. S., Lewis, G. D., DeCarli, C., Vasan, R. S., & Seshadri, S. (2016). Midlife exercise blood pressure, heart rate, and fitness relate to brain volume 2 decades later. *Neurology, 86*(14), 1313–1319.

Spirduso, W. W. (1975). Reaction and movement time as a function of age and physical activity level. *Journal of Gerontology, 30*(4), 435–440.

Spirduso, W. W., & Clifford, P. (1978). Replication of age and physical activity effects on reaction and movement time. *Journal of Gerontology, 33*(1), 26–30.

Steves, C. J., Mehta, M. M., Jackson, S. H. D., & Spector, T. D. (2016). Kicking back cognitive ageing: leg power predicts cognitive ageing after ten years in older female twins. *Gerontology, 62*(2), 138–149.

Stothart, C. R., Simons, D. J., Boot, W. R., & Kramer, A. F. (2014). Is the effect of aerobic exercise on cognition a placebo effect? *PLoS ONE, 9*(10), e109557.

Suri, D., & Vaidya, V. A. (2013). Glucocorticoid regulation of brain-derived neurotrophic factor: relevance to hippocampal structural and functional plasticity. *Neuroscience, 239,* 196–213.

Swain, R. A., Harris, A. B., Wiener, E. C., Dutka, M. V., Morris, H. D., Theien, B. E., ... Greenough, W. T. (2003). Prolonged exercise induces angiogenesis and increases cerebral blood volume in primary motor cortex of the rat. *Neuroscience, 117*(4), 1037–1046.

Szuhany, K., Bugatti, M., & Otto, M.W. (2015). A meta-analytic review of the effects of exercise on brain-derived neurotrophic factor. *Journal of Psychiatric Research, 60*, 56–64.

UCI Media. (2015, Oct. 25). Carl Cotman, "Exercise and Alzheimer's disease research." [Video file]. Retrieved from https://www.youtube.com/watch?v=cuo_YJv4kIk

Uda, M., Ishido, M., Kami, K., & Masuhara, M. (2006). Effects of chronic treadmill running on neurogenesis in the dentate gyrus of the hippocampus of adult rat. *Brain Research, 1104*(1), 64–72.

Um, H. S., Kang, E. B., Leem, Y. H., Cho, I. H., Yang, C. H., Chae, K. R., ... Cho, J. Y. (2008). Exercise training acts as a therapeutic strategy for reduction of the pathogenic phenotypes for Alzheimer's disease in an NSE/APPsw-transgenic model. *International Journal of Molecular Medicine, 22*(4), 529–5.

Underwood, E. (2018, Mar. 9) Study undercuts claims of new neurons in adult brains. *Science, 359*(6380), 1083.

van Gelder, B. M., Tijhuis, M. A. R., Kalmijn, S., Giampaoli, S., Nissinen, A., & Kromhout, D. (2004). Physical activity in relation to cognitive decline in elderly men: the FINE Study. *Neurology, 63*(12), 2316–2321.

van Praag, H., Kempermann, G., & Gage, F. H. (1999). Running increases cell proliferation and neurogenesis in the adult mouse dentate gyrus. *Nature Neuroscience, 2*(3), 266–270.

van Praag, H., Shubert, T., Zhao, C., & Gage, F. H. (2005). Exercise enhances learning and hippocampal neurogenesis in aged mice. *Journal of Neuroscience: The Official Journal of the Society for Neuroscience, 25*(38), 8680–8685.

Vaynman, S., Ying, Z., & Gomez-Pinilla, F. (2003). Interplay between brain-derived neurotrophic factor and signal transduction modulators in the regulation of the effects of exercise on synaptic-plasticity. *Neuroscience, 122*(3), 647–657.

Vaynman, S., Ying, Z., & Gómez-Pinilla, F. (2004a). Exercise induces BDNF and synapsin I to specific hippocampal subfields. *Journal of Neuroscience Research, 76*(3), 356–362.

Vaynman, S., Ying, Z., & Gomez-Pinilla, F. (2004b). Hippocampal BDNF mediates the efficacy of exercise on synaptic plasticity and cognition. *European Journal of Neuroscience, 20*(10), 2580–2590.

Vidoni, E. D., Johnson, D. K., Morris, J. K., Van Sciver, A., Greer, C. S., Billinger, S. A., ... Burns, J. M. (2015). Dose-response of aerobic exercise on cognition: a community-based, pilot randomized controlled trial. *PLoS ONE, 10*(7), e0131647.

Vivar, C., Peterson, B. D., & van Praag, H. (2016). Running rewires the neuronal network of adult-born dentate granule cells. *NeuroImage, 131*, 29–41.

Voss, M. W., Vivar, C., Kramer, A. F., & van Praag, H. (2013). Bridging animal and human models of exercise-induced brain plasticity. *Trends in Cognitive Sciences, 17*(10), 525–544.

Voytek, B. (2013, May 20). Are there really as many neurons in the human brain as stars in the Milky Way? [Web log post] Brain metrics, Scitable. Retrieved from http://www.nature.com/scitable/blog/brain-metrics/are_there_really_as_many

Waterhouse, E. G., An, J. J., Orefice, L. L., Baydyuk, M., Liao, G.-Y., Zheng, K., ... Xu, B. (2012). Brain-derived neurotrophic factor promotes differentiation and maturation of adult-born neurons through GABAergic transmission. *Journal of Neuroscience: The Official Journal of the Society for Neuroscience, 32*(41), 14318–14330.

Weiler, N. (2018, Mar. 7). The adult human brain doesn't produce new neurons to renew itself, study finds. *UCSF News.* Retrieved from https://www.ucsf.edu/news/2018/03/409986/birth-new-neurons-human-hippocampus-ends-childhood

White, L. J., & Castellano, V. (2008). Exercise and brain health—implications for multiple sclerosis: Part 1—neuronal growth factors. *Sports Medicine (Auckland, NZ), 38*(2), 91–100.

Winter, B., Breitenstein, C., Mooren, F. C., Voelker, K., Fobker, M., Lechtermann, A., . . . Knecht, S. (2007). High-impact running improves learning. *Neurobiology of Learning and Memory, 87*(4), 597–609.

Wrann, C. D., White, J. P., Salogiannnis, J., Laznik-Bogoslavski, D., Wu, J., Ma, D., . . . Spiegelman, B. M. (2013). Exercise induces hippocampal BDNF through a PGC-1α/FNDC5 pathway. *Cell Metabolism, 18*(5), 649–659.

Yaffe, K., Barnes, D., Nevitt, M., Lui, L. Y., & Covinsky, K. (2001). A prospective study of physical activity and cognitive decline in elderly women: women who walk. *Archives of Internal Medicine, 161*(14), 1703–1708.

Yuste, R., & Church, G. M. (2014). The new century of the brain. *Scientific American, 310*(3), 38–45.

Zhu, N., Jacobs, D. R., Schreiner, P. J., Yaffe, K., Bryan, N., Launer, L. J., . . . Sternfeld, B. (2014). Cardiorespiratory fitness and cognitive function in middle age: the CARDIA Study. *Neurology, 82*(15), 1339–1346.

CHAPTER 9

Abu-Omar, K., Rütten, A., & Lehtinen, V. (2004). Mental health and physical activity in the European Union. *Sozial- Und Praventivmedizin, 49*(5), 301–309.

Agudelo, L. Z., Femenía, T., Orhan, F., Porsmyr-Palmertz, M., Goiny, M., Martinez-Redondo, V., . . . Ruas, J. L. (2014). Skeletal muscle PGC-1α1 modulates kynurenine metabolism and mediates resilience to stress-induced depression. *Cell, 159*(1), 33–45.

Alderman, B. L., Olson, R. L., Brush, C. J., & Shors, T. J. (2016). MAP training: combining meditation and aerobic exercise reduces depression and rumination while enhancing synchronized brain activity. *Translational Psychiatry, 6*(2), e726.

Aldred, J., Astell, A., Behr, R., Cochrane, L., Hind, J., Pickard, A., . . . Wiseman, E. (2008, Mar. 9). The world's 50 most powerful blogs. *The Guardian.* Retrieved from https://www.theguardian.com/technology/2008/mar/09/blogs

Anderson, E., & Shivakumar, G. (2013). Effects of exercise and physical activity on anxiety. *Frontiers in Psychiatry, 4*, 27.

Anxiety and Depression Association of America. (2016, Aug.). *Facts and statistics.* Retrieved from https://www.adaa.org/about-adaa/press-room/facts-statistics

Arent, S. M., Landers, D. M., & Etnier, J. L. (2000). The effects of exercise on mood in older adults: a meta-analytic review. *Journal of Aging and Physical Activity, 8*(4), 407–430.

Babyak, M., Blumenthal, J. A., Herman, S., Khatri, P., Doraiswamy, M., Moore, K., . . . Krishnan, K. R. (2000). Exercise treatment for major depression: maintenance of therapeutic benefit at 10 months. *Psychosomatic Medicine, 62*(5), 633–638.

Berchtold, N. C., Cesslak, J. P., Cotman, C. W. (2002), Hippocampal brain-derived neurotrophic factor gene regulation by exercise and the medial septum. *Trends in Neuroscience, 25,* 295–301.

Bernstein, E. E., & McNally, R. J. (2017). Acute aerobic exercise helps overcome emotion regulation deficits. *Cognition & Emotion, 31*(4), 834–843.

Bjørnebekk, A. (2007). *On antidepressant effects of running and SSRI: Focus on hippocampus and striatal dopamine pathways.* (Doctoral dissertation, Karolinska Institutet). Retrieved from https://openarchive.ki.se/xmlui/handle/10616/38952

Blake, H., Mo, P., Malik, S., & Thomas, S. (2009). How effective are physical activity interventions for alleviating depressive symptoms in older people? A systematic review. *Clinical Rehabilitation, 23*(10), 873–887.

Blumenthal, J. A., Babyak, M. A., Moore, K. A., Craighead, W. E., Herman, S., Khatri, P., . . . Krishnan, K. R. (1999). Effects of exercise training on older patients with major depression. *Archives of Internal Medicine, 159*(19), 2349–2356.

Blumenthal, J. A., Babyak, M. A., Murali Doraiswamy, P., Watkins, L., Hoffman, B. M., Barbour, K. A., . . . Sherwood, A. (2007). Exercise and pharmacotherapy in the treatment of major depressive disorder. *Psychosomatic Medicine, 69*(7), 587–596.

Blumenthal, J. A., Smith, P. J., & Hoffman, B. M. (2012). Is exercise a viable treatment for depression? *ACSM's Health & Fitness Journal, 16*(4), 14–21.

Boecker, H., & Dishman R. K. (2015). Physical activity and reward: the role of endogenous opioids. In Ekkekekis, P. (Ed.), *Routledge handbook of physical activity and mental health* (pp. 57–70). London, England: Routledge, Taylor and Francis Group.

Boecker, H., Sprenger, T., Spilker, M. E., Henriksen, G., Koppenhoefer, M., Wagner, K. J., . . . Tolle, T. R. (2008). The runner's high: opioidergic mechanisms in the human brain. *Cerebral Cortex (New York, NY: 1991), 18*(11), 2523–2531.

Bortz, W. M., Angwin, P., Mefford, I. N., Boarder, M. R., Noyce, N., & Barchas, J. D. (1981). Catecholamines, dopamine, and endorphin levels during extreme exercise. *New England Journal of Medicine, 305*(8), 466–467.

Bremner, J. D., Narayan, M., Anderson, E. R., Staib, L. H., Miller, H. L., & Charney, D. S. (2000). Hippocampal volume reduction in major depression. *American Journal of Psychiatry, 157*(1), 115–118.

Brezun, J. M., & Daszuta, A. (1999). Depletion in serotonin decreases neurogenesis in the dentate gyrus and the subventricular zone of adult rats. *Neuroscience, 89*(4), 999–1002.

Brezun, J. M., & Daszuta, A. (2000). Serotonin may stimulate granule cell proliferation in the adult hippocampus, as observed in rats grafted with foetal raphe neurons. *European Journal of Neuroscience, 12*(1), 391–396.

Broocks, A., Bandelow, B., Pekrun, G., George, A., Meyer, T., Bartmann, U., . . . Rüther, E. (1998). Comparison of aerobic exercise, clomipramine, and placebo in the treatment of panic disorder. *American Journal of Psychiatry, 155*(5), 603–609.

Brown, E. S., Rush, A. J., & McEwen, B. S. (1999). Hippocampal remodeling and damage by corticosteroids: implications for mood disorders. *Neuropsychopharmacology, 21*(4), 474–484.

Brown, W. J., Ford, J. H., Burton, N. W., Marshall, A. L., & Dobson, A. J. (2005). Prospective study of physical activity and depressive symptoms in middle-aged women. *American Journal of Preventive Medicine, 29*(4), 265–272.

Campbell, S., Marriott, M., Nahmias, C., & MacQueen, G. M. (2004). Lower hippocampal volume in patients suffering from depression: a meta-analysis. *American Journal of Psychiatry, 161*(4), 598–607.

Carek, P. J., Laibstain, S. E., & Carek, S. M. (2011). Exercise for the treatment of depression and anxiety. *International Journal of Psychiatry in Medicine, 41*(1), 15–28.

Carr, D. B., Bullen, B. A., Skrinar, G. S., Arnold, M. A., Rosenblatt, M., Beitins, I. Z., . . . McArthur, J. W. (1981). Physical conditioning facilitates the exercise-induced secretion of beta-endorphin and beta-lipotropin in women. *New England Journal of Medicine, 305*(10), 560–563.

Centers for Disease Control and Prevention, National Center for Health Statistics. (2016, Oct. 6). Depression. Retrieved from https://www.cdc.gov/nchs/fastats/depression.htm

Chaouloff, F., Elghozi, J. L., Guezennec, Y., & Laude, D. (1985). Effects of conditioned running on plasma, liver and brain tryptophan and on brain 5-hydroxytryptamine metabolism of the rat. *British Journal of Pharmacology, 86*(1), 33–41.

Cooney, G. M., Dwan, K., Greig, C. A., Lawlor, D. A., Rimer, J., Waugh, F. R., . . . Mead, G. E. (2013). Exercise for depression. *Cochrane Database of Systematic Reviews,* (9), CD004366.

Cotman, C. W., Berchtold, N. C., & Christie, L.-A. (2007). Exercise builds brain health: key roles of growth factor cascades and inflammation. *Trends in Neurosciences, 30*(9), 464–472.

Cox, R. H., Thomas, T. R., Hinton, P. S., & Donahue, O. M. (2004). Effects of acute 60 and 80% VO2max bouts of aerobic exercise on state anxiety of women of different age groups across time. *Research Quarterly for Exercise and Sport, 75*(2), 165–175.

Craft, L. L., & Landers, D. M. (1998). The effect of exercise on clinical depression and depression resulting from mental illness: a meta-analysis. *Journal of Sport and Exercise Psychology, 20*(4), 339–357.

Craft, L. L., & Perna, F. M. (2004). The benefits of exercise for the clinically depressed. *Primary Care Companion to the Journal of Clinical Psychiatry, 6*(3), 104–111.

Delgado, P. L. (2000). Depression: the case for a monoamine deficiency. *Journal of Clinical Psychiatry, 61*(Suppl 6), 7–11.

Dimeo, F., Bauer, M., Varahram, I., Proest, G., & Halter, U. (2001). Benefits from aerobic exercise in patients with major depression: a pilot study. *British Journal of Sports Medicine, 35*(2), 114–117.

Dishman, R. K. (1997). Brain monoamines, exercise, and behavioral stress: animal models. *Medicine and Science in Sports and Exercise, 29*(1), 63–74.

Dishman, R. K., Berthoud, H.-R., Booth, F. W., Cotman, C. W., Edgerton, V. R., Fleshner, M. R., . . . Zigmond, M. J. (2006). Neurobiology of exercise. *Obesity, 14*(3), 345–356.

Dishman, R. K., & O'Connor, P.J. (2009). Lessons in exercise neurobiology: the case of endorphins. *Mental Health and Physical Activity, 2*(1), 4–9.

Doyne, E. J., Ossip-Klein, D. J., Bowman, E. D., Osborn, K. M., McDougall-Wilson, I. B., & Neimeyer, R. A. (1987). Running versus weight lifting in the treatment of depression. *Journal of Consulting and Clinical Psychology, 55*(5), 748–754.

Droge-Young, E. (2017, Mar. 14). Personal communication.

Duke Today Staff. (2000, Sept. 22). Study: exercise has long-lasting effect on depression. *Duke Today.* Retrieved from https://today.duke.edu/2000/09/exercise922.html

Duman, C. H., Schlesinger, L., Russell, D. S., & Duman, R. S. (2008). Voluntary exercise produces antidepressant and anxiolytic behavioral effects in mice. *Brain Research, 1199*, 148–158.

Duman, R. (2017, Mar. 29). Personal communication.

Duman, R. S. (2004). Depression: a case of neuronal life and death? *Biological Psychiatry, 56*(3), 140–145.

Duman, R. S., Aghajanian, G. K., Sanacora, G., & Krystal, J. H. (2016). Synaptic plasticity and depression: new insights from stress and rapid-acting antidepressants. *Nature Medicine, 22*(3), 238–249.

Duman, R. S., Heninger, G. R., & Nestler, E. J. (1997). A molecular and cellular theory of depression. *Archives of General Psychiatry, 54*(7), 597–606.

Duman, R. S., Nakagawa, S., & Malberg, J. (2001). Regulation of adult neurogenesis by antidepressant treatment. *Neuropsychopharmacology, 25*(6), 836–844.

Dunn, A. L., Reigle, T. G., Youngstedt, S. D., Armstrong, R. B., & Dishman, R. K. (1996). Brain norepinephrine and metabolites after treadmill training and wheel running in rats. *Medicine and Science in Sports and Exercise, 28*(2), 204–209.

Dunn, A. L., Trivedi, M. H., Kampert, J. B., Clark, C. G., & Chambliss, H. O. (2005). Exercise treatment for depression: efficacy and dose response. *American Journal of Preventive Medicine, 28*(1), 1–8.

Dunn, A. L., Trivedi, M. H., & O'Neal, H. A. (2001). Physical activity dose-response effects on outcomes of depression and anxiety. *Medicine and Science in Sports and Exercise, 33*(6 Suppl), S587–597–610.

Erickson, K. I., Miller, D. L., & Roecklein, K. A. (2012). The aging hippocampus: interactions between exercise, depression, and BDNF. *The Neuroscientist, 18*(1), 82–97.

Ernst, C., Olson, A. K., Pinel, J. P. J., Lam, R. W., & Christie, B. R. (2006). Antidepressant effects of exercise: evidence for an adult-neurogenesis hypothesis? *Journal of Psychiatry & Neuroscience, 31*(2), 84–92.

Fabel, K., Fabel, K., Tam, B., Kaufer, D., Baiker, A., Simmons, N., . . . Palmer, T. D. (2003). VEGF is necessary for exercise-induced adult hippocampal neurogenesis. *European Journal of Neuroscience, 18*(10), 2803–2812.

Farmer, M. E., Locke, B. Z., Mościcki, E. K., Dannenberg, A. L., Larson, D. B., & Radloff, L. S. (1988). Physical activity and depressive symptoms: the NHANES I Epidemiologic Follow-up Study. *American Journal of Epidemiology, 128*(6), 1340–1351.

Farrell, P. A., Gates, W. K., Maksud, M. G., & Morgan, W. P. (1982). Increases in plasma beta-endorphin/beta-lipotropin immunoreactivity after treadmill running in humans. *Journal of Applied Physiology: Respiratory, Environmental and Exercise Physiology, 52*(5), 1245–1249.

Franz, S. I., & Hamilton, G. V. (1905). The effects of exercise upon the retardation in conditions of depression. *American Journal of Psychiatry, 62*(2), 239–256.

Fremont, J., & Craighead, L. W. (1987). Aerobic exercise and cognitive therapy in the treatment of dysphoric moods. *Cognitive Therapy and Research, 11*(2), 241–251.

Fuss, J., Steinle, J., Bindila, L., Auer, M. K., Kirchherr, H., Lutz, B., & Gass, P. (2015). A runner's high depends on cannabinoid receptors in mice. *Proceedings of the National Academy of Sciences of the United States of America, 112*(42), 13105–13108.

Galper, D. I., Trivedi, M. H., Barlow, C. E., Dunn, A. L., & Kampert, J. B. (2006). Inverse association between physical inactivity and mental health in men and women. *Medicine and Science in Sports and Exercise, 38*(1), 173–178.

Gómez-Pinilla, F., Ying, Z., Roy, R. R., Molteni, R., & Edgerton, V. R. (2002). Voluntary exercise induces a BDNF-mediated mechanism that promotes neuroplasticity. *Journal of Neurophysiology, 88*(5), 2187–2195.

Goodwin, R. D. (2003). Association between physical activity and mental disorders among adults in the United States. *Preventive Medicine, 36*(6), 698–703.

Gould, E., & Tanapat, P. (1999). Stress and hippocampal neurogenesis. *Biological Psychiatry, 46*(11), 1472–1479.

Greer, T. L., Grannemann, B. D., Chansard, M., Karim, A. I., & Trivedi, M. H. (2015). Dose-dependent changes in cognitive function with exercise augmentation for major depression: results from the TREAD study. *European Neuropsychopharmacology, 25*(2), 248–256.

Greer, T. L., Trombello, J. M., Rethorst, C. D., Carmody, T. J., Jha, M. K., Liao, A., . . . Trivedi, M. H. (2016). Improvements in psychosocial function and health related quality of life following exercise augmentation in patients with treatment response but non-remitted major depressive disorder: results from the TREAD study. *Depression and Anxiety, 33*(9), 870–881.

Greist, J. H., Klein, M. H., Eischens, R. R., Faris, J., Gurman, A. S., & Morgan, W. P. (1979). Running as treatment for depression. *Comprehensive Psychiatry, 20*(1), 41–54.

Harber, V. J., & Sutton, J. R. (1984). Endorphins and exercise. *Sports Medicine, 1*(2), 154–171.

Harvey, S. B., Overland, S., Hatch, S. L., Wessley, S., Mykletun, A., & Hotopf, J. (2017). Exercise and the prevention of depression: results of the HUNT cohort study. *American Journal of Psychiatry, 175*(1), 28–36.

Herring, M. P., O'Connor, P. J., & Dishman, R. K. (2010). The effect of exercise training on anxiety symptoms among patients: a systematic review. *Archives of Internal Medicine, 170*(4), 321–331.

Heyman, E., Gamelin, F.-X., Goekint, M., Piscitelli, F., Roelands, B., Leclair, E., . . . Meeusen, R. (2012). Intense exercise increases circulating endocannabinoid and BDNF levels in humans: possible implications for reward and depression. *Psychoneuroendocrinology, 37*(6), 844–851.

Hirschfeld, R. M. (2000). History and evolution of the monoamine hypothesis of depression. *Journal of Clinical Psychiatry, 61*(Suppl 6), 4–6.

Hogan, C. L., Mata, J., & Carstensen, L. L. (2013). Exercise holds immediate benefits for affect and cognition in younger and older adults. *Psychology and Aging, 28*(2), 587–594.

Hunsberger, J. G., Newton, S. S., Bennett, A. H., Duman, C. H., Russell, D. S., Salton, S. R., & Duman, R. S. (2007). Antidepressant actions of the exercise-regulated gene VGF. *Nature Medicine, 13*(12), 1476–1482.

Jabr, F. (2017, Jan.). Head strong. *Scientific American Mind, 28*(1), 27–31.

Jin, K., Zhu, Y., Sun, Y., Mao, X. O., Xie, L., & Greenberg, D. A. (2002). Vascular endothelial growth factor (VEGF) stimulates neurogenesis in vitro and in vivo. *Proceedings of the National Academy of Sciences of the United States of America, 99*(18), 11946–11950.

Josefsson, T., Lindwall, M., & Archer, T. (2014). Physical exercise intervention in depressive disorders: meta-analysis and systematic review. *Scandinavian Journal of Medicine & Science in Sports, 24*(2), 259–272.

Karten, Y. J. G., Olariu, A., & Cameron, H. A. (2005). Stress in early life inhibits neurogenesis in adulthood. *Trends in Neurosciences, 28*(4), 171–172.

Keeney, B. K., Raichlen, D. A., Meek, T. H., Wijeratne, R. S., Middleton, K. M., Gerdeman, G. L., & Garland, T. (2008). Differential response to a selective cannabinoid receptor antagonist (SR141716: rimonabant) in female mice from lines selectively bred for high voluntary wheel-running behaviour. *Behavioural Pharmacology, 19*(8), 812–820.

Khazan, O. (2014, Mar. 24). For depression, prescribing exercise before medication. *The Atlantic.* Retrieved from https://www.theatlantic.com/health/archive/2014/03/for-depression-prescribing-exercise-before-medication/284587/

Klein, M. H., Greist, J. H., Gurman, A. S., Neimeyer, R. A., Lesser, D. P., Bushnell, N. J., & Smith, R. E. (1984). A comparative outcome study of group psychotherapy vs. exercise treatments for depression. *International Journal of Mental Health, 13*(3–4), 148–176.

Knapen, J., & Vancampfort, D. (2013). Evidence for exercise therapy in the treatment of depression and anxiety. *International Journal of Psychosocial Rehabilitation, 17*(2), 75–87.

Kodama, M., Fujioka, T., & Duman, R. S. (2004). Chronic olanzapine or fluoxetine administration increases cell proliferation in hippocampus and prefrontal cortex of adult rat. *Biological Psychiatry, 56*(8), 570–580.

Kramer, A. F., Erickson, K. I., & Colcombe, S. J. (2006). Exercise, cognition, and the aging brain. *Journal of Applied Physiology (Bethesda, MD: 1985), 101*(4), 1237–1242.

Krogh, J., Nordentoft, M., Sterne, J. A. C., & Lawlor, D. A. (2011). The effect of exercise in clinically depressed adults: systematic review and meta-analysis of randomized controlled trials. *Journal of Clinical Psychiatry, 72*(4), 529–538.

Kuhn, S. L., Raichlen, D. A., & Clark, A. E. (2016). What moves us? How mobility and movement are at the center of human evolution. *Evolutionary Anthropology, 25*(3), 86–97.

Lampinen, P., Heikkinen, R. L., & Ruoppila, I. (2000). Changes in intensity of physical exercise as predictors of depressive symptoms among older adults: an eight-year follow-up. *Preventive Medicine, 30*(5), 371–380.

Laske, C., Banschbach, S., Stransky, E., Bosch, S., Straten, G., Machann, J., . . . Eschweiler, G. W. (2010). Exercise-induced normalization of decreased BDNF serum concentration in elderly women with remitted major depression. *International Journal of Neuropsychopharmacology, 13*(5), 595–602.

Lathia, N., Sandstrom, G. M., Mascolo, C., & Rentfrow, P. J. (2017). Happier people live more active lives: using smartphones to link happiness and physical activity. *PLoS ONE, 12*(1), e0160589.

Lavelle, J. (2015, Oct. 8). New brain effects behind "runner's high." *Scientific American.* Retrieved from https://www.scientificamerican.com/article/new-brain-effects-behind-runner-s-high/

LeBouthillier, D. M., & Asmundson, G. J. G. (2015). A single bout of aerobic exercise reduces anxiety sensitivity but not intolerance of uncertainty or distress tolerance: a randomized controlled trial. *Cognitive Behaviour Therapy, 44*(4), 252–263.

Lee, Y., & Park, K. (2008). Does physical activity moderate the association between depressive symptoms and disability in older adults? *International Journal of Geriatric Psychiatry, 23*(3), 249–256.

Li, N., Lee, B., Liu, R.-J., Banasr, M., Dwyer, J. M., Iwata, M., . . . Duman, R. S. (2010). mTOR-dependent synapse formation underlies the rapid antidepressant effects of NMDA antagonists. *Science, 329*(5994), 959–964.

Long, B. C., & Stavel, R. van. (1995). Effects of exercise training on anxiety: a meta-analysis. *Journal of Applied Sport Psychology, 7*(2), 167–189.

Maddock, R. J., Casazza, G. A., Fernandez, D. H., & Maddock, M. I. (2016). Acute modulation of cortical glutamate and GABA content by physical activity. *Journal of Neuroscience, 36*(8), 2449–2457.

Malberg, J. E., & Duman, R. S. (2003). Cell proliferation in adult hippocampus is decreased by inescapable stress: reversal by fluoxetine treatment. *Neuropsychopharmacology, 28*(9), 1562–1571.

Malberg, J. E., Eisch, A. J., Nestler, E. J., & Duman, R. S. (2000). Chronic antidepressant treatment increases neurogenesis in adult rat hippocampus. *Journal of Neuroscience, 20*(24), 9104–9110.

Mammen, G., & Faulkner, G. (2013). Physical activity and the prevention of depression: a systematic review of prospective studies. *American Journal of Preventive Medicine, 45*(5), 649–657.

Margolis, Z. (n.d.). Bio. *Zoe Margolis.* Retrieved from http://www.zoemargolis.co.uk/bio/

Margolis, Z. (n.d.). *Zoe Margolis.* Retrieved from http://www.zoemargolis.co.uk/

Margolis, Z. (2015, Aug. 24). Running saved my life. *The Guardian*. Retrieved from https://www.theguardian.com/lifeandstyle/2015/aug/24/running-saved-my-life-depression-doctors-pills-therapy-did-nothing

Markoff, R. A., Ryan, P., & Young, T. (1982). Endorphins and mood changes in long-distance running. *Medicine and Science in Sports and Exercise, 14*(1), 11–15.

Martinowich, K., & Lu, B. (2008). Interaction between BDNF and serotonin: role in mood disorders. *Neuropsychopharmacology, 33*(1), 73–83.

Martinsen, E. W. (2008). Physical activity in the prevention and treatment of anxiety and depression. *Nordic Journal of Psychiatry, 62*(Suppl 47), 25–29.

Martinsen, E. W., Hoffart, A., & Solberg, O. (1989). Comparing aerobic with nonaerobic forms of exercise in the treatment of clinical depression: a randomized trial. *Comprehensive Psychiatry, 30*(4), 324–331.

Martinsen, E. W., Medhus, A., & Sandvik, L. (1985). Effects of aerobic exercise on depression: a controlled study. *British Medical Journal (Clinical Research Ed.), 291*(6488), 109.

Massart, R., Mongeau, R., & Lanfumey, L. (2012). Beyond the monoaminergic hypothesis: neuroplasticity and epigenetic changes in a transgenic mouse model of depression. *Philosophical Transactions of the Royal Society B: Biological Sciences, 367*(1601), 2485–2494.

Mather, A. S., Rodriguez, C., Guthrie, M. F., McHarg, A. M., Reid, I. C., & McMurdo, M. E. T. (2002). Effects of exercise on depressive symptoms in older adults with poorly responsive depressive disorder: randomised controlled trial. *British Journal of Psychiatry: The Journal of Mental Science, 180*, 411–415.

Mattson, M. P., Maudsley, S., & Martin, B. (2004). BDNF and 5-HT: a dynamic duo in age-related neuronal plasticity and neurodegenerative disorders. *Trends in Neurosciences, 27*(10), 589–594.

McMurray, R. G., Berry, M. J., Hardy, C. J., Sheps, D. (1988). Physiologic and psychologic responses to a low dose of naloxone administered during prolonged running. *Annals of Sports Medicine and Research, 4*, 21–25.

Mervaala, E., Föhr, J., Könönen, M., Valkonen-Korhonen, M., Vainio, P., Partanen, K., . . . Lehtonen, J. (2000). Quantitative MRI of the hippocampus and amygdala in severe depression. *Psychological Medicine, 30*(1), 117–125.

Morgan, A. J., Parker, A. G., Alvarez-Jimenez, M., & Jorm, A. F. (2013). Exercise and mental health: an Exercise and Sports Science Australia commissioned review. *Journal of Exercise Physiology Online, 16*(4).

Mura, G., Moro, M. F., Patten, S. B., & Carta, M. G. (2014). Exercise as an add-on strategy for the treatment of major depressive disorder: a systematic review. *CNS Spectrums, 19*(6), 496–508.

Neeper, S. A., Gómez-Pinilla, F., Choi, J., & Cotman, C. W. (1996). Physical activity increases mRNA for brain-derived neurotrophic factor and nerve growth factor in rat brain. *Brain Research, 726*(1–2), 49–56.

North, T. C., McCullagh, P., & Tran, Z. V. (1990). Effect of exercise on depression. *Exercise and Sport Sciences Reviews, 18*, 379–415.

Paffenbarger, R. S., Lee, I. M., & Leung, R. (1994). Physical activity and personal characteristics associated with depression and suicide in American college men. *Acta Psychiatrica Scandinavica Supplementum, 377*, 16–22.

Penedo, F. J., & Dahn, J. R. (2005). Exercise and well-being: a review of mental and physical health benefits associated with physical activity. *Current Opinion in Psychiatry, 18*(2), 189–193.

Perraton, L. G., Kumar, S., & Machotka, Z. (2010). Exercise parameters in the treatment of clinical depression: a systematic review of randomized controlled trials. *Journal of Evaluation in Clinical Practice, 16*(3), 597–604.

Raichlen, D. (2016, Nov. 3). Exercise and endocannabinoid signaling in humans. In M. Mattson & M. Fleshner (Chairs), *Exercise triggers adaptive brain cell stress responses*. Symposium conducted at the meeting of the American Physiological Society, Phoenix, AZ.

Raichlen, D. A., Foster, A. D., Gerdeman, G. L., Seillier, A., & Giuffrida, A. (2012). Wired to run: exercise-induced endocannabinoid signaling in humans and cursorial mammals with implications for the "runner's high." *Journal of Experimental Biology, 215*, 1331–1336.

Raichlen, D. A., & Polk, J. D. (2013). Linking brains and brawn: exercise and the evolution of human neurobiology. *Proceedings of the Royal Society B: Biological Sciences, 280*(1750), 20122250.

Rebar, A. L., Stanton, R., Geard, D., Short, C., Duncan, M. J., & Vandelanotte, C. (2015). A meta-meta-analysis of the effect of physical activity on depression and anxiety in non-clinical adult populations. *Health Psychology Review, 9*(3), 366–378.

Rethorst, C. D., Moynihan, J., Lyness, J. M., Heffner, K. L., & Chapman, B. P. (2011). Moderating effects of moderate-intensity physical activity in the relationship between depressive symptoms and interleukin-6 in primary care patients. *Psychosomatic Medicine, 73*(3), 265–269.

Rethorst, C. D., Sunderajan, P., Greer, T. L., Grannemann, B. D., Nakonezny, P. A., Carmody, T. J., & Trivedi, M. H. (2013). Does exercise improve self-reported sleep quality in non-remitted major depressive disorder? *Psychological Medicine, 43*(4), 699–709.

Rethorst, C. D., Toups, M. S., Greer, T. L., Nakonezny, P. A., Carmody, T. J., Grannemann, B. D., . . . Trivedi, M. H. (2013). Pro-inflammatory cytokines as predictors of antidepressant effects of exercise in major depressive disorder. *Molecular Psychiatry, 18*(10), 1119–1124.

Rethorst, C. D., Wipfli, B. M., & Landers, D. M. (2009). The antidepressive effects of exercise: a meta-analysis of randomized trials. *Sports Medicine, 39*(6), 491–511.

Reynolds, G. (2012, Apr. 25). The evolution of the runner's high. *New York Times*. Retrieved from https://well.blogs.nytimes.com/2012/04/25/the-evolution-of-the-runners-high/

Reynolds, G. (2014, Oct. 1). How exercise may protect against depression. *New York Times*. Retrieved from https://well.blogs.nytimes.com/2014/10/01/how-exercise-may-protect-against-depression/

Reynolds, G. O., Otto, M. W., Ellis, T. D., & Cronin-Golomb, A. (2016). The therapeutic potential of exercise to improve mood, cognition, and sleep in Parkinson's disease. *Movement Disorders, 31*(1), 23–38.

Rosenbrock, H., Koros, E., Bloching, A., Podhorna, J., & Borsini, F. (2005). Effect of chronic intermittent restraint stress on hippocampal expression of marker proteins for synaptic plasticity and progenitor cell proliferation in rats. *Brain Research, 1040*(1–2), 55–63.

Russo-Neustadt, A. A., Beard, R. C., Huang, Y. M., & Cotman, C. W. (2000). Physical activity and antidepressant treatment potentiate the expression of specific brain-derived neurotrophic factor transcripts in the rat hippocampus. *Neuroscience, 101*(2), 305–312.

Ruuskanen, J. M., & Ruoppila, I. (1995). Physical activity and psychological well-being among people aged 65 to 84 years. *Age and Ageing, 24*(4), 292–296.

Schobersberger, W., Hobisch-Hagen, P., Fries, D., Wiedermann, F., Rieder-Scharinger, J., Villiger, B., . . . Jelkmann, W. (2000). Increase in immune activation, vascular endothelial growth factor and erythropoietin after an ultramarathon run at moderate altitude. *Immunobiology, 201*(5), 611–620.

Schoenfeld, T. J., Rada, P., Pieruzzini, P. R., Hsueh, B., & Gould, E. (2013). Physical exercise prevents stress-induced activation of granule neurons and enhances local inhibitory mechanisms in the dentate gyrus. *Journal of Neuroscience, 33*(18), 7770–7777.

Schuch, F. B., Vancampfort, D., Richards, J., Rosenbaum, S., Ward, P. B., & Stubbs, B. (2016). Exercise as a treatment for depression: a meta-analysis adjusting for publication bias. *Journal of Psychiatric Research, 77*, 42–51.

Schuch, F. B., Vancampfort, D., Sui, X., Rosenbaum, S., Firth, J., Richards, J., . . . Stubbs, B. (2016). Are lower levels of cardiorespiratory fitness associated with incident depression? A systematic review of prospective cohort studies. *Preventive Medicine, 93*, 159–165.

Sciolino, N. R., Dishman, R. K., & Holmes, P. V. (2012). Voluntary exercise offers anxiolytic potential and amplifies galanin gene expression in the locus coeruleus of the rat. *Behavioural Brain Research, 233*(1), 191–200.

Sheline, Y. I., Sanghavi, M., Mintun, M. A., & Gado, M. H. (1999). Depression duration but not age predicts hippocampal volume loss in medically healthy women with recurrent major depression. *Journal of Neuroscience: The Official Journal of the Society for Neuroscience, 19*(12), 5034–5043.

Sheline, Y. I., Wang, P. W., Gado, M. H., Csernansky, J. G., & Vannier, M. W. (1996). Hippocampal atrophy in recurrent major depression. *Proceedings of the National Academy of Sciences of the United States of America, 93*(9), 3908–3913.

Shirayama, Y., Chen, A. C.-H., Nakagawa, S., Russell, D. S., & Duman, R. S. (2002). Brain-derived neurotrophic factor produces antidepressant effects in behavioral models of depression. *Journal of Neuroscience, 22*(8), 3251–3261.

Sims, J., Galea, M., Taylor, N., Dodd, K., Jespersen, S., Joubert, L., & Joubert, J. (2009). Regenerate: assessing the feasibility of a strength-training program to enhance the physical and mental health of chronic post stroke patients with depression. *International Journal of Geriatric Psychiatry, 24*(1), 76–83.

Singh, N. A., Clements, K. M., & Singh, M. A. (2001). The efficacy of exercise as a long-term antidepressant in elderly subjects: a randomized, controlled trial. *Journals of Gerontology Series A: Biological Sciences and Medical Sciences, 56*(8), M497–504.

Singh, N. A., Stavrinos, T. M., Scarbek, Y., Galambos, G., Liber, C., & Fiatarone Singh, M. A. (2005). A randomized controlled trial of high- versus low-intensity weight training versus general practitioner care for clinical depression in older adults. *Journals of Gerontology Series A: Biological Sciences and Medical Sciences, 60*(6), 768–776.

Siuciak, J. A., Lewis, D. R., Wiegand, S. J., & Lindsay, R. M. (1997). Antidepressant-like effect of brain-derived neurotrophic factor (BDNF). *Pharmacology, Biochemistry, and Behavior, 56*(1), 131–137.

Smith, J. C. (2013). Effects of emotional exposure on state anxiety after acute exercise. *Medicine and Science in Sports and Exercise, 45*(2), 372–378.

Smits, J. A. J., Berry, A. C., Rosenfield, D., Powers, M. B., Behar, E., & Otto, M. W. (2008). Reducing anxiety sensitivity with exercise. *Depression and Anxiety, 25*(8), 689–699.

Stanton, R., & Reaburn, P. (2014). Exercise and the treatment of depression: a review of the exercise program variables. *Journal of Science and Medicine in Sport, 17*(2), 177–182.

Stathopoulou, G., Powers, M. B., Berry, A., & Otto, M. W. (2006). Exercise interventions for mental health: a quantitative and qualitative review. *Clinical Psychology: Science and Practice*, 13(2), 179–193.

Steffens, D. C., Byrum, C. E., McQuoid, D. R., Greenberg, D. L., Payne, M. E., Blitchington, T. F., . . . Krishnan, K. R. (2000). Hippocampal volume in geriatric depression. *Biological Psychiatry*, 48(4), 301–309.

Stockmeier, C. A., Mahajan, G. J., Konick, L. C., Overholser, J. C., Jurjus, G. J., Meltzer, H. Y., . . . Rajkowska, G. (2004). Cellular changes in the postmortem hippocampus in major depression. *Biological Psychiatry*, 56(9), 640–650.

Strawbridge, W. J., Deleger, S., Roberts, R. E., & Kaplan, G. A. (2002). Physical activity reduces the risk of subsequent depression for older adults. *American Journal of Epidemiology*, 156(4), 328–334.

Ströhle, A. (2009). Physical activity, exercise, depression and anxiety disorders. *Journal of Neural Transmission*, 116(6), 777–784.

Ströhle, A., Feller, C., Onken, M., Godemann, F., Heinz, A., & Dimeo, F. (2005). The acute antipanic activity of aerobic exercise. *American Journal of Psychiatry*, 162(12), 2376–2378.

Stubbs, B., Vancampfort, D., Rosenbaum, S., Ward, P. B., Richards, J., Soundy, A., . . . Schuch, F. B. (2016). Dropout from exercise randomized controlled trials among people with depression: a meta-analysis and meta regression. *Journal of Affective Disorders*, 190, 457–466.

Szuhany, K. L., Bugatti, M., & Otto, M. W. (2015). A meta-analytic review of the effects of exercise on brain-derived neurotrophic factor. *Journal of Psychiatric Research*, 60, 56–64.

Ten Have, M., de Graaf, R., & Monshouwer, K. (2011). Physical exercise in adults and mental health status findings from the Netherlands mental health survey and incidence study (NEMESIS). *Journal of Psychosomatic Research*, 71(5), 342–348.

Thayer, R. E., Newman, J. R., & McClain, T. M. (1994). Self-regulation of mood: strategies for changing a bad mood, raising energy, and reducing tension. *Journal of Personality and Social Psychology*, 67(5), 910–925.

Tkachuk, G. A., & Martin, G. L. (1999). Exercise therapy for patients with psychiatric disorders: research and clinical implications. *Professional Psychology: Research and Practice*, 3(3), 275–282.

Trivedi, M. H., Greer, T. L., Church, T. S., Carmody, T. J., Grannemann, B. D., Galper, D. I., . . . Blair, S. N. (2011). Exercise as an augmentation treatment for nonremitted major depressive disorder: a randomized, parallel dose comparison. *Journal of Clinical Psychiatry*, 72(5), 677–684.

Trivedi, M. H., Greer, T. L., Grannemann, B. D., Chambliss, H. O., & Jordan, A. N. (2006). Exercise as an augmentation strategy for treatment of major depression. *Journal of Psychiatric Practice*, 12(4), 205–213.

US Department of Health and Human Services, National Institutes of Health, National Institute of Mental Health. (n.d.). *Major depression among adults*. Retrieved from https://www.nimh.nih.gov/health/statistics/prevalence/major-depression-among-adults.shtml

van Uffelen, J. G. Z., van Gellecum, Y. R., Burton, N. W., Peeters, G., Heesch, K. C., & Brown, W. J. (2013). Sitting-time, physical activity, and depressive symptoms in mid-aged women. *American Journal of Preventive Medicine*, 45(3), 276–281.

Wedekind, D., Broocks, A., Weiss, N., Engel, K., Neubert, K., & Bandelow, B. (2010). A randomized, controlled trial of aerobic exercise in combination with paroxetine in the treatment of panic disorder. *World Journal of Biological Psychiatry*, 11(7), 904–913.

Weir, K. (2011). The exercise effect. *American Psychological Association Monitor on Psychology, 42*(11), 48. Retrieved from http://www.apa.org/monitor/2011/12/exercise.aspx

Wipfli, B. M., Rethorst, C. D., & Landers, D. M. (2008). The anxiolytic effects of exercise: a meta-analysis of randomized trials and dose-response analysis. *Journal of Sport & Exercise Psychology, 30*(4), 392–410.

World Health Organization, Media Centre. (2016, Apr. 13). *Investing in treatment for depression and anxiety leads to fourfold return.* [News release]. Retrieved from http://www.who.int/mediacentre/news/releases/2016/depression-anxiety-treatment/en/

World Health Organization, Media Centre. (2017, Feb.). *Depression* [Fact sheet]. Retrieved from http://www.who.int/mediacentre/factsheets/fs369/en/

Yale University. (2007, Dec. 3). Newly-identified exercise gene could help with depression. *ScienceDaily.* Retrieved from www.sciencedaily.com/releases/2007/12/071202155304.htm

Yeung, R. R. (1996). The acute effects of exercise on mood state. *Journal of Psychosomatic Research, 40*(2), 123–141.

CHAPTER 10

Allen, J. M., Mailing, L. J., Cohrs, J., Salmonson, C., Fryer, J. D., Nehra, V., . . . Woods, J. A. (2018). Exercise training-induced modification of the gut microbiota persists after microbiota colonization and attenuates the response to chemically-induced colitis in gnotobiotic mice. *Gut Microbes, 9*(2), 115–130.

Allen, J. M., Mailing, L. J., Niemiro, G. M., Moore, R., Cook, M. D., White, B. A., . . . Woods, J.A. (2017). Exercise alters gut microbiota composition and function in lean and obese humans. *Medicine and Science in Sports and Exercise, 50*(4), 747–757.

Barton, W., Penney, N. C., Cronin, O., Garcia-Perez, I., Molloy, M. G., Holmes, E., . . . O'Sullivan, O. (2018). The microbiome of professional athletes differs from that of more sedentary subjects in composition and particularly at the functional metabolic level. *Gut, 67*(4), 625–633.

Benakis, C., Brea, D., Caballero, S., Faraco, G., Moore, J., Murphy, M., . . . Anrather, J. (2016). Commensal microbiota affects ischemic stroke outcome by regulating intestinal γδT cells. *Nature Medicine, 22*(5), 516–523.

Bergland, C. (2016, Jan. 4). Exercise alters gut microbes that promote brain health. *Psychology Today.* Retrieved from https://www.psychologytoday.com/blog/the-athletes-way/201601/exercise-alters-gut-microbes-promote-brain-health

Bermon, S., Petriz, B., Kajėnienė, A., Prestes, J., Castell, L., & Franco, O. L. (2015). The microbiota: an exercise immunology perspective. *Exercise Immunology Review, 21*, 70–79.

Bik, E. M. (2016). The hoops, hopes, and hypes of human microbiome research. *Yale Journal of Biology and Medicine, 89*(3), 363–373.

Braniste, V., Al-Asmakh, M., Kowal, C., Anuar, F., Abbaspour, A., Tóth, M., . . . Pettersson, S. (2014). The gut microbiota influences blood-brain barrier permeability in mice. *Science Translational Medicine, 6*(263), 263ra158.

Bressa, C., Bailén-Andrino, M., Pérez-Santiago, J., González-Soltero, R., Pérez, M., Montalvo-Lominchar, M. G., . . . Larrosa, M. (2017). Differences in gut microbiota profile between women with active lifestyle and sedentary women. *PLoS ONE, 12*(2), e0171352.

Burokas, A., Moloney, R. D., Dinan, T. G., & Cryan, J. F. (2015). Microbiota regulation of the mammalian gut-brain axis. *Advances in Applied Microbiology, 91*, 1–62.

Cantarel, B. L., Lombard, V., & Henrissat, B. (2012). Complex carbohydrate utilization by the healthy human microbiome. *PLoS ONE, 7*(6), e28742.

Cerdá, B., Pérez, M., Pérez-Santiago, J. D., Tornero-Aguilera, J. F., González-Soltero, R., & Larrosa, M. (2016). Gut microbiota modification: another piece in the puzzle of the benefits of physical exercise in health? *Frontiers in Physiology, 7*, 51.

Choi, J. J., Eum, S. Y., Rampersaud, E., Daunert, S., Abreu, M. T., & Toborek, M. (2013). Exercise attenuates PCB-induced changes in the mouse gut microbiome. *Environmental Health Perspectives, 121*(6), 725–730.

Claesson, M. J., Jeffery, I. B., Conde, S., Power, S. E., O'Connor, E. M., Cusack, S., ... O'Toole, P. W. (2012). Gut microbiota composition correlates with diet and health in the elderly. *Nature, 488*(7410), 178–184.

Clarke, S. F., Murphy, E. F., O'Sullivan, O., Lucey, A. J., Humphreys, M., Hogan, A., ... Cotter, P. D. (2014). Exercise and associated dietary extremes impact on gut microbial diversity. *Gut, 63*(12), 1913–1920.

Conlon, M. A., & Bird, A. R. (2015). The impact of diet and lifestyle on gut microbiota and human health. *Nutrients, 7*(1), 17–44.

Cook, M. D., Allen, J. M., Pence, B. D., Wallig, M. A., Gaskins, H. R., White, B. A., & Woods, J. A. (2016). Exercise and gut immune function: evidence of alterations in colon immune cell homeostasis and microbiome characteristics with exercise training. *Immunology and Cell Biology, 94*(2), 158–163.

Cronin, O., Molloy, M. G., & Shanahan, F. (2016). Exercise, fitness, and the gut. *Current Opinion in Gastroenterology, 32*(2), 67–73.

Cryan, J. F., & Dinan, T. G. (2015). More than a gut feeling: the microbiota regulates neurodevelopment and behavior. *Neuropsychopharmacology, 40*(1), 241–242.

David, L. A., Maurice, C. F., Carmody, R. N., Gootenberg, D. B., Button, J. E., Wolfe, B. E., ... Turnbaugh, P. J. (2014). Diet rapidly and reproducibly alters the human gut microbiome. *Nature, 505*(7484), 559–563.

De Palma, G., Blennerhassett, P., Lu, J., Deng, Y., Park, A. J., Green, W., ... Bercik, P. (2015). Microbiota and host determinants of behavioural phenotype in maternally separated mice. *Nature Communications, 6*, 7735.

Estaki, M., Pither, J., Baumeister, P., Little, J. P., Gill, S. K., Ghosh, S., ... Gibson, D. L. (2016). Cardiorespiratory fitness as a predictor of intestinal microbial diversity and distinct metagenomic functions. *Microbiome, 4*, 42.

Evans, C. C., LePard, K. J., Kwak, J. W., Stancukas, M. C., Laskowski, S., Dougherty, J., ... Ciancio, M. J. (2014). Exercise prevents weight gain and alters the gut microbiota in a mouse model of high fat diet-induced obesity. *PLoS ONE, 9*(3), e92193.

Fierer, N., Lauber, C. L., Zhou, N., McDonald, D., Costello, E. K., & Knight, R. (2010). Forensic identification using skin bacterial communities. *Proceedings of the National Academy of Sciences of the United States of America, 107*(14), 6477–6481.

Filippis, F. D., Pellegrini, N., Vannini, L., Jeffery, I. B., Storia, A. L., Laghi, L., ... Ercolini, D. (2016). High-level adherence to a Mediterranean diet beneficially impacts the gut microbiota and associated metabolome. *Gut, 65*(11), 1812–1821.

Gleeson, M. (2016). Immunological aspects of sport nutrition. *Immunology and Cell Biology, 94*(2), 117–123.

Hair, M., & Sharpe, J. (2014). The human microbiome. *Center for Ecogenetics, University of Washington.* Retrieved from https://depts.washington.edu/ceeh/downloads/FF_Microbiome.pdf

Handelsman, J. (2016, May 13). Announcing the National Microbiome Initiative [Blogpost]. *The White House: President Barack Obama.* Retrieved from https://obamawhitehouse.archives.gov/blog/2016/05/13/announcing-national-microbiome-initiative

Ho, P., & Ross, D. A. (2017). More than a gut feeling: the implications of the gut microbiota in psychiatry. *Biological Psychiatry, 81*(5), e35–e37.

Hoban, A. E., Stilling, R. M., Moloney, G., Shanahan, F., Dinan, T. G., & Clarke, G. (2018). The microbiome regulates amygdala-dependent fear recall. *Molecular Psychiatry, 23*(5), 1134–1144.

Hold, G. L. (2014). The gut microbiota, dietary extremes and exercise. *Gut, 63*(12), 1838–1839.

Huurre, A., Kalliomäki, M., Rautava, S., Rinne, M., Salminen, S., & Isolauri, E. (2008). Mode of delivery: effects on gut microbiota and humoral immunity. *Neonatology, 93*(4), 236–240.

Jackson, M., Jeffrey, I. B., Beaumont, M., Bell, J. T., Clark, A. G., Ley, R. E. (2016). Signatures of early frailty in the gut microbiota. *Genome Medicine, 8*(1), 8.

Janssen, A. W. F., & Kersten, S. (2015). The role of the gut microbiota in metabolic health. *FASEB Journal, 29*(8), 3111–3123.

Jeffery, I. B., Lynch, D. B., & O'Toole, P.W. (2016). Composition and temporal stability of the gut microbiota in older persons. *ISME Journal, 10*, 170–182.

Kelly, D., King, T., & Aminov, R. (2007). Importance of microbial colonization of the gut in early life to the development of immunity. *Mutation Research, 622*(1–2), 58–69.

Mariat, D., Firmesse, O., Levenez, F., Guimaraes, V. D., Sokol, H., Dore, J., . . . Furet, J. P. (2009). The Firmicutes/Bacteroidetes ratio of the human microbiota changes with age. *BMC Microbiology, 9*, 123.

Matsumoto, M., Inoue, R., Tsukahara, T., Ushida, K., Chiji, H., Matsubara, N., & Hara, H. (2008). Voluntary running exercise alters microbiota composition and increases n-butyrate concentration in the rat cecum. *Bioscience, Biotechnology, and Biochemistry, 72*(2), 572–576.

Mayer, E. A., Tillisch, K., & Gupta, A. (2015). Gut/brain axis and the microbiota. *Journal of Clinical Investigation, 125*(3), 926–938.

Mika, A., & Fleshner, M. (2016). Early-life exercise may promote lasting brain and metabolic health through gut bacterial metabolites. *Immunology and Cell Biology, 94*(2), 151–157.

Mika, A., Van Treuren, W., González, A., Herrera, J. J., Knight, R., & Fleshner, M. (2015). Exercise is more effective at altering gut microbial composition and producing stable changes in lean mass in juvenile versus adult male F344 Rats. *PLoS ONE, 10*(5), e0125889.

Morrison, D. J., & Preston, T. (2016). Formation of short chain fatty acids by the gut microbiota and their impact on human metabolism. *Gut Microbes, 7*(3), 189–200.

Murphy, K., Curley, D., O'Callaghan, T. F., O'Shea, C.-A., Dempsey, E. M., O'Toole, P. W., . . . Stanton, C. (2017). The composition of human milk and infant faecal microbiota over the first three months of life: a pilot study. *Scientific Reports, 7*, 40597.

Nicholson, J. K., Holmes, E., Kinross, J., Burcelin, R., Gibson, G., Jia, W., & Pettersson, S. (2012). Host-gut microbiota metabolic interactions. *Science, 336*(6086), 1262–1267.

O'Keefe, S. J. D., Li, J. V., Lahti, L., Ou, J., Carbonero, F., Mohammed, K., . . . Zoetendal, E. G. (2015). Fat, fiber and cancer risk in African Americans and rural Africans. *Nature Communications, 6*, 6342.

O'Sullivan, O., Cronin, O., Clarke, S. F., Murphy, E. F., Molloy, M. G., Shanahan, F., & Cotter, P. D. (2015). Exercise and the microbiota. *Gut Microbes, 6*(2), 131–136.

O'Toole, P. W., & Jeffery, I. B. (2015). Gut microbiota and aging. *Science (New York, NY), 350*(6265), 1214–1215.

Panigrahi, P., Parida, S., Nanda, N.C., Satpathy, R., Pradhan, L., Chandel, D. S., . . . Gewold, I. H. (2017). A randomized symbiotic trial to prevent sepsis among infants in rural India. *Nature, 548*(7668), 407–412.

Perry, R. J., Peng, L., Barry, N. A., Cline, G. W., Zhang, D., Cardone, R. L., . . . Shulman, G. I. (2016). Acetate mediates a microbiome-brain-β cell axis promoting metabolic syndrome. *Nature, 534*(7606), 213–217.

Peters, H., De Vries, W.R., Vanberge-Henegouw, G., & Akkermans, L. (2001). Potential benefits and hazards of physical activity and exercise on the gastrointestinal tract. *Gut, 48*(3), 435–439.

Petriz, B. A., Castro, A. P., Almeida, J. A., Gomes, C. P., Fernandes, G. R., Kruger, R. H., . . . Franco, O. L. (2014). Exercise induction of gut microbiota modifications in obese, non-obese and hypertensive rats. *BMC Genomics, 15*(1), 511.

Rankin, A., O'Donavon, C., Madigan, S. M., O'Sullivan, O., & Cotter, P. D. (2017). "Microbes in sport": the potential role of the gut microbiota in athlete health and performance. *British Journal of Sports Medicine, 51*(9), 698–699.

Reynolds, G. (2014, June 18). Exercise and the "good" bugs in our gut. *New York Times*. Retrieved from https://well.blogs.nytimes.com/2014/06/18/exercise-and-the-good-bugs-in-our-gut/

Roduit, C., Scholtens, S., Jongste, J. C. de, Wijga, A. H., Gerritsen, J., Postma, D. S., . . . Smit, H. A. (2009). Asthma at 8 years of age in children born by caesarean section. *Thorax, 64*(2), 107–113.

Rossen, N. G., MacDonald, J. K., de Vries, E. M., D'Haens, G. R., de Vos, W. M., Zoetendal, E. G., & Ponsioen, C. Y. (2015). Fecal microbiota transplantation as novel therapy in gastroenterology: a systematic review. *World Journal of Gastroenterology, 21*(17), 5359–5371.

Schardt, D. (2016, Dec. 1). Microbiome: it takes a village. *Nutrition Action Healthletter, 44*(10), 9–11.

Sekirov, I., Russell, S. L., Antunes, L. C. M., & Finlay, B. B. (2010). Gut microbiota in health and disease. *Physiological Reviews, 90*(3), 859–904.

Sender, R., Fuchs, S., & Milo, R. (2016). Are we really vastly outnumbered? Revisiting the ratio of bacterial to host cells in humans. *Cell, 164*(3), 337–340.

Shell, E. R. (2015, April 1). Artificial sweetners may change our gut bacteria in dangerous ways. *Scientific American*. Retrieved from https://www.scientificamerican.com/article/artificial-sweeteners-may-change-our-gut-bacteria-in-dangerous-ways/

Smith, P. A. (2015). The tantalizing links between gut microbes and the brain. *Nature, 526*(7573), 312–314.

Smits, S. A., Leach, J., Sonnenburg, E. D., Gonzalez, C. G., Lichtman, J. S., Reid, G., . . . Sonnenburg, J. L. (2017). Seasonal cycling in the gut microbiome of the Hadza hunter-gatherers of Tanzania. *Science, 357*(6353), 802–806.

Sommer, F., & Bäckhed, F. (2013). The gut microbiota: masters of host development and physiology. *Nature Reviews Microbiology, 11*(4), 227–238.

Stilling, R. M., Bordenstein, S. R., Dinan, T. G., & Cryan, J. F. (2014). Friends with social benefits: host-microbe interactions as a driver of brain evolution and development? *Frontiers in Cellular and Infection Microbiology, 4*, 147.

Stulberg, E., Fravel, D., Proctor, L. M., Murray, D. M., LoTempio, J., Chrisey, L., . . . Records, A. (2016). An assessment of US microbiome research. *Nature Microbiology, 1*, 15015.

Suez, J., Korem, T., Silberman-Schapira, G., Segal, E., & Elinav, E. (2015). Non-caloric artificial sweeteners and the microbiome: findings and challenges. *Gut Microbes, 6*(2), 149–155.

Suez, J., Korem, T. Zeevi, D., Zilberman-Schapira, G., Thaiss, C. A., & Maza, O. (2014). Artificial sweeteners induce glucose intolerance by altering the gut microbiota. *Nature, 514*(7521), 181–186.

Thaiss, C. A., Zmora, N., Levy, M., & Elinav, E. (2016). The microbiome and innate immunity. *Nature, 535*(7610), 65–74.

Thevaranjan, N., Puchta, A., Schulz, C., Naidoo, A., Szamosi, J. C., Vershoor, C. P. (2017). Age-associated microbial dysbiosis promotes intestinal permeability, systemic inflammation, and macrophage dysfunction. *Cell Host & Microbe, 21,* 455–466.

Trompette, A., Gollwitzer, E. S., Yadava, K., Sichelstiel, A. K., Sprenger, N., Ngom-Bru, C., . . . Marsland, B. J. (2014). Gut microbiota metabolism of dietary fiber influences allergic airway disease and hematopoiesis. *Nature Medicine, 20*(2), 159–166.

Weill Cornell Medical College. (2016, Mar. 28). GI tract bacteria help decrease stroke. *Science Newsline/Medicine.* Retrieved from http://www.sciencenewsline.com/news/2016032821220050.html

West, N. P., Pyne, D. B., Peake, J. M., & Cripps, A. W. (2009). Probiotics, immunity and exercise: a review. *Exercise Immunology Review, 15,* 107–126.

Wu, G. D., Chen, J., Hoffmann, C., Bittinger, K., Chen, Y.-Y., Keilbaugh, S. A., . . . Lewis, J. D. (2011). Linking long-term dietary patterns with gut microbial enterotypes. *Science 334*(6052), 105–108.

Wu, H., Tremaroli, V., & Bäckhed, F. (2015). Linking microbiota to human diseases: a systems biology perspective. *Trends in Endocrinology & Metabolism, 26*(12), 758–770.

Wu, H.-J., & Wu, E. (2012). The role of gut microbiota in immune homeostasis and autoimmunity. *Gut Microbes, 3*(1), 4–14.

Yong, E. (2016, July 22). Breast-feeding the micro-biome. *The New Yorker.* Retrieved from http://www.newyorker.com/tech/elements/breast-feeding-the-microbiome

Zimmer, C. (2012, June 18). Tending the body's microbial garden. *New York Times.*

Zimmer, C. (2017, Aug. 29). Gut bacteria can change with the seasons. *New York Times.*

CHAPTER 11

Abramson, J. L., & Vaccarino, V. (2002). Relationship between physical activity and inflammation among apparently healthy middle-aged and older US adults. *Archives of Internal Medicine, 162*(11), 1286–1292.

Balducci, S., Zanuso, S., Nicolucci, A., Fernando, F., Cavallo, S., Cardelli, P., . . . Pugliese, G. (2010). Anti-inflammatory effect of exercise training in subjects with type 2 diabetes and the metabolic syndrome is dependent on exercise modalities and independent of weight loss. *Nutrition, Metabolism, and Cardiovascular Diseases, 20*(8), 608–617.

Bermon, S. (2007). Airway inflammation and upper respiratory tract infection in athletes: is there a link? *Exercise Immunology Review, 13,* 6–14.

Bermon, S., Petriz, B., Kajénienè, A., Prestes, J., Castell, L., & Franco, O. L. (2015). The microbiota: an exercise immunology perspective. *Exercise Immunology Review, 21,* 70–79.

Bishop, N. C., & Gleeson, M. (2009). Acute and chronic effects of exercise on markers of mucosal immunity. *Frontiers in Bioscience (Landmark Ed.), 14,* 4444–4456.

Campbell, J. P., & Turner, J. E. (2018). Debunking the myth of exercise-induced immune suppression: redefining the impact of exercise on immunological health across the lifespan. *Frontiers in Immunology, 9,* 648.

Campisi, J., & Fleshner, M. (2003). The role of extracellular HSP72 in acute stress-induced potentiation of innate immunity in physically active rats. *Journal of Applied Physiology, 94,* 43–52.

Cronin, O., Keohane, D. M., Molloy, M. G., & Shanahan, F. (2017). The effect of exercise interventions on inflammatory biomarkers in healthy, physically inactive subjects: a systematic review. *QJM, A Monthly Journal of the Association of Physicians, 119*(10), 629–637.

Dimitrov, S., Hulteng, E., & Hong, S. (2017). Inflammation and exercise: inhibition of monocytic intracellular TNF production by acute exercise via B2-adrenergic activation. *Brain, Behavior and Immunity, 61*, 60–68.

Duggal, N. A., Pollock, R. D., Lazarus, N. R., Harridge, S., & Lord, J. M. (2018). Major features of immunesenescence, including reduced thymic output, are ameliorated by high levels of physical activity in adulthood, *Aging Cell, 17*(2).

Febbraio, M. A. (2007). Exercise and inflammation. *Journal of Applied Physiology, 103*(1), 376.

Febbraio, M. A., Hiscock, N., Sacchetti, M., Fischer, C. P., & Pedersen, B. K. (2004). Interleukin-6 is a novel factor mediating glucose homeostasis during skeletal muscle contraction. *Diabetes, 53*(7), 1643–1648.

Fleshner, M. (2005). Physical activity and stress resistance: sympathetic nervous system adaptations prevent stress-induced immunosuppression. *Exercise and Sport Sciences Reviews, 33*(3), 120–126.

Fleshner, M., Campisi, J., Deak, T., Greenwood, B. N., Kintzel, J., Leem, T. H., Smith, T. P., & Sorensen, B. (2002). Acute stressor exposure facilitates innate immunity more in physically active than in sedentary rats. *American Journal of Physiology, Regulatory, Integrative and Comparative Physiology, 282*(6), R1680–1686.

Fleshner, M., Greenwood, B. N., & Yirmiya, R. (2014). Neuronal-glial mechanisms of exercise-evoked stress robustness. *Current Topics in Behavioral Neurosciences, 18*, 1–12.

Ford, E. S. (2002). Does exercise reduce inflammation? Physical activity and C-reactive protein among U.S. adults. *Epidemiology, 13*(5), 561–568.

Francaux, M. (2009). Toll-like receptor signalling induced by endurance exercise. *Applied Physiology, Nutrition, and Metabolism, 34*(3), 454–458.

Freidenreich, D. J., & Volek, J. S. (2012). Immune responses to resistance exercise. *Exercise Immunology Review, 18*, 8–41.

Geffken, D. F., Cushman, M., Burke, G. L., Polak, J. F., Sakkinen, P. A., & Tracy, R. P. (2001). Association between physical activity and markers of inflammation in a healthy elderly population. *American Journal of Epidemiology, 153*(3), 242–250.

Gleeson, M. (2007). Immune function in sport and exercise. *Journal of Applied Physiology, 103*(2), 693–699.

Gleeson, M., McFarlin, B., & Flynn, M. (2006). Exercise and toll-like receptors. *Exercise Immunology Review, 12*, 34–53.

Gleeson, M., & Pyne, D. B. (2016). Respiratory inflammation and infections in high-performance athletes. *Immunology and Cell Biology, 94*(2), 124–131.

Gleeson, M., Pyne, D. B., Elkington, L. J., Hall, S. T., Attia, J. R., Oldmeadow, C., . . . Callister, R. (2017). Developing a multi-component immune model for evaluating the risk of respiratory illness in athletes. *Exercise Immunology Review, 23*, 52–64.

Grant, R. W., Mariani, R. A., Vieira, V. J., Fleshner, M., Smith, T. P., Keylock, K. T., . . . Woods, J. A. (2008). Cardiovascular exercise intervention improves the primary antibody response to keyhole limpet hemocyanin (KLH) in previously sedentary older adults. *Brain, Behavior, and Immunity, 22*(6), 923–932.

Haaland, D. A., Sabljic, T. F., Baribeau, D. A., Mukovozov, I. M., & Hart, L. E. (2008). Is regular exercise a friend or foe of the aging immune system? A systematic review. *Clinical Journal of Sport Medicine, 18*(6), 539–548.

Hamer, M. (2007). The relative influences of fitness and fatness on inflammatory factors. *Preventive Medicine, 44*(1), 3–11.

Hamer, M., Sabia, S., Batty, G. D., Shipley, M. J., Tabák, A. G., Singh-Manoux, A., & Kivimaki, M. (2012). Physical activity and inflammatory markers over 10 years follow up in men and women from the Whitehall II cohort study. *Circulation, 126*(8), 928–933.

Handschin, C., & Spiegelman, B. M. (2008). The role of exercise and PGC1α in inflammation and chronic disease. *Nature, 454*(7203), 463–469.

Ho, S. S., Dhaliwal, S. S., Hills, A. P., & Pal, S. (2013). Effects of chronic exercise training on inflammatory markers in Australian overweight and obese individuals in a randomized controlled trial. *Inflammation, 36*(3), 625.

Hotamisligil, G. S., Murray, D. L., Choy, L. N., & Spiegelman, B. M. (1994). Tumor necrosis factor alpha inhibits signaling from the insulin receptor. *Proceedings of the National Academy of Sciences of the United States of America, 91*(11), 4854–4858.

Khan Academy. (n.d.). Innate immunity. Retrieved from https://www.khanacademy.org/test-prep/mcat/organ-systems/the-immune-system/a/innate-immunity

Janeway, C. A., Travers, P., Walport, M., & Shlomchik, M. J. (2001). Principles of innate and adaptive immunity. *Immunobiology: The immune system in health and disease,* 5th ed. New York, NY: Garland Science. Retrieved from https://www.ncbi.nlm.nih.gov/books/NBK27090/

Kakanis, M. W., Peake, J., Brenu, E. W., Simmonds, M., Gray, B., Hooper, S. L., & Marshall-Gradisnik, S. M. (2010). The open window of susceptibility to infection after acute exercise in healthy young male elite athletes. *Exercise Immunology Review, 16,* 119–137.

Karstoft, K., & Pedersen, B. K. (2016). Exercise and type 2 diabetes: focus on metabolism and inflammation. *Immunology and Cell Biology, 94*(2), 146–150.

Kohut, M. L., Cooper, M. M., Nickolaus, M. S., Russell, D. R., & Cunnick, J. E. (2002). Exercise and psychosocial factors modulate immunity to influenza vaccine in elderly individuals. *Journals of Gerontology Series A: Biological Sciences and Medical Sciences, 57*(9), M557–562.

Kohut, M. L., & Senchina, D. S. (2004). Reversing age-associated immunosenescence via exercise. *Exercise Immunology Review, 10,* 6–41.

Kramer, H. F., & Goodyear, L. J. (2007). Exercise, MAPK, and NF-κB signaling in skeletal muscle. *Journal of Applied Physiology, 103*(1), 388–395.

Lancaster, G. I., & Febbraio, M. A. (2016). Exercise and the immune system: implications for elite athletes and the general population. *Immunology and Cell Biology, 94*(2), 115–116.

Lancaster, G. I., Khan, Q., Drysdale, P., Wallace, F., Jeukendrup, A. E., Drayson, M. T., & Gleeson, M. (2005). The physiological regulation of toll-like receptor expression and function in humans. *Journal of Physiology, 563*(Pt 3), 945–955.

Lara Fernandes, J., Serrano, C. V., Toledo, F., Hunziker, M. F., Zamperini, A., Teo, F. H., . . . Negrão, C. E. (2011). Acute and chronic effects of exercise on inflammatory markers and B-type natriuretic peptide in patients with coronary artery disease. *Clinical Research in Cardiology, 100*(1), 77–84.

Lawrence, T. (2009). The nuclear factor NF-κB pathway in inflammation. *Cold Spring Harbor Perspectives in Biology, 1*(6), a001651.

MacKinnon, L. T. (2000). Overtraining effects on immunity and performance in athletes. *Immunology and Cell Biology, 78*(5), 502–509.

Martins, R. A., Neves, A. P., Coelho-Silva, M. J., Veríssimo, M. T., & Teixeira, A. M. (2010). The effect of aerobic versus strength-based training on high-sensitivity C-reactive protein in older adults. *European Journal of Applied Physiology, 110*(1), 161–169.

Mika, A., Van Treuren, W., González, A., Herrera, A. J., Knight, R., & Fleshner, M. (2015). Exercise is more effective at altering gut microbial composition and producing stable changes in lean mass in juvenile versus adult male F344 rats. *PLoS ONE, 10*(5), e0125889.

Moraska, A., & Fleshner, M. (2001). Voluntary physical activity prevents stress-induced behavioral depression and anti-KLH antibody suppression. *American Journal of Physiology. Regulatory, Integrative and Comparative Physiology, 281*(2), R484–R489.

Nickerson, M., Elphick, G. F., Campisi, J., & Fleshner, M. (2005). Physical activity alters the brain Hsp72 and IL1beta responses to peripheral *E. coli* challenge. *American Journal of Physiology, 289*, 1665–1674.

Nieman, D. C. (1994). Exercise, infection, and immunity. *International Journal of Sports Medicine, 15*(Suppl 3), S131–S141.

Nieman, D. C. (2000). Exercise effects on systemic immunity. *Immunology and Cell Biology, 78*(5), 496–501.

Nieman, D. C. (2003). Current perspective on exercise immunology. *Current Sports Medicine Reports, 2*(5), 239–242.

Nieman, D. C., Henson, D. A., Austin, M. D., & Sha, W. (2011). Upper respiratory tract infection is reduced in physically fit and active adults. *British Journal of Sports Medicine, 45*(12), 987–992.

Nieto-Vazquez, I., Fernández-Veledo, S., Krämer, D. K., Vila-Bedmar, R., Garcia-Guerra, L., & Lorenzo, M. (2008). Insulin resistance associated to obesity: the link TNF-alpha. *Archives of Physiology and Biochemistry, 114*(3), 183–194.

Pedersen, B. K., Akerström, T. C. A., Nielsen, A. R., & Fischer, C. P. (2007). Role of myokines in exercise and metabolism. *Journal of Applied Physiology, 103*(3), 1093–1098.

Pedersen, B. K., & Bruunsgaard, H. (2003). Possible beneficial role of exercise in modulating low-grade inflammation in the elderly. *Scandinavian Journal of Medicine & Science in Sports, 13*(1), 56–62.

Pedersen, B. K., & Hoffman-Goetz, L. (2000). Exercise and the immune system: regulation, integration, and adaptation. *Physiological Reviews, 80*(3), 1055–1081.

Pedersen, L., Idorn, M., Olofsson, G. H., Lauenborg, B., Nookaew, I., Hansen, R. H., . . . Hojman, P. (2016). Voluntary running suppresses tumor growth through epinephrine- and IL-6-dependent NK cell mobilization and redistribution. *Cell Metabolism, 23*(3), 554–562.

Petersen, A. M. W., & Pedersen, B. K. (2005). The anti-inflammatory effect of exercise. *Journal of Applied Physiology, 98*(4), 1154–1162.

Phillips, M. D., Flynn, M. G., McFarlin, B. K., Stewart, L. K., & Timmerman, K. L. (2010). Resistance training at eight-repetition maximum reduces the inflammatory milieu in elderly women. *Medicine and Science in Sports and Exercise, 42*(2), 314–325.

Plaisance, E. P., & Grandjean, P. W. (2006). Physical activity and high-sensitivity C-reactive protein. *Sports Medicine, 36*(5), 443–458.

Retief, F. P., & Cilliers, L. (1998). The epidemic of Athens, 430–426 BC. *South African Medical Journal, 88*(1), 50–53.

Reynolds, G. (2018, Mar. 14). How exercise can keep aging muscles and immune systems "young." *New York Times.*

Reynolds, G. (2018, Apr. 25). How strenuous exercise affects our immune system. *New York Times.*

Shephard, R. J. (2010). Development of the discipline of exercise immunology. *Exercise Immunology Review, 16,* 194–222.

Silverman, M. N., & Deuster, P. A. (2014). Biological mechanisms underlying the role of physical fitness in health and resilience. *Interface Focus, 4*(5), 20140040.

Simpson, R. J., Lowder, T. W., Spielmann, G., Bigley, A. B., LaVoy, E. C., & Kunz, H. (2012). Exercise and the aging immune system. *Ageing Research Reviews, 11*(3), 404–420.

Smith, T. P., Kennedy, S. L., & Fleshner, M. (2004). Influence of age and physical activity on the primary in vivo antibody and T cell-mediated responses in men. *Journal of Applied Physiology, 97*(2), 491–498.

Speaker, K. J., Cox, S. S., Paton, M. M., Serebrakian, A., Maslanik, T., Greenwood, B. N., & Fleshner, M. (2014). Six weeks of voluntary wheel running modulates inflammatory protein (MCP-1, IL-6, and IL-10) and DAMP (Hsp72) responses to acute stress in white adipose tissue of lean rats. *Brain, Behavior, and Immunity, 39,* 87–98.

Starkie, R., Ostrowski, S. R., Jauffred, S., Febbraio, M., & Pedersen, B. K. (2003). Exercise and IL-6 infusion inhibit endotoxin-induced TNF-alpha production in humans. *FASEB Journal, 17*(8), 884–886.

Steensberg, A., van Hall, G., Osada, T., Sacchetti, M., Saltin, B., & Pedersen, B. K. (2000). Production of interleukin-6 in contracting human skeletal muscles can account for the exercise-induced increase in plasma interleukin-6. *Journal of Physiology, 529*(Pt 1), 237–242.

Tiainen, K., Hurme, M., Hervonen, A., Luukkaala, T., & Jylhä, M. (2010). Inflammatory markers and physical performance among nonagenarians. *Journals of Gerontology Series A: Biological Sciences and Medical Sciences, 65*(6), 658–663.

Timmerman, K. L., Flynn, M. G., Coen, P. M., Markofski, M. M., & Pence, B. D. (2008). Exercise training-induced lowering of inflammatory (CD14+CD16+) monocytes: a role in the anti-inflammatory influence of exercise? *Journal of Leukocyte Biology, 84*(5), 1271–1278.

Timmons, B. W., & Cieslak, T. (2008). Human natural killer cell subsets and acute exercise: a brief review. *Exercise Immunology Review, 14,* 8–23.

University of California, San Diego. (2017, Jan. 13). Exercise . . . it does a body good: 20 minutes can act as anti-inflammatory. *Science Newsline, Medicine.* Retrieved from http://www.sciencenewsline.com/news/2017011316450051.html

Vaisberg, M., Suguri, V. M., Gregorio, L. C., Lopes, J. D., & Bachi, A. L. L. (2013). Cytokine kinetics in nasal mucosa and sera: new insights in understanding upper-airway disease of marathon runners. *Exercise Immunology Review, 19,* 49–59.

Walsh, N. P., Gleeson, M., Shephard, R. J., Gleeson, M., Woods, J. A., Bishop, N. C., . . . Simon, P. (2011). Position statement. Part one: immune function and exercise. *Exercise Immunology Review, 17,* 6–63.

CHAPTER 12

Abrahamson, P. E., Gammon, M. D., Lund, M. J., Britton, J. A., Marshall, S. W., Flagg, E. W., . . . Coates, R. J. (2006). Recreational physical activity and survival among young women with breast cancer. *Cancer, 107*(8), 1777–1785.

American Cancer Society. (2015). *Global cancer facts & figures,* 3rd ed. Retrieved from https://www.cancer.org/research/cancer-facts-statistics/global.html

American Cancer Society. (2017, Jan. 5). How common is breast cancer? Breast cancer survivors Retrieved from https://www.cancer.org/cancer/breast-cancer/about/how-common-is-breast-cancer.html

Ballantyne, C. (2009, Jan. 2). Does exercise really make you healthier? *Scientific American.* Retrieved from https://www.scientificamerican.com/article/does-exercise-really-make/

Ballard-Barbash, R., Friedenreich, C. M., Courneya, K. S., Siddiqi, S. M., McTiernan, A., & Alfano, C. M. (2012). Physical activity, biomarkers, and disease outcomes in cancer survivors: a systematic review. *Journal of the National Cancer Institute, 104*(11), 815–840.

Beasley, J. M., Kwan, M. L., Chen, W. Y., Weltzien, E. K., Kroenke, C. H., Lu, W., . . . Caan, B. J. (2012). Meeting the physical activity guidelines and survival after breast cancer: findings from the After Breast Cancer Pooling Project. *Breast Cancer Research and Treatment, 131*(2), 637–643.

Betof, A. S., Lascola, C. D., Weitzel, D., Landon, C., Scarbrough, P. M., Devi, G. R., . . . Dewhirst, M. W. (2015). Modulation of murine breast tumor vascularity, hypoxia, and chemotherapeutic response by exercise. *Journal of the National Cancer Institute, 107*(5), djv040.

Bradshaw, P. T., Ibrahim, J. G., Stevens, J., Cleveland, R., Abrahamson, P. E., Satia, J. A., . . . Gammon, M. D. (2012). Post-diagnosis change in bodyweight and survival after breast cancer diagnosis. *Epidemiology, 23*(2), 320–327.

Buffart, L. M., Kalter, J., Sweegers, M. G., Courneya, K. S., Newton, R. U., Aaronson, N. K., . . . Brug, J. (2017). Effects and moderators of exercise on quality of life and physical function in patients with cancer: an individual patient data meta-analysis of 34 RCTs. *Cancer Treatment Reviews, 52*, 91–104.

Burfoot, A. (2015, May 19). Exercise fights cancer tumors directly. *Runner's World.* Retrieved from https://www.runnersworld.com/health/exercise-fights-cancer-tumors-directly

Camoriano, J. K., Loprinzi, C. L., Ingle, J. N., Therneau, T. M., Krook, J. E., & Veeder, M. H. (1990). Weight change in women treated with adjuvant therapy or observed following mastectomy for node-positive breast cancer. *Journal of Clinical Oncology, 8*(8), 1327–1334.

Cannioto, R. A., LaMonte, M. J., Kelemen, L. E., Risch, H. A., Eng, K. H., Minlikeeva, A. N., . . . Moysich, K. B. (2016). Recreational physical inactivity and mortality in women with invasive epithelial ovarian cancer: evidence from the Ovarian Cancer Association Consortium. *British Journal of Cancer, 115*(1), 95–101.

Cannioto, R., LaMonte, M. J., Risch, H. A., Hong, C. C., Sucheston-Campbell, L. E., Eng, K. H., . . . Moysich, K. B. (2016). Chronic recreational physical inactivity and epithelial ovarian cancer risk: evidence from the Ovarian Cancer Association Consortium. *Cancer Epidemiology, Biomarkers & Prevention, 25*(7), 1114–1124.

Chan, D. S. M., Vieira, A. R., Aune, D., Bandera, E. V., Greenwood, D. C., McTiernan, A., . . . Norat, T. (2014). Body mass index and survival in women with breast cancer: systematic literature review and meta-analysis of 82 follow-up studies. *Annals of Oncology, 25*(10), 1901–1914.

Chao, A., Connell, C. J., Jacobs, E. J., McCullough, M. L., Patel, A. V., Calle, E. E., . . . Thun, M. J. (2004). Amount, type, and timing of recreational physical activity in relation to colon and rectal cancer in older adults: the Cancer Prevention Study II Nutrition Cohort. *Cancer Epidemiology, Biomarkers & Prevention, 13*(12), 2187–2195.

Chasen, M., Bhargava, R., & MacDonald, N. (2014). Rehabilitation for patients with advanced cancer. *Canadian Medical Association Journal, 186*(14), 1071–1075.

Chen, X., Lu, W., Zheng, W., Gu, K., Matthews, C. E., Chen, Z., . . . Shu, X. O. (2011). Exercise after diagnosis of breast cancer in association with survival. *Cancer Prevention Research, 4*(9), 1409–1418.

Chen, X., Zheng, Y., Zheng, W., Gu, K., Chen, Z., Lu, W., & Shu, X. O. (2009). The effect of regular exercise on quality of life among breast cancer survivors. *American Journal of Epidemiology, 170*(7), 854–862.

Cormie, P., Newton, R. U., Taaffe, D. R., Spry, N., Joseph, D., Akhlil Hamid, M., & Galvão, D. A. (2013). Exercise maintains sexual activity in men undergoing androgen suppression for prostate cancer: a randomized controlled trial. *Prostate Cancer and Prostatic Diseases, 16*(2), 170–175.

Courneya, K. S. (2003). Exercise in cancer survivors: an overview of research. *Medicine and Science in Sports and Exercise, 35*(11), 1846–1852.

Courneya, K. S., Booth, C. M., Gill, S., O'Brien, P., Vardy, J., Friedenreich, C. M., . . . Meyer, R. M. (2008). The Colon Health and Life-Long Exercise Change trial: a randomized trial of the National Cancer Institute of Canada Clinical Trials Group. *Current Oncology, 15*(6), 271–278.

Courneya, K. S., Friedenreich, C. M., Sela, R. A., Quinney, H. A., Rhodes, R. E., & Handman, M. (2003). The group psychotherapy and home-based physical exercise (group-hope) trial in cancer survivors: physical fitness and quality of life outcomes. *Psycho-Oncology, 12*(4), 357–374.

Courneya, K. S., Segal, R. J., Mackey, J. R., Gelmon, K., Reid, R. D., Friedenreich, C. M., . . . McKenzie, D. C. (2007). Effects of aerobic and resistance exercise in breast cancer patients receiving adjuvant chemotherapy: a multicenter randomized controlled trial. *Journal of Clinical Oncology, 25*(28), 4396–4404.

Cramer, H., Lauche, R., Klose, P., Dobos, G., & Langhorst, J. (2014). A systematic review and meta-analysis of exercise interventions for colorectal cancer patients. *European Journal of Cancer Care, 23*(1), 3–14.

Cramp, F., & Byron-Daniel, J. (2012). Exercise for the management of cancer-related fatigue in adults. *Cochrane Database of Systematic Reviews, *(11), CD006145.

Dana Farber Cancer Institute. (2017, May 18). How does exercise reduce cancer risk? [Blog post]. Retrieved from http://blog.dana-farber.org/insight/2016/05/how-does-exercise-reduce-cancer-risk/

DeNoon, D. J. (2010, June 16). Why does diabetes raise cancer risk? *WebMD.* Retrieved from http://www.webmd.com/diabetes/news/20100616/why-does-diabetes-increase-cancer-risk

Emaus, A., Veierød, M. B., Tretli, S., Finstad, S. E., Selmer, R., Furberg, A.-S., . . . Thune, I. (2010). Metabolic profile, physical activity, and mortality in breast cancer patients. *Breast Cancer Research and Treatment, 121*(3), 651–660.

Friedenreich, C. M., Gregory, J., Kopciuk, K. A., Mackey, J. R., & Courneya, K. S. (2009). Prospective cohort study of lifetime physical activity and breast cancer survival. *International Journal of Cancer, 124*(8), 1954–1962.

Friedenreich, C. M., Neilson, H. K., & Lynch, B. M. (2010). State of the epidemiological evidence on physical activity and cancer prevention. *European Journal of Cancer, 46*(14), 2593–2604.

Friedenreich, C. M., Wang, Q., Neilson, H. K., Kopciuk, K. A., McGregor, S. E., & Courneya, K. S. (2016). Physical activity and survival after prostate cancer. *European Urology, 70*(4), 576–585.

Galvão, D. A., & Newton, R. U. (2005). Review of exercise intervention studies in cancer patients. *Journal of Clinical Oncology, 23*(4), 899–909.

Galvão, D. A., Taaffe, D. R., Spry, N., Gardiner, R. A., Taylor, R., Risbridger, G. P., . . . Newton, R. U. (2016). Enhancing active surveillance of prostate cancer: the potential of exercise medicine. *Nature Reviews Urology, 13*(5), 258–265.

Galvão, D. A., Taaffe, D. R., Spry, N., Joseph, D., & Newton, R. U. (2010). Combined resistance and aerobic exercise program reverses muscle loss in men undergoing androgen suppression therapy for prostate cancer without bone metastases: a randomized controlled trial. *Journal of Clinical Oncology, 28*(2), 340–347.

Gardner, J. R., Livingston, P. M., & Fraser, S. F. (2014). Effects of exercise on treatment-related adverse effects for patients with prostate cancer receiving androgen-deprivation therapy: a systematic review. *Journal of Clinical Oncology, 32*(4), 335–346.

Gerritsen, J. K. W., & Vincent, A. J. P. E. (2016). Exercise improves quality of life in patients with cancer: a systematic review and meta-analysis of randomised controlled trials. *British Journal of Sports Medicine, 50*(13), 796–803.

Hacker, E. (2009). Exercise and quality of life: strengthening the connections. *Clinical Journal of Oncology Nursing, 13*(1), 31–39.

Hamer, J., & Warner, E. (2017). Lifestyle modifications for patients with breast cancer to improve prognosis and optimize overall health. *Canadian Medical Association Journal, 189*(7), E268–E274.

Hardy, O. T., Czech, M. P., & Corvera, S. (2012). What causes the insulin resistance underlying obesity? *Current Opinion in Endocrinology, Diabetes, and Obesity, 19*(2), 81–87.

Holick, C. N., Newcomb, P. A., Trentham-Dietz, A., Titus-Ernstoff, L., Bersch, A. J., Stampfer, M. J., . . . Willett, W. C. (2008). Physical activity and survival after diagnosis of invasive breast cancer. *Cancer Epidemiology, Biomarkers & Prevention, 17*(2), 379–386.

Holmes, M. D., Chen, W. Y., Feskanich, D., Kroenke, C. H., & Colditz, G. A. (2005). Physical activity and survival after breast cancer diagnosis. *Journal of the American Medical Association, 293*(20), 2479–2486.

Inoue, M., Yamamoto, S., Kurahashi, N., Iwasaki, M., Sasazuki, S., Tsugane, S., & Japan Public Health Center-Based Prospective Study Group. (2008). Daily total physical activity level and total cancer risk in men and women: results from a large-scale population-based cohort study in Japan. *American Journal of Epidemiology, 168*(4), 391–403.

Irwin, M. L., Crumley, D., McTiernan, A., Bernstein, L., Baumgartner, R., Gilliland, F. D., . . . Ballard-Barbash, R. (2003). Physical activity levels before and after a diagnosis of breast cancer: the Health, Eating, Activity, and Lifestyle (HEAL) Study. *Cancer, 97*(7), 1746–1757.

Irwin, M. L., Smith, A. W., McTiernan, A., Ballard-Barbash, R., Cronin, K., Gilliland, F. D., . . . Bernstein, L. (2008). Influence of pre- and postdiagnosis physical activity on mortality in breast cancer survivors: the Health, Eating, Activity, and Lifestyle Study. *Journal of Clinical Oncology, 26*(24), 3958–3964.

Jacobsen, P. B., Donovan, K. A., Vadaparampil, S. T., & Small, B. J. (2007). Systematic review and meta-analysis of psychological and activity-based interventions for cancer-related fatigue. *Health Psychology, American Psychological Association, 26*(6), 660–667.

Jones, L. W., Viglianti, B. L., Tashjian, J. A., Kothadia, S. M., Keir, S. T., Freedland, S. J., . . . Dewhirst, M. W. (2010). Effect of aerobic exercise on tumor physiology in an animal model of human breast cancer. *Journal of Applied Physiology, 108*(2), 343–348.

Kasznicki, J., Sliwinska, A., & Drzewoski, J. (2014). Metformin in cancer prevention and therapy. *Annals of Translational Medicine, 2*(6), 57.

Kenfield, S. A., Stampfer, M. J., Giovannucci, E., & Chan, J. M. (2011). Physical activity and survival after prostate cancer diagnosis in the Health Professionals Follow-Up Study. *Journal of Clinical Oncology, 29*(6), 726–732.

King, M.-C., Marks, J. H., Mandell, J. B., & New York Breast Cancer Study Group. (2003). Breast and ovarian cancer risks due to inherited mutations in BRCA1 and BRCA2. *Science, 302*(5645), 643–646.

Knols, R., Aaronson, N. K., Uebelhart, D., Fransen, J., & Aufdemkampe, G. (2005). Physical exercise in cancer patients during and after medical treatment: a systematic review of randomized and controlled clinical trials. *Journal of Clinical Oncology, 23*(16), 3830–3842.

Kroenke, C. H., Chen, W. Y., Rosner, B., & Holmes, M. D. (2005). Weight, weight gain, and survival after breast cancer diagnosis. *Journal of Clinical Oncology, 23*(7), 1370–1378.

Kushi, L. H., Doyle, C., McCullough, M., Rock, C. L., Demark-Wahnefried, W., Bandera, E. V., . . . American Cancer Society 2010 Nutrition and Physical Activity Guidelines Advisory Committee. (2012). American Cancer Society Guidelines on nutrition and physical activity for cancer prevention: reducing the risk of cancer with healthy food choices and physical activity. *CA: A Cancer Journal for Clinicians, 62*(1), 30–67.

Lahart, I. M., Metsios, G. S., Nevill, A. M., & Carmichael, A. R. (2015). Physical activity, risk of death and recurrence in breast cancer survivors: a systematic review and meta-analysis of epidemiological studies. *Acta Oncologica, 54*(5), 635–654.

Laukkanen, J. A., Rauramaa, R., Mäkikallio, T. H., Toriola, A. T., & Kurl, S. (2011). Intensity of leisure-time physical activity and cancer mortality in men. *British Journal of Sports Medicine, 45*(2), 125–129.

Lee, I.-M. (2003). Physical activity and cancer prevention: data from epidemiologic studies. *Medicine and Science in Sports and Exercise, 35*(11), 1823–1827.

Lemanne, D., Cassileth, B., & Gubili, J. (2013). The role of physical activity in cancer prevention, treatment, recovery, and survivorship. *Oncology (Williston Park), 27*(6), 580–585.

Ligibel, J. A., Campbell, N., Partridge, A., Chen, W. Y., Salinardi, T., Chen, H., . . . Winer, E. P. (2008). Impact of a mixed strength and endurance exercise intervention on insulin levels in breast cancer survivors. *Journal of Clinical Oncology, 26*(6), 907–912.

Lønning, P. E., Helle, S. I., Johannessen, D. C., Ekse, D., & Adlercreutz, H. (1996). Influence of plasma estrogen levels on the length of the disease-free interval in postmenopausal women with breast cancer. *Breast Cancer Research and Treatment, 39*(3), 335–341.

Lowe, S. S., Watanabe, S. M., & Courneya, K. S. (2009). Physical activity as a supportive care intervention in palliative cancer patients: a systematic review. *Journal of Supportive Oncology, 7*(1), 27–34.

MacVicar, M. G., Winningham, M. L., & Nickel, J. L. (1989). Effects of aerobic interval training on cancer patients' functional capacity. *Nursing Research, 38*(6), 348–351.

McCullough, D. J., Nguyen, L. M.-D., Siemann, D. W., & Behnke, B. J. (2013). Effects of exercise training on tumor hypoxia and vascular function in the rodent preclinical orthotopic prostate cancer model. *Journal of Applied Physiology, 115*(12), 1846–1854.

McCullough, D. J., Stabley, J. N., Siemann, D. W., & Behnke, B. J. (2014). Modulation of blood flow, hypoxia, and vascular function in orthotopic prostate tumors during exercise. *Journal of the National Cancer Institute, 106*(4), dju036.

McNeely, M. L., Campbell, K. L., Rowe, B. H., Klassen, T. P., Mackey, J. R., & Courneya, K. S. (2006). Effects of exercise on breast cancer patients and survivors: a systematic review and meta-analysis. *Canadian Medical Association Journal, 175*(1), 34–41.

McTiernan, A. (2004). Physical activity after cancer: physiologic outcomes. *Cancer Investigation, 22*(1), 68–81.

McTiernan, A. (Ed.). (2005). *Cancer prevention and management through exercise and weight control.* Boca Raton, FL: CRC Press.

McTiernan, A., Rajan, B., Tworoger, S. S., Irwin, M., Bernstein, L., Baumgartner, R., . . . Ballard-Barbash, R. (2003). Adiposity and sex hormones in postmenopausal breast cancer survivors. *Journal of Clinical Oncology, 21*(10), 1961–1966.

Meyerhardt, J. A., Giovannucci, E. L., Holmes, M. D., Chan, A. T., Chan, J. A., Colditz, G. A., & Fuchs, C. S. (2006). Physical activity and survival after colorectal cancer diagnosis. *Journal of Clinical Oncology, 24*(22), 3527–3534.

Mock, V., Pickett, M., Ropka, M. E., Muscari Lin, E., Stewart, K. J., Rhodes, V. A., . . . McCorkle, R. (2001). Fatigue and quality of life outcomes of exercise during cancer treatment. *Cancer Practice, 9*(3), 119–127.

Moore, S. C., Lee, I.-M., Weiderpass, E., Campbell, P. T., Sampson, J. N., Kitahara, C. M., . . . Patel, A. V. (2016). Association of leisure-time physical activity with risk of 26 types of cancer in 1.44 million adults. *JAMA Internal Medicine, 176*(6), 816–825.

Mustian, K. M., Alfano, C. M., Heckler, C., Kleckner, A. S., Kleckner, I. R., Leach, C. R., . . . Miller, S. M. (2017). Comparison of pharmaceutical, psychological, and exercise treatments for cancer-related fatigue: a meta-analysis. *JAMA Oncology, 3*(7), 961–968.

Mustian, K. M., Morrow, G. R., Carroll, J. K., Figueroa-Moseley, C. D., Jean-Pierre, P., & Williams, G. C. (2007). Integrative nonpharmacologic behavioral interventions for the management of cancer-related fatigue. *The Oncologist, 12*(Suppl 1), 52–67.

Mustian, K. M., Peppone, L. J., Palesh, O. G., Janelsins, M. C., Mohile, S. G., Purnell, J. Q., & Darling, T. V. (2009). Exercise and cancer-related fatigue. *US Oncology, 5*(2), 20–23.

Mustian, K. M., Sprod, L. K., Janelsins, M., Peppone, L. J., & Mohile, S. (2012). Exercise recommendations for cancer-related fatigue, cognitive impairment, sleep problems, depression, pain, anxiety, and physical dysfunction: a review. *Oncology & Hematology Review, 8*(2), 81–88.

Mustian, K. M., Sprod, L. K., Palesh, O. G., Peppone, L. J., Janelsins, M. C., Mohile, S. G., & Carroll, J. (2009). Exercise for the management of side effects and quality of life among cancer survivors. *Current Sports Medicine Reports, 8*(6), 325–330.

National Cancer Institute. (2017, Jan. 27). *Physical activity and cancer* [Fact Sheet]. Retrieved from https://www.cancer.gov/about-cancer/causes-prevention/risk/obesity/physical-activity-fact-sheet

National Cancer Institute. (2017, Mar. 22). *Cancer statistics.* Retrieved from https://www.cancer.gov/about-cancer/understanding/statistics

Newton, R. U., & Galvão, D. A. (2016). Accumulating evidence for physical activity and prostate cancer survival: time for a definitive trial of exercise medicine? *European Urology, 70*(4), 586–587.

Oldervoll, L. M., Kaasa, S., Hjermstad, M. J., Lund, J. A., & Loge, J. H. (2004). Physical exercise results in the improved subjective well-being of a few or is effective rehabilitation for all cancer patients? *European Journal of Cancer, 40*(7), 951–962.

Oldervoll, L. M., Loge, J. H., Lydersen, S., Paltiel, H., Asp, M. B., Nygaard, U. V., . . . Kaasa, S. (2011). Physical exercise for cancer patients with advanced disease: a randomized controlled trial. *The Oncologist, 16*(11), 1649–1657.

Oncology Nursing Society. (n.d.). Research on exercise and QOL in cancer populations spans three decades. Retrieved from https://www.ons.org/practice-resources/clinical-practice/research-exercise-and-qol-cancer-populations-spans-three

Patel, A. V., Hildebrand, J. S., Campbell, P. T., Teras, L. R., Craft, L. L., McCullough, M. L., & Gapstur, S. M. (2015). Leisure-time spent sitting and site-specific cancer incidence in a large U.S. cohort. *Cancer Epidemiology, Biomarkers & Prevention,* 24(9), 1350–1359.

Patterson, S. (2014, Nov.–Dec.). Metformin may have broad utility in cancer. *Oncolog— The University of Texas MD Anderson Cancer Center,* 59(11–12). Retrieved from https://www.mdanderson.org/publications/oncolog/november-december-2014/ beyond-diabetes-metformin-may-have-broad-utility-in-cancer.html

Pedersen, L., Idorn, M., Olofsson, G. H., Lauenborg, B., Nookaew, I., Hansen, R. H., . . . Hojman, P. (2016). Voluntary running suppresses tumor growth through epinephrine- and IL-6-dependent NK cell mobilization and redistribution. *Cell Metabolism,* 23(3), 554–562.

Pierce, J. P., Stefanick, M. L., Flatt, S. W., Natarajan, L., Sternfeld, B., Madlensky, L., . . . Rock, C. L. (2007). Greater survival after breast cancer in physically active women with high vegetable-fruit intake regardless of obesity. *Journal of Clinical Oncology,* 25(17), 2345–2351.

Rajarajeswaran, P., & Vishnupriya, R. (2009). Exercise in cancer. *Indian Journal of Medical and Paediatric Oncology,* 30(2), 61–70.

Rapaport, L. (2017, Mar. 6). Exercise better than drugs for cancer fatigue. *Health News, Reuters.* Retrieved from http://www.reuters.com/article/ us-health-cancer-fatigue-idUSKBN16D2DY

Reynolds, G. (2009, Aug. 18). Phys ed: does exercise reduce your cancer risk? *Well, New York Times.* Retrieved from https://well.blogs.nytimes.com/2009/08/18/ phys-ed-does-exercise-reduce-your-cancer-risk/

Reynolds, G. (2015, Mar. 25). How exercise may aid cancer treatment. *Well, New York Times.* Retrieved from https://well.blogs.nytimes.com/2015/03/25/how-exercise-may- aid-cancer-treatment/

Reynolds, G. (2016, Feb. 24). How exercise may lower cancer risk. *Well, New York Times.* Retrieved from https://well.blogs.nytimes.com/2016/02/24/how-exercise- may-lower-cancer-risk/

Richman, E. L., Kenfield, S. A., Stampfer, M. J., Paciorek, A., Carroll, P. R., & Chan, J. M. (2011). Physical activity after diagnosis and risk of prostate cancer progression: data from the Cancer of the Prostate Strategic Urologic Research Endeavor. *Cancer Research,* 71(11), 3889–3895.

Roswell Park Cancer Institute. (2016, May 10). Exercise may reduce the risk of cervical cancer. [Press release]. Retrieved from https://www.roswellpark.org/media/ news/exercise-may-reduce-risk-cervical-cancer

Rundqvist, H., Augsten, M., Strömberg, A., Rullman, E., Mijwel, S., Kharaziha, P., . . . Östman, A. (2013). Effect of acute exercise on prostate cancer cell growth. *PLoS ONE,* 8(7), e67579.

Schmitz, K. H., Holtzman, J., Courneya, K. S., Mâsse, L. C., Duval, S., & Kane, R. (2005). Controlled physical activity trials in cancer survivors: a systematic review and meta-analysis. *Cancer Epidemiology, Biomarkers & Prevention,* 14(7), 1588–1595.

Segal, R. J., Reid, R. D., Courneya, K. S., Malone, S. C., Parliament, M. B., Scott, C. G., . . . Wells, G. A. (2003). Resistance exercise in men receiving androgen deprivation therapy for prostate cancer. *Journal of Clinical Oncology,* 21(9), 1653–1659.

Simon, S. (2017, Jan. 5). Cancer facts and figures: death rate down 25% since 1991. *American Cancer Society.* Retrieved from https://www.cancer.org/latest-news/ cancer-facts-and-figures-death-rate-down-25-since-1991.html

Slattery, M. L. (2004). Physical activity and colorectal cancer. *Sports Medicine,* 34(4), 239–252.

Smith, A. J., Phipps, W. R., Thomas, W., Schmitz, K. H., & Kurzer, M. S. (2013). The effects of aerobic exercise on estrogen metabolism in healthy premenopausal women. *Cancer Epidemiology, Biomarkers & Prevention, 22*(5), 756–764.

Song, M., & Giovannucci, E. (2016). Preventable incidence and mortality of carcinoma associated with lifestyle factors among white adults in the United States. *JAMA Oncology, 2*(9), 1154–1161.

Sternfeld, B., Weltzien, E., Quesenberry, C. P., Castillo, A. L., Kwan, M., Slattery, M. L., & Caan, B. J. (2009). Physical activity and risk of recurrence and mortality in breast cancer survivors: findings from the LACE Study. *Cancer Epidemiology, Biomarkers & Prevention, 18*(1), 87–95.

Szender, J. B., Cannioto, R., Gulati, N. R., Schmitt, K., Friel, G., Minlikeeva, A., . . . Moysich, K. B. (2016). Impact of physical inactivity on risk of developing cancer of the uterine cervix: a case-control study. *Journal of Lower Genital Tract Disease, 20*(3), 230–233.

Taaffe, D. R., Newton, R. U., Spry, N., Joseph, D., Chambers, S. K., Gardiner, R. A., . . . Galvão, D. A. (2017). Effects of different exercise modalities on fatigue in prostate cancer patients undergoing androgen deprivation therapy: a year-long randomised controlled trial. *European Urology, 72*(2), 293–299.

Thomas, G. A., Cartmel, B., Harrigan, M., Fiellin, M., Capozza, S., Zhou, Y., . . . Irwin, M. L. (2017). The effect of exercise on body composition and bone mineral density in breast cancer survivors taking aromatase inhibitors. *Obesity, 25*(2), 346–351.

Thune, I., & Furberg, A. S. (2001). Physical activity and cancer risk: dose-response and cancer, all sites and site-specific. *Medicine and Science in Sports and Exercise, 33*(6 Suppl), S530–550.

Tomasetti, C., & Vogelstein, B. (2015). Variation in cancer risk among tissues can be explained by the number of stem cell divisions. *Science, 347*(6217), 78–81.

Valenti, M., Porzio, G., Aielli, F., Verna, L., Cannita, K., Manno, R., . . . Ficorella, C. (2008). Physical exercise and quality of life in breast cancer survivors. *International Journal of Medical Sciences, 5*(1), 24–28.

Vashistha, V., Singh, B., Kaur, S., Prokop, L. J., & Kaushik, D. (2016). The effects of exercise on fatigue, quality of life, and psychological function for men with prostate cancer: systematic review and meta-analyses. *European Urology Focus, 2*(3), 284–295.

West-Wright, C. N., Henderson, K. D., Sullivan-Halley, J., Ursin, G., Deapen, D., Neuhausen, S., . . . Bernstein, L. (2009). Long-term and recent recreational physical activity and survival after breast cancer: the California Teachers Study. *Cancer Epidemiology, Biomarkers & Prevention, 18*(11), 2851–2859.

Winningham, M. L., MacVicar, M. G., & Burke, C. A. (1986). Exercise for cancer patients: guidelines and precautions. *The Physician and Sportsmedicine, 14*(10), 125–134.

Wolin, K. Y., Yan, Y., Colditz, G. A., & Lee, I.-M. (2009). Physical activity and colon cancer prevention: a meta-analysis. *British Journal of Cancer, 100*(4), 611–616.

World Cancer Research Fund/American Institute for Cancer Research. (2007). *Nutrition, physical activity and the prevention of cancer: a global perspective.* Washington DC: American Institute for Cancer Research.

CHAPTER 13

American Federation for Aging Research. (2016). Biomarkers of aging, Infoaging guides. Retrieved from https://www.afar.org/docs/AFAR_BIOMARKERS_OF_AGING_2016.pdf

American Psychological Association. (n.d.) Stress: the different kinds of stress. Retrieved from http://www.apa.org/helpcenter/stress-kinds.aspx

Armanios, M. Y., Chen, J. J.-L., Cogan, J. D., Alder, J. K., Ingersoll, R. G., Markin, C., . . . Loyd, J. E. (2007). Telomerase mutations in families with idiopathic pulmonary fibrosis. *New England Journal of Medicine, 356*(13), 1317–1326.

Arsenis, N. C., You, T., Ogawa, E. F., Tinsley, G. M., & Zuo, L. (2017). Physical activity and telomere length: impact of aging and potential mechanisms of action. *Oncotarget, 8*(27), 45008–45019.

Artandi, S. E., Chang, S., Lee, S. L., Alson, S., Gottlieb, G. J., Chin, L., & DePinho, R. A. (2000). Telomere dysfunction promotes non-reciprocal translocations and epithelial cancers in mice. *Nature, 406*(6796), 641–645.

Artandi, S. E., & DePinho, R. A. (2010). Telomeres and telomerase in cancer. *Carcinogenesis, 31*(1), 9–18.

Babizhayev, M. A., Savel'yeva, E. L., Moskvina, S. N., & Yegorov, Y. E. (2011). Telomere length is a biomarker of cumulative oxidative stress, biologic age, and an independent predictor of survival and therapeutic treatment requirement associated with smoking behavior. *American Journal of Therapeutics, 18*(6), e209–226.

Barnett, R. (2017, Apr. 27). The puzzle of aging: Elizabeth Blackburn speaks at TED2017. [Web log post]. Retrieved from https://blog.ted.com/the-puzzle-of-aging-elizabeth-blackburn-speaks-at-ted2017/

Bernardes de Jesus, B., Vera, E., Schneeberger, K., Tejera, A. M., Ayuso, E., Bosch, F., & Blasco, M. A. (2012). Telomerase gene therapy in adult and old mice delays aging and increases longevity without increasing cancer. *EMBO Molecular Medicine, 4*(8), 691–704.

Blackburn, E. H. (2009, Dec. 7). Telomeres and telomerase: the means to the end. [Nobel lecture]. Retrieved from https://www.nobelprize.org/nobel_prizes/medicine/laureates/2009/blackburn_lecture.pdf

Blackburn, E., & Epel, E. (2017). *The telomere effect.* New York, NY: Grand Central Publishing, Hachette Book Group.

Blackburn, E. H., Epel, E. S., & Lin, J. (2015). Human telomere biology: a contributory and interactive factor in aging, disease risks, and protection. *Science 350*(6265), 1193–1198.

Blasco, M. A., Lee, H. W., Hande, M. P., Samper, E., Lansdorp, P. M., DePinho, R. A., & Greider, C. W. (1997). Telomere shortening and tumor formation by mouse cells lacking telomerase RNA. *Cell, 91*(1), 25–34.

Bodnar, A. G., Ouellette, M., Frolkis, M., Holt, S. E., Chiu, C. P., Morin, G. B., . . . Wright, W. E. (1998). Extension of life-span by introduction of telomerase into normal human cells. *Science, 279*(5349), 349–352.

Boks, M. P., van Mierlo, H. C., Rutten, B. P. F., Radstake, T. R. D. J., De Witte, L., Geuze, E., . . . Vermetten, E. (2015). Longitudinal changes of telomere length and epigenetic age related to traumatic stress and post-traumatic stress disorder. *Psychoneuroendocrinology, 51*, 506–512.

Boonekamp, J. J., Mulder, G. A., Salomons, H. M., Dijkstra, C., & Verhulst, S. (2014). Nestling telomere shortening, but not telomere length, reflects developmental stress and predicts survival in wild birds. *Proceedings of the Royal Society B: Biological Sciences, 281*(1785), 20133287.

Borghini, A., Giardini, G., Tonacci, A., Mastorci, F., Mercuri, A., Mrakic-Sposta, S., . . . Pratali, L. (2015). Chronic and acute effects of endurance training on telomere length. *Mutagenesis, 30*(5), 711–716.

Bouchard, C., Blair, S. N., & Katzmarzyk, P. T. (2015). Less sitting, more physical activity, or higher fitness? *Mayo Clinic Proceedings, 90*(11), 1533–1540.

Breitling, L. P., Saum, K.-U., Perna, L., Schöttker, B., Holleczek, B., & Brenner, H. (2016). Frailty is associated with the epigenetic clock but not with telomere length in a German cohort. *Clinical Epigenetics, 8*, 21.

Brigham Young University. (2017, May 10). High levels of exercise linked to nine years of less aging at the cellular level: new research shows a major advantage for those who are highly active. *ScienceDaily.* Retrieved from www.sciencedaily.com/releases/2017/05/170510115211.htm

Burfoot, A. (2006, Sept. 7). Should you be afraid of free radicals? *Runner's World.* Retrieved from https://www.runnersworld.com/health/should-you-be-afraid-of-free-radicals

Cawthon, R. M., Smith, K. R., O'Brien, E., Sivatchenko, A., & Kerber, R. A. (2003). Association between telomere length in blood and mortality in people aged 60 years or older. *Lancet, 361*(9355), 393–395.

Chen, S. H., Epel, E. S., Mellon, S. H., Lin, J., Reus, V. I., Rosser, R., . . . Wolkowitz, O. M. (2014). Adverse childhood experiences and leukocyte telomere maintenance in depressed and healthy adults. *Journal of Affective Disorders, 169*, 86–90.

Cherkas, L. F., Hunkin, J. L., Kato, B. S., Richards, J. B., Gardner, J. P., Surdulescu, G. L., . . . Aviv, A. (2008). The association between physical activity in leisure time and leukocyte telomere length. *Archives of Internal Medicine, 168*(2), 154–158.

Clopton, J. (2017, Apr. 19). What tiny telomeres may tell us about aging. *WebMD.* Retrieved from https://www.webmd.com/special-reports/anti-aging-science/20170419/telomere-aging-link

Codd, V., Nelson, C. P., Albrecht, E., Mangino, M., Deelen, J., Buxton, J. L., . . . Samani, N. J. (2013). Identification of seven loci affecting mean telomere length and their association with disease. *Nature Genetics, 45*(4), 422–427e2.

Conger, K. (2015, Jan. 22). *Telomere extension turns back the aging clock in cultured human cells, study finds.* [Press release]. Retrieved from https://med.stanford.edu/news/all-news/2015/01/telomere-extension-turns-back-aging-clock-in-cultured-cells.html

Correia-Melo, C., Hewitt, G., & Passos, J. F. (2014). Telomeres, oxidative stress and inflammatory factors: partners in cellular senescence?. *Longevity & Healthspan, 3*, 1.

Damjanovic, A. K., Yang, Y., Glaser, R., Kiecolt-Glaser, J. K., Nguyen, H., Laskowski, B., . . . Weng, N. (2007). Accelerated telomere erosion is associated with a declining immune function of caregivers of Alzheimer's disease patients. *Journal of Immunology, 179*(6), 4249–4254.

Darrow, S. M., Verhoeven, J. E., Révész, D., Lindqvist, D., Penninx, B. W., Delucchi, K. L., . . . Mathews, C. A. (2016). The association between psychiatric disorders and telomere length: a meta-analysis involving 14,827 persons. *Psychosomatic Medicine, 78*(7), 776–787.

Denham, J., Nelson, C. P., O'Brien, B. J., Nankervis, S. A., Denniff, M., Harvey, J. T., . . . Charchar, F. J. (2013). Longer leukocyte telomeres are associated with ultra-endurance exercise independent of cardiovascular risk factors. *PLoS ONE, 8*(7), e69377.

Diman, A., Boros, J., Poulain, F., Rodriguez, J., Purnelle, M., Episkopou, H., . . . Decottignies, A. (2016). Nuclear respiratory factor 1 and endurance exercise promote human telomere transcription. *Science Advances, 2*(7), e1600031.

Douglas, S. (2013, Aug. 5). Ultrarunners have longer telomeres (which is good). *Runner's World.* Retrieved from https://www.runnersworld.com/newswire/ultrarunners-have-longer-telomeres-which-is-good

Drury, S., Theall, K., Gleason, M., Smyke, A., De Vivo, I., Wong, J., . . . Nelson, C. (2012). Telomere length and early severe social deprivation: linking early adversity and cellular aging. *Molecular Psychiatry, 17*(7), 719–727.

Du, M., Prescott, J., Kraft, P., Han, J., Giovannucci, E., Hankinson, S. E., & De Vivo, I. (2012). Physical activity, sedentary behavior, and leukocyte telomere length in women. *American Journal of Epidemiology, 175*(5), 414–422.

Eitan, E., Hutchison, E. R., & Mattson, M. P. (2014). Telomere shortening in neurological disorders: an abundance of unanswered questions. *Trends in Neurosciences, 37*(5), 256–263.

Entringer, S., Epel, E. S., Kumsta, R., Lin, J., Hellhammer, D. H., Blackburn, E. H., . . . Wadhwa, P. D. (2011). Stress exposure in intrauterine life is associated with shorter telomere length in young adulthood. *Proceedings of the National Academy of Sciences of the United States of America, 108*(33), E513–E518.

Entringer, S., Epel, E. S., Lin, J., Buss, C., Shahbaba, B., Blackburn, E. H., . . . Wadhwa, P. D. (2013). Maternal psychosocial stress during pregnancy is associated with newborn leukocyte telomere length. *American Journal of Obstetrics and Gynecology, 208*(2), 134.e1–134.e7.

Epel, E. S., Blackburn, E. H., Lin, J., Dhabhar, F. S., Adler, N. E., Morrow, J. D., & Cawthon, R. M. (2004). Accelerated telomere shortening in response to life stress. *Proceedings of the National Academy of Sciences of the United States of America, 101*(49), 17312–17315.

Epel, E., Daubenmier, J., Moskowitz, J. T., Folkman, S., & Blackburn, E. (2009). Can meditation slow rate of cellular aging? Cognitive stress, mindfulness, and telomeres. *Annals of the New York Academy of Sciences, 1172*, 34–53.

Epel, E. S., & Prather, A. A. (2018). Stress, telomeres and psychopathology: towards a deeper understanding of a triad of early aging. *American Review of Clinical Psychology, 14*, 371–397.

Fernandez, E. (2013, Sept. 16). Lifestyle changes may lengthen telomeres, a measure of cell aging. *UCSF News Center.* Retrieved from https://www.ucsf.edu/news/2013/09/108886/lifestyle-changes-may-lengthen-telomeres-measure-cell-aging

Foreman, J. (2003, Mar. 25). Telomerase: a promising cancer drug stuck in patent hell? *Boston Globe.* Retrieved from http://judyforeman.com/columns/telomerase-promising-cancer-drug-stuck-patent-hell/

Fouquerel, E., Lormand, J., Bose, A., Lee, H.-T., Kim, G. S., Li, J., . . . Opresko, P. L. (2016). Oxidative guanine base damage regulates human telomerase activity. *Nature Structural & Molecular Biology, 23*(12), 1092–1100.

Genetic Science Learning Center. (n.d.). Are telomeres the key to aging and cancer? *Learn. Genetics, University of Utah.* Retrieved from http://learn.genetics.utah.edu/content/basics/telomeres/

Gotlib, I. H., LeMoult, J., Colich, N. L., Foland-Ross, L. C., Hallmayer, J., Joormann, J., . . . Wolkowitz, O. M. (2015). Telomere length and cortisol reactivity in children of depressed mothers. *Molecular Psychiatry, 20*(5), 615–620.

Greider, C. W., & Blackburn, E. H. (1996). Telomeres, telomerase and cancer. *Scientific American, 274*(2), 92–97.

Hanssen, L. M., Schutte, N. S., Malouff, J. M., & Epel, E. S. (2017). The relationship between childhood psychosocial stressor level and telomere length: a meta-analysis. *Health Psychology Research, 5*(1), 6378.

Hau, M., Haussmann, M. F., Greives, T. J., Matlack, C., Costantini, D., Quetting, M., . . . Partecke, J. (2015). Repeated stressors in adulthood increase the rate of biological ageing. *Frontiers in Zoology, 12*, 4.

Haussmann, M. F., & Heidinger, B. J. (2015). Telomere dynamics may link stress exposure and ageing across generations. *Biology Letters, 11*(11), 20150396.

Haycock, P. C., Heydon, E. E., Kaptoge, S., Butterworth, A. S., Thompson, A., & Willeit, P. (2014). Leucocyte telomere length and risk of cardiovascular disease: systematic review and meta-analysis. *British Medical Journal, 349*, g4227.

Heidinger, B. J., Blount, J. D., Boner, W., Griffiths, K., Metcalfe, N. B., & Monaghan, P. (2012). Telomere length in early life predicts lifespan. *Proceedings of the National Academy of Sciences of the United States of America, 109*(5), 1743–1748.

Herborn, K. A., Heidinger, B. J., Boner, W., Noguera, J. C., Adam, A., Daunt, F., & Monaghan, P. (2014). Stress exposure in early post-natal life reduces telomere length: an experimental demonstration in a long-lived seabird. *Proceedings of the Royal Society B: Biological Sciences, 281*(1782), 20133151.

Hjelmborg, J. B., Dalgård, C., Möller, S., Steenstrup, T., Kimura, M., Christensen, K., . . . Aviv, A. (2015). The heritability of leucocyte telomere length dynamics. *Journal of Medical Genetics, 52*(5), 297–302.

Ho, R. T. H., Chan, J. S. M., Wang, C.-W., Lau, B. W. M., So, K. F., Yuen, L. P., . . . Chan, C. L. W. (2012). A randomized controlled trial of qigong exercise on fatigue symptoms, functioning, and telomerase activity in persons with chronic fatigue or chronic fatigue syndrome. *Annals of Behavioral Medicine, 44*(2), 160–170.

Hoge, E. A., Chen, M. M., Orr, E., Metcalf, C. A., Fischer, L. E., Pollack, M. H., . . . Simon, N. M. (2013). Loving-kindness meditation practice associated with longer telomeres in women. *Brain, Behavior, and Immunity, 32*, 159–163.

Holysz, H., Lipinska, N., Paszel-Jaworska, A., & Rubis, B. (2013). Telomerase as a useful target in cancer fighting: the breast cancer case. *Tumor Biology, 34*(3), 1371–1380.

Houben, J. M. J., Moonen, H. J. J., van Schooten, F. J., & Hageman, G. J. (2008). Telomere length assessment: biomarker of chronic oxidative stress? *Free Radical Biology & Medicine, 44*(3), 235–246.

Hu, J., Hwang, S. S., Liesa, M., Gan, B., Sahin, E., Jaskelioff, M., . . . DePinho, R. A. (2012). Anti-telomerase therapy provokes ALT and mitochondrial adaptive mechanisms in cancer. *Cell, 148*(4), 651–663.

Jacobs, T. L., Epel, E. S., Lin, J., Blackburn, E. H., Wolkowitz, O. M., Bridwell, D. A., . . . Saron, C. D. (2011). Intensive meditation training, immune cell telomerase activity, and psychological mediators. *Psychoneuroendocrinology, 36*(5), 664–681.

Jäger, K., & Walter, M. (2016). Therapeutic targeting of telomerase. *Genes, 7*(7), 39.

Jodczyk, S., Fergusson, D. M., Horwood, L. J., Pearson, J. F., & Kennedy, M. A. (2014). No association between mean telomere length and life stress observed in a 30 year birth cohort. *PLoS ONE, 9*(5), e97102.

Kawanishi, S., & Oikawa, S. (2004). Mechanism of telomere shortening by oxidative stress. *Annals of the New York Academy of Sciences, 1019*, 278–284.

Khan, S., Naidoo, D. P., & Chuturgoon, A. A. (2012). Telomeres and atherosclerosis. *Cardiovascular Journal of Africa, 23*(10), 563–571.

Kim, J.-H., Ko, J.-H., Lee, D., Lim, I., & Bang, H. (2012). Habitual physical exercise has beneficial effects on telomere length in postmenopausal women. *Menopause, 19*(10), 1109–1115.

Knight, M. (2015, Mar. 25). Buy your telomere testing kit here! Evidence based or pseudo-science? *Genetic Literacy Project.* Retrieved from https://geneticliteracyproject.org/2015/03/25/buy-your-telomere-testing-kit-here-evidence-based-or-psuedo-science/

Lanhan, B. (2017, June 28). BYU research suggests exercise reverses cellular aging process. *Daily Universe*. Retrieved from http://universe.byu.edu/2017/06/28/byu-research-suggests-exercise-reverses-cellular-aging-process1/

Lapham, K., Kvale, M. N., Lin, J., Connell, S., Croen, L. A., Dispensa, B. P., . . . Blackburn, E. H. (2015). Automated assay of telomere length measurement and informatics for 100,000 subjects in the Genetic Epidemiology Research on Adult Health and Aging (GERA) Cohort. *Genetics, 200*(4), 1061–1072.

LaRocca, T. J., Seals, D. R., & Pierce, G. L. (2010). Leukocyte telomere length is preserved with aging in endurance exercise-trained adults and related to maximal aerobic capacity. *Mechanisms of Ageing and Development, 131*(2), 165–167.

Latifovic, L., Peacock, S. D., Massey, T. E., & King, W. D. (2016). The influence of alcohol consumption, cigarette smoking, and physical activity on leukocyte telomere length. *Cancer Epidemiology, Biomarkers & Prevention, 25*(2), 374–380.

Li, Q., Du, J., Feng, R., Xu, Y., Wang, H., Sang, Q., . . . Wang, L. (2014). A possible new mechanism in the pathophysiology of polycystic ovary syndrome (PCOS): the discovery that leukocyte telomere length is strongly associated with PCOS. *Journal of Clinical Endocrinology and Metabolism, 99*(2), E234–240.

Li, X., Wang, J., Zhou, J., Huang, P., & Li, J. (2017). The association between post-traumatic stress disorder and shorter telomere length: a systematic review and meta-analysis. *Journal of Affective Disorders, 218*, 322–326.

Li, Y., Zhou, G., Bruno, I.G, Cooke, J.P. (2017). Telomerase mRNA reverses senescence in progeria cells. *Journal of the American College of Cardiology, 70*(6), 804–805.

Li, Z., He, Y., Wang, D., Tang, J., & Chen, X. (2017). Association between childhood trauma and accelerated telomere erosion in adulthood: a meta-analytic study. *Journal of Psychiatric Research, 93*, 64–71.

Lin, J., Blalock, J. A., Chen, M., Ye, Y., Gu, J., Cohen, L., . . . Wu, X. (2015). Depressive symptoms and short telomere length are associated with increased mortality in bladder cancer patients. *Cancer Epidemiology, Biomarkers & Prevention, 24*(2), 336–343.

Lin, J., Epel, E., & Blackburn, E. (2012). Telomeres and lifestyle factors: roles in cellular aging. *Mutation Research, 730*(1–2), 85–89.

Loprinzi, P. D. (2015). Cardiorespiratory capacity and leukocyte telomere length among adults in the United States. *American Journal of Epidemiology, 182*(3), 198–201.

Loprinzi, P. D., Loenneke, J. P., & Blackburn, E. H. (2015). Movement-based behaviors and leukocyte telomere length among US adults. *Medicine and Science in Sports and Exercise, 47*(11), 2347–2352.

Loprinzi, P. D., & Sng, E. (2016). Mode-specific physical activity and leukocyte telomere length among U.S. adults: implications of running on cellular aging. *Preventive Medicine, 85*, 17–19.

Lu, A. T., Salfati, E. L., Chen, B. H., Ferrucci, L., Levy, D., Joehanes, R., . . . Horvath, S. (2018). GWAS of epigenetic aging rates in blood reveals a critical role for TERT. *Nature Communications, 9*(1), 387.

Ludlow, A. T., Zimmerman, J. B., Witkowski, S., Hearn, J. W., Hatfield, B. D., & Roth, S. M. (2008). Relationship between physical activity level, telomere length, and telomerase activity. *Medicine and Science in Sports and Exercise, 40*(10), 1764–1771.

Ma, H., Zhou, Z., Wei, S., Liu, Z., Pooley, K. A., Dunning, A. M., . . . Wei, Q. (2011). Shortened telomere length is associated with increased risk of cancer: a meta-analysis. *PLoS ONE, 6*(6), e20466.

Marioni, R. E., Harris, S. E., Shah, S., McRae, A. F., von Zglinicki, T., Martin-Ruiz, C., . . . Deary, I. J. (2016). The epigenetic clock and telomere length are independently associated with chronological age and mortality. *International Journal of Epidemiology, 45*(2), 424–432.

Martin-Ruiz, C. M., Gussekloo, J., van Heemst, D., von Zglinicki, T., & Westendorp, R. G. J. (2005). Telomere length in white blood cells is not associated with morbidity or mortality in the oldest old: a population-based study. *Aging Cell, 4*(6), 287–290.

Mason, C., Risques, R.-A., Xiao, L., Duggan, C. R., Imayama, I., Campbell, K. L., . . . McTiernan, A. (2013). Independent and combined effects of dietary weight loss and exercise on leukocyte telomere length in postmenopausal women. *Obesity (Silver Spring, MD), 21*(12), E549–E554.

Mather, K. A., Jorm, A. F., Parslow, R. A., & Christensen, H. (2011). Is telomere length a biomarker of aging? A review. *Journals of Gerontology Series A: Biological Sciences and Medical Sciences, 66*(2), 202–213.

Mathur, M. B., Epel, E., Kind, S., Desai, M., Parks, C. G., Sandler, D. P., & Khazeni, N. (2016). Perceived stress and telomere length: a systematic review, meta-analysis, and methodologic considerations for advancing the field. *Brain, Behavior, and Immunity, 54*, 158–169.

Mathur, S., Ardestani, A., Parker, B., Cappizzi, J., Polk, D., & Thompson, P. D. (2013). Telomere length and cardiorespiratory fitness in marathon runners. *Journal of Investigative Medicine, 61*(3), 613–615.

Merville, S. (2012, Feb. 20). Blocking telomerase kills cancer cells but provokes resistance, progression. [Press release]. *University of Texas MD Anderson Cancer Center.* Retrieved from https://www.mdanderson.org/newsroom/2012/02/blocking-telomerase-kills-cancer-but-provokes-progression.html

Mishra, S., Kumar, R., Malhotra, N., Singh, N., & Dada, R. (2016). Mild oxidative stress is beneficial for sperm telomere length maintenance. *World Journal of Methodology, 6*(2), 163–170.

Mundstock, E., Zatti, H., Louzada, F. M., Oliveira, S. G., Guma, F. T. C. R., Paris, M. M., . . . Mattiello, R. (2015). Effects of physical activity in telomere length: systematic review and meta-analysis. *Ageing Research Reviews, 22*, 72–80.

National Cancer Institute. (2017, Mar. 22). Cancer statistics. Retrieved from https://www.cancer.gov/about-cancer/understanding/statistics

Nautiyal, S., DeRisi, J. L., & Blackburn, E. H. (2002). The genome-wide expression response to telomerase deletion in *Saccharomyces cerevisiae. Proceedings of the National Academy of Sciences of the United States of America, 99*(14), 9316–9321.

Needham, B. L., Fernandez, J. R., Lin, J., Epel, E. S., & Blackburn, E. H. (2012). Socioeconomic status and cell aging in children. *Social Science & Medicine (1982), 74*(12), 1948–1951.

Oliveira, B. S., Zunzunegui, M. V., Quinlan, J., Fahmi, H., Tu, M. T., & Guerra, R. O. (2016). Systematic review of the association between chronic social stress and telomere length: a life course perspective. *Ageing Research Reviews, 26*, 37–52.

Ornish, D., Lin, J., Chan, J. M., Epel, E., Kemp, C., Weidner, G., . . . Blackburn, E. H. (2013). Effect of comprehensive lifestyle changes on telomerase activity and telomere length in men with biopsy-proven low-risk prostate cancer: 5-year follow-up of a descriptive pilot study. *Lancet Oncology, 14*(11), 1112–1120.

Østhus, I. B. Ø., Sgura, A., Berardinelli, F., Alsnes, I. V., Brønstad, E., Rehn, T., . . . Nauman, J. (2012). Telomere length and long-term endurance exercise: does exercise training affect biological age? A pilot study. *PLoS ONE, 7*(12), e52769.

O'Sullivan, R. J., & Almouzni, G. (2014). Assembly of telomeric chromatin to create ALTernative endings. *Trends in Cell Biology, 24*(11), 675–685.

Pollack, A. (2011, May 18). A blood test offers clues to longevity. *New York Times*. Retrieved from http://www.nytimes.com/2011/05/19/business/19life.html?mcubz=1

Price, L. H., Kao, H.-T., Burgers, D. E., Carpenter, L. L., & Tyrka, A. R. (2013). Telomeres and early-life stress: an overview. *Biological Psychiatry, 73*(1), 15–23.

Puterman, E., Gemmill, A., Karasek, D., Weir, D., Adler, N. E., Prather, A. A., & Epel, E. S. (2016). Lifespan adversity and later adulthood telomere length in the nationally representative US Health and Retirement Study. *Proceedings of the National Academy of Sciences of the United States of America, 113*(42), E6335–E6342.

Puterman, E., Lin, J., Blackburn, E., O'Donovan, A., Adler, N., & Epel, E. (2010). The power of exercise: buffering the effect of chronic stress on telomere length. *PLoS ONE, 5*(5), e10837.

Puterman, E., Lin, J., Krauss, J., Blackburn, E. H., & Epel, E. S. (2015). Determinants of telomere attrition over one year in healthy older women: stress and health behaviors matter. *Molecular Psychiatry, 20*(4), 529–535.

Puterman, E., Weiss, J., Lin, J., Schillf, S., Slusher, A. L., Johansen, K. L., & Epel, E. S. (2018). Aerobic exercise lengthens telomeres and reduces stress in family caregivers: a randomized controlled trial—Curt Richter Award Paper 2018. *Psychoneuroendocrinology, 98*, 245–252.

Rae, D. E., Vignaud, A., Butler-Browne, G. S., Thornell, L.-E., Sinclair-Smith, C., Derman, E. W., . . . Collins, M. (2010). Skeletal muscle telomere length in healthy, experienced, endurance runners. *European Journal of Applied Physiology, 109*(2), 323–330.

Ramunas, J., Yakubov, E., Brady, J. J., Corbel, S. Y., Holbrook, C., Brandt, M., . . . Blau, H. M. (2015). Transient delivery of modified mRNA encoding TERT rapidly extends telomeres in human cells. *FASEB Journal, 29*(5), 1930–1939.

Raynaud, C. M., Sabatier, L., Philipot, O., Olaussen, K. A., & Soria, J.-C. (2008). Telomere length, telomeric proteins and genomic instability during the multistep carcinogenic process. *Critical Reviews in Oncology/Hematology, 66*(2), 99–117.

Révész, D., Milaneschi, Y., Terpstra, E. M., & Penninx, B. W. J. H. (2016). Baseline biopsychosocial determinants of telomere length and 6-year attrition rate. *Psychoneuroendocrinology, 67*, 153–162.

Ridout, K. K., Levandowski, M., Ridout, S. J., Gantz, L., Goonan, K., Palermo, D., . . . Tyrka, A. R. (2018). Early life adversity and telomere length: a meta-analysis. *Molecular Psychiatry, 23*(4), 858–871.

Ridout, K. K., Ridout, S. J., Price, L. H., Sen, S., & Tyrka, A. R. (2016). Depression and telomere length: a meta-analysis. *Journal of Affective Disorders, 191*, 237–247.

Rode, L., Nordestgaard, B. G., & Bojesen, S. E. (2015). Peripheral blood leukocyte telomere length and mortality among 64,637 individuals from the general population. *Journal of the National Cancer Institute, 107*(6), djv074.

Saretzki, G. (2003). Telomerase inhibition as cancer therapy. *Cancer Letters, 194*(2), 209–219.

Saßenroth, D., Meyer, A., Salewsky, B., Kroh, M., Norman, K., Steinhagen-Thiessen, E., & Demuth, I. (2015). Sports and exercise at different ages and leukocyte telomere length in later life—data from the Berlin Aging Study II (BASE-II). *PLoS ONE, 10*(12), e0142131.

Schaakxs, R., Verhoeven, J. E., Oude Voshaar, R. C., Comijs, H. C., & Penninx, B. W. J. H. (2015). Leukocyte telomere length and late-life depression. *American Journal of Geriatric Psychiatry, 23*(4), 423–432.

Schneper, L. M., Brooks-Gunn, J., Notterman, D. A., & Suomi, S. J. (2016). Early life experiences and telomere length in adult rhesus monkeys: an exploratory study. *Psychosomatic Medicine, 78*(9), 1066–1071.

Shadyab, A. H., LaMonte, M. J., Kooperberg, C., Reiner, A. P., Carty, C. L., Manini, T. M., ... LaCroix, A. Z. (2017a). Leisure-time physical activity and leukocyte telomere length among older women. *Experimental Gerontology, 95*, 141–147.

Shadyab, A. H., LaMonte, M. J., Kooperberg, C., Reiner, A. P., Carty, C. L., Manini, T. M., ... LaCroix, A. Z. (2017b). Association of accelerometer-measured physical activity with leukocyte telomere length among older women. *Journals of Gerontology Series A: Biological Sciences and Medical Sciences, 72*(11), 1532–1537.

Shadyab, A. H., Macera, C. A., Shaffer, R. A., Jain, S., Gallo, L. C., LaMonte, M. J., ... LaCroix, A. Z. (2017). Associations of accelerometer-measured and self-reported sedentary time with leukocyte telomere length in older women. *American Journal of Epidemiology, 185*(3), 172–184.

Shalev, I., Entringer, S., Wadhwa, P. D., Wolkowitz, O. M., Puterman, E., Lin, J., & Epel, E. S. (2013). Stress and telomere biology: a lifespan perspective. *Psychoneuroendocrinology, 38*(9), 1835–1842.

Shalev, I., Moffitt, T., Sugden, K., Williams, B., Houts, R., Danese, A., ... Caspi, A. (2013). Exposure to violence during childhood is associated with telomere erosion from 5 to 10 years of age: a longitudinal study. *Molecular Psychiatry, 18*(5), 576–581.

Shammas, M. A. (2011). Telomeres, lifestyle, cancer, and aging. *Current Opinion in Clinical Nutrition and Metabolic Care, 14*(1), 28–34.

Shay, J. W., & Wright, W. E. (2011). Role of telomeres and telomerase in cancer. *Seminars in Cancer Biology, 21*(6), 349–353.

Shin, Y.-A., Lee, J.-H., Song, W., & Jun, T.-W. (2008). Exercise training improves the antioxidant enzyme activity with no changes of telomere length. *Mechanisms of Ageing and Development, 129*(5), 254–260.

Silva, L. C. R., de Araújo, A. L., Fernandes, J. R., Matias, M. de S. T., Silva, P. R., Duarte, A. J. S., ... Benard, G. (2016). Moderate and intense exercise lifestyles attenuate the effects of aging on telomere length and the survival and composition of T cell subpopulations. *Age, 38*(1), 24.

Simon, N. M., Smoller, J. W., McNamara, K. L., Maser, R. S., Zalta, A. K., Pollack, M. H., ... Wong, K.-K. (2006). Telomere shortening and mood disorders: preliminary support for a chronic stress model of accelerated aging. *Biological Psychiatry, 60*(5), 432–435.

Song, Z., von Figura, G., Liu, Y., Kraus, J. M., Torrice, C., Dillon, P., ... Rudolph, K. L. (2010). Lifestyle impacts on the aging associated expression of biomarkers of DNA damage and telomere dysfunction in human blood. *Aging Cell, 9*(4), 607–615.

Strong, W. (2013, Mar. 24). Telomeres: should you measure yours with TeloMe? [Web blog post]. *Biohack Yourself.* Retrieved from http://biohackyourself.com/telomeres-should-you-measure-yours-with-telome/

Surtees, P. G., Wainwright, N. W. J., Pooley, K. A., Luben, R. N., Khaw, K.-T., Easton, D. F., & Dunning, A. M. (2011). Life stress, emotional health, and mean telomere length in the European Prospective Investigation into Cancer (EPIC)-Norfolk population study. *Journals of Gerontology Series A: Biological Sciences and Medical Sciences, 66*(11), 1152–1162.

Telomere Diagnostics Inc. (2013, Oct. 24). *Telomere Diagnostics, Inc. (TDx), previously known as Telome Health, Inc., announces its name change.* [Press release]. Retrieved from http://www.evaluategroup.com/Universal/View.aspx?type=Story&id=464272

TeloYears. (n.d.). *Telomere Diagnostics Inc.* Retrieved from https://www.teloyears.com/home/

TeloYears Reviews. (n.d.). *TeloYears.* Retrieved from https://www.highya.com/teloyears-reviews

Tucey, T. M., & Lundblad, V. (2014). Regulated assembly and disassembly of the yeast telomerase quaternary complex. *Genes & Development, 28*(19), 2077–2089.

Tucker, L. A. (2017). Physical activity and telomere length in U.S. men and women: an NHANES investigation. *Preventive Medicine, 100*, 145–151.

University of Pittsburgh Schools of the Health Sciences. (2016, Nov. 8). Key mechanisms of cancer, aging and inflammation uncovered. *ScienceDaily*. Retrieved from www.sciencedaily.com/releases/2016/11/161108111356.htm

US National Library of Medicine. (2017, Nov. 14). Dyskeratosis congenital. *Genetics Home Reference*. Retrieved from https://ghr.nlm.nih.gov/condition/dyskeratosis-congenita#genes

US National Library of Medicine. (2017, Nov. 14). TERT gene. *Genetics Home Reference*. Retrieved from https://ghr.nlm.nih.gov/gene/TERT

Verhoeven, J. E., Révész, D., van Oppen, P., Epel, E. S., Wolkowitz, O. M., & Penninx, B. W. J. H. (2015). Anxiety disorders and accelerated cellular ageing. *British Journal of Psychiatry, 206*(5), 371–378.

Verhoeven, J. E., van Oppen, P., Puterman, E., Elzinga, B., & Penninx, B. W. J. H. (2015). The association of early and recent psychosocial life stress with leukocyte telomere length. *Psychosomatic Medicine, 77*(8), 882–891.

von Zglinicki, T. (2002). Oxidative stress shortens telomeres. *Trends in Biochemical Sciences, 27*(7), 339–344.

von Zglinicki, T., & Martin-Ruiz, C. M. (2005). Telomeres as biomarkers for ageing and age-related diseases. *Current Molecular Medicine, 5*(2), 197–203.

Weischer, M., Bojesen, S. E., & Nordestgaard, B. G. (2014). Telomere shortening unrelated to smoking, body weight, physical activity, and alcohol intake: 4,576 general population individuals with repeat measurements 10 years apart. *PLoS Genetics, 10*(3), e1004191.

Wentzensen, I. M., Mirabello, L., Pfeiffer, R. M., & Savage, S. A. (2011). The association of telomere length and cancer: a meta-analysis. *Cancer Epidemiology, Biomarkers & Prevention, 20*(6), 1238–1250.

Werner, C., Fürster, T., Widmann, T., Pöss, J., Roggia, C., Hanhoun, M., . . . Laufs, U. (2009). Physical exercise prevents cellular senescence in circulating leukocytes and in the vessel wall. *Circulation, 120*(24), 2438–2447.

Werner, C., Hanhoun, M., Widmann, T., Kazakov, A., Semenov, A., Pöss, J., . . . Laufs, U. (2008). Effects of physical exercise on myocardial telomere-regulating proteins, survival pathways, and apoptosis. *Journal of the American College of Cardiology, 52*(6), 470–482.

Willeit, P., Willeit, J., Mayr, A., Weger, S., Oberhollenzer, F., Brandstätter, A., . . . Kiechl, S. (2010). Telomere length and risk of incident cancer and cancer mortality. *Journal of the American Medical Association, 304*(1), 69–75.

Williams, S. C. P. (2013). No end in sight for telomerase-targeted cancer drugs. *Nature Medicine, 19*(1), 6.

Wojcicki, J. M., Heyman, M. B., Elwan, D., Shiboski, S., Lin, J., Blackburn, E., & Epel, E. (2015). Telomere length is associated with oppositional defiant behavior and maternal clinical depression in Latino preschool children. *Translational Psychiatry, 5*(6), e581.

Wojcicki, J. M., Olveda, R., Heyman, M. B., Elwan, D., Lin, J., Blackburn, E., & Epel, E. (2016). Cord blood telomere length in Latino infants: relation with maternal education and infant sex. *Journal of Perinatology, 36*(3), 235–241.

Wolinsky, H. (2011). Testing time for telomeres: telomere length can tell us something about disease susceptibility and ageing, but are commercial tests ready for prime time? *EMBO Reports, 12*(9), 897–900.

Wolkowitz, O. M., Epel, E. S., Reus, V. I., & Mellon, S. H. (2010). Depression gets old fast: do stress and depression accelerate cell aging? *Depression and Anxiety, 27*(4), 327–338.

Wolkowitz, O. M., Mellon, S. H., Epel, E. S., Lin, J., Dhabhar, F. S., Su, Y., . . . Blackburn, E. H. (2011). Leukocyte telomere length in major depression: correlations with chronicity, inflammation and oxidative stress—preliminary findings. *PLoS ONE, 6*(3), e17837.

Zalli, A., Carvalho, L. A., Lin, J., Hamer, M., Erusalimsky, J. D., Blackburn, E. H., & Steptoe, A. (2014). Shorter telomeres with high telomerase activity are associated with raised allostatic load and impoverished psychosocial resources. *Proceedings of the National Academy of Sciences of the United States of America, 111*(12), 4519–4524.

Zhan, Y., Song, C., Karlsson, R., Tillander, A., Reynolds, C. A., Pedersen, N. L., & Hägg, S. (2015). Telomere length shortening and alzheimer disease: a Mendelian randomization study. *JAMA Neurology, 72*(10), 1202–1203.

Zhang, J., Rane, G., Dai, X., Shanmugam, M. K., Arfuso, F., Samy, R. P., . . . Sethi, G. (2016). Ageing and the telomere connection: an intimate relationship with inflammation. *Ageing Research Reviews, 25,* 55–69.

CHAPTER 14

Acarbose. (2018). *WebMD.* Retrieved from https://www.webmd.com/drugs/2/drug-5207/acarbose-oral/details

Aliper, A., Jellen, L., Cortese, F., Artemov, A., Karpinskky-Semper, D., Moskalve, A., . . . Zhavoronkov, A. (2017). Towards natural mimetics of metformin and rapamycin. *Aging, 9*(11), 2245–2268.

American Federation for Aging Research. (2011). *Theories of aging.* Retrieved from http://www.afar.org/docs/migrated/111121_INFOAGING_GUIDE_THEORIES_OF_AGINGFR.pdf

American Federation for Aging Research. (2018). TAME—Targeting aging with metformin. Retrieved from https://www.afar.org/natgeo/

Arnquist, S. (2009, Aug. 17). With resveratrol, buyer beware. *New York Times.*

Artificial intelligence for drug discovery, biomarker development and aging research. (2018). *Insilico Medicine.* Retrieved from http://www.insilico.com

Baker, D. J., Wijshake, T., Tchkonia, T., LeBrasseur, N.K., Childs, B.G., van de Sluis, B., & van Deursen, J. M. (2011). Clearance of p16 INK4a-positive senescent cells delays ageing-associated disorders. *Nature, 469,* 232–236.

Bannister, C. A., Holden, S. E., Jenkins-Jones, S., Morgan, C. L., Halcox, J. P., Schernthaner, G., . . . Currie, C. J. (2014). Can people with type 2 diabetes live longer than those without? A comparison of mortality in people initiated with metformin or sulphonylurea monotherapy and matched, non-diabetic controls. *Diabetes, Obesity and Metabolism, 16*(11), 1165–1173.

Barger, J. L., Kayo, T., Vann, J. M., Arias, E. B., Wang, J., Hacker, T. A., . . . Prolla, T. A. (2008). A low dose of dietary resveratrol partially mimics caloric restriction and retards aging parameters in mice. *PLoS ONE, 3*(6), e2264.

Beil, L. (2017, May 10). "Exercise pill" turns couch potato mice into marathoners. *Science News.* Retrieved from https://www.sciencenews.org/article/exercise-pill-turns-couch-potato-mice-marathoners

Bonkowski, M. S., & Sinclair, D. A. (2016). Slowing ageing by design: the rise of NAD+ and sirtuin activating compounds. *Nature Reviews Molecular Cell Biology, 11*(11), 679–690.

Borel, R. (2016, Mar. 28). Who will be first to "hack the code" of aging? *Popular Science.* Retrieved from https://www.popsci.com/who-will-be-first-to-hack-code-aging

Boström, P., Wu, J., Jedrychowski, M. P., Korde, A., Ye, L., Lo, J. C., . . . Spiegelman, B. M. (2012). A PGC1-α-dependent myokine that drives brown-fat-like development of white fat and thermogenesis. *Nature, 481*(7382), 463–468.

Buhr, S. (2017). A new lawsuit alleges anti-aging startup Elysium Health hasn't paid its sole supplier. *Oath Tech Network.* Retrieved from https://techcrunch.com/2017/01/16/a-new-lawsuit-alleges-anti-aging-startup-elysium-health-hasnt-paid-its-supplier-and-is-in-breach-of-agreement/

Calico, LLC. (2018). Retrieved from https://www.calicolabs.com

Callaway, E. (2010, Aug. 16). GlaxoSmithKline strikes back over anti-aging pills. *Nature.* Retrieved from doi:10.1038/news.2010.412

Carroll, J. (2016, Apr. 21). Novartis' "breakthrough" muscle drug bimagrumab flunks a late-stage trial. *FierceBiotech.* Retrieved from https://www.fiercebiotech.com/biotech/novartis-breakthrough-muscle-drug-bimagrumab-flunks-a-late-stage-trial

Casebourne, C., (2017). Scientists find natural mimetics of anti-cancer and anti-aging drugs metformin and rapamycin. *Biogerontology Research Foundation.* [Press release]. Retrieved from http://www.sciencenewsline.com/news/2017112921320015.html

Chalkiadaki, A., & Guarente, L. (2015). The multifaceted functions of sirtuins in cancer. *Nature Reviews Cancer, 15,* 608–624.

Colaianni, G., Cuscito, C., Mongelli, T., Pignataro, P., Buccoliero, C., Liu, P., . . . Grano, M. (2015). The myokine irisin increases cortical bone mass. *Proceedings of the National Academy of Sciences of the United States of America, 112*(39), 12157–12162.

Dai, H., Kustigian, L., Carney, D., Case, A., Considine, T., & Hubbard, B. P. (2010). SIRT1 activation by small molecules: kinetic and biophysical evidence for direct interaction of enzyme and activator. *Journal of Biological Chemistry, 285*(43), 32695–32703.

Dang, W. (2014). The controversial world of sirtuins. *Drug Discovery Today, Technologies, 12,* e9–e17.

Das, A., Huang, G. X., Bonkowski, M. S., Longchamp, A., Li, C., Schultz, M. B., . . . Sinclair, D. A. (2018), Impairment of an endothelial NAD+ signaling network is a reversible cause of vascular aging, *Cell, 173*(1)., 74–89.

Dentico, M. J. (2016, Sept. 4). Basis, the anti-aging pill that freezes the clock and preserves your health. *Inquisitr.* Retrieved from http://www.inquisitr.com/3475008/basis-the-anti-aging-pill-that-freezes-the-clock-and-preserves-your-health/

Ehninger, D., Neff, F., & Xie, K. (2014). Longevity, aging and rapamycin. *Cellular and Molecular Life Sciences, 71*(22), 4325–4346.

Elysium Health. (2018). Living healthier, longer through extraordinary science. Retrieved from https://www.elysiumhealth.com/mission

Fan, W., Waizenegger, W., Lin, C. S., Sorrentino, V., He, M.-X., & Wall, C. E. (2017). PPARdelta promotes running endurance by preserving glucose. *Cell Metabolism, 25*(5), 1186–1193.

Fiuza-Luces, C., Garatachea, N., Berger, N. A., & Lucia, A. (2013). Exercise is the real polypill. *Physiology (Bethesda, MD), 28*(5), 330–358.

Gershgorn, D. (2015, Oct. 6). Billionaire Peter Thiel invests in the war on aging, detecting spoiled food, and more. *Popular Science.* Retrieved from https://www.popsci.com/billionaire-peter-thiel-invests-in-war-on-aging-and-spoiled-meat#page-2

Harmon, A. (2016, May 16). Dogs test drug aimed at humans' biggest killer: age. *New York Times.* Retrieved from https://www.nytimes.com/2016/05/17/us/aging-research-disease-dogs.html

Harrison, D. E., Strong, R., Sharp, Z. D., Nelson, J. F., Astle, C. M., & Nadon, N. L. (2009). Rapamycin fed late in life extends lifespan in genetically heterogeneous mice. *Nature, 460*(7253), 392–395.

Hawley, J. A., Hargreaves, M., Joyner, M. J., & Zierath, J. R. (2014). Integrative biology of exercise. *Cell, 159*(4), 738–749.

Higashi, Y., Sukhanov, S., Anwar, A., Shai, S.-Y., & Delafontaine, P. (2012). Aging, atherosclerosis, and IGF-1. *Journals of Gerontology Series A: Biological Sciences and Medical Sciences, 67A*(6), 626–639.

Higashida, K., Kim, S. H., Jung, S. R., Asaka, M., Holloszy, J. O., & Han, D.-H. (2013). Effects of resveratrol and SIRT1 on PGC-1alpha activity and mitochondrial biogenesis: a reevaluation. *PLoS Biology, 11*(7), e1001603.

Hoffman, N. J, Parker, B. L., Chaudhuri, R., Fisher-Wellman, K. H., Kleinert, M., & Humphrey, S. J. (2015). Global phosphoproteomic analysis of human skeletal muscled reveals a network of exercise-related kinases and AMPK substrates. *Cell Metabolism, 22*(5), 922–935.

Hubbard, B. P., Gomes, A. P., Dai, H., Li, J., Case, A. W., Considine, T., . . . Sinclair, D. A. (2013). Evidence for a common mechanism of SIRT1 regulation by allosteric activators. *Science, 339*(6124), 1216–1219.

Hubbard, B. P., & Sinclair, D. A. (2013). Small molecular SIRT1 activators for the treatment of aging and age-related diseases. *Trends in Pharmacological Sciences, 35*(3), 146–154.

Human Longevity Institute. (2018). Retrieved from https://www.humanlongevity.com/management-team/

Imai, S., & Guarente, L. (2014). NAD$^+$ and sirtuins in aging and disease. *Trends in Cell Biology, 24*(8), 464–471.

Imai, S.-I., & Guarente, L. (2016). It takes two to tango: NAD+ and sirtuins in aging/longevity control. *NPJ Aging and Mechanisms of Disease, 2,* 16017.

Jedrychowski, M. P., Wrann, C. D., Paulo, J. A., Gerber, K. K., Szpyt, J., Robinson, M. M., . . . Spiegelman, B. M. (2015). Detection and quantitation of circulating human irisin by tandem mass spectrometry. *Cell Metabolism, 22*(4), 734–740.

Jin, K. (2010). Modern biological theories of aging. *Aging and Disease, 1*(2), 72–74.

Johnson, S. C., Rabinovitch, P. S., and Kaeberlein, M. (2013). mTOR is a key modulator of ageing and age-related disease. *Nature, 493,* 338–345.

Kaeberlein, M., Rabinovitch, P. S., & Martin, G. M. (2015). Healthy aging: the ultimate preventative medicine, geroscience interventions with translational potential. *Science, 350*(6265), 1192.

Karlin-Smith, S. (2017). Why a drug for aging would challenge Washington. *POLITICO, The Agenda.* Retrieved from https://www.google.com/search?source=hp&ei=Y1F OWu2gJaypggfuz72w

Kennedy, B. K., & Pennypacker, J. K. (2015). Aging interventions get human. *Oncotarget, 6*(2), 590–591.

Kirkland, J. L., Tchkonia, T., Zhu, Y., Niedernhofer, L. J., & Robbins, P. D. (2017). The clinical potential of senolytic drugs. *Journal of the American Geriatrics Society, 65*(10), 2297–2301.

Krueger, J. G., Suarez-Farinas, M., Cueto, I., Khacherian, A., Matheson, R., Parish, L. C., . . . Jacobson, E. W. (2015). A randomized, placebo-controlled study of SRT2104, a SIRT1 activator, in patients with moderate to severe psoriasis. *PLoS ONE, 10*(11), e0142081.

Lagouge, M., Argmann, C., Gerhart-Hines, Z., Meziane, H., Lerin, C., Messadeq, N., . . . Auwerx, J. (2006). Resveratrol improves mitochondrial function and protects against metabolic disease by activating SIRT1 and PGC-1 alpha. *Cell,* *127*(6), 1109–1122.

Li, J., Bonkowski, M. S., Moniot, S., Zhang, D., Hubbard, B. P., Ling, A. J. Y., . . . Sinclair, D. A. (2017). A conserved NAD(+) binding pocket that regulates protein-protein interactions during aging. *Science, 355*(6331), 1312–1317.

Li, J., Kim, S. G., & Blenis, J. (2014). Rapamycin: one drug, many effects. *Cell Metabolism, 19*(3), 373–379.

Li, S., & Laher, I. (2015). Exercise pills: at the starting line. *Trends in Pharmacological Sciences, 36*(12), 906–917.

Libri, V., Brown, A. P., Gambarota, G., Haddad, J., Shields, G. S., Dawes, W., . . . Matthews, P. M. (2012). A pilot randomized, placebo-controlled, double blind phase 1 trial of the novel SIRT1 activator SRT2104 in elderly volunteers. *PLoS ONE, 7*(12), e51395.

Lloyd, B. A., Hake, H. S., Ishiwata, T., Farmer, C. E., Loetz, E. C., Fleshner, M., . . . Greenwood, B. N. (2017). Exercise increases mTOR signaling in brain regions involved in cognition and emotional behavior. *Behavioural Brain Research, 323,* 56–67.

Lorenzetti, L. (2016, Mar. 7). The obsession with "curing" aging is now big business. *Fortune.*

MacDonald, F. (2017). It's happening: scientists can now reverse DNA ageing in mice—humans are next. *Science Alert.* Retrieved from http://www.sciencealert.com/scientists-have-successfully-reversed-dna-ageing-in-mice

Makin, S. (2017, Apr. 21). Fountain of youth? Young blood infusions "rejuvenate" old mice. *Scientific American.* Retrieved from https://www.scientificamerican.com/article/fountain-of-youth-young-blood-infusions-ldquo-rejuvenate-rdquo-old-mice/

Mannick, J. B., Del Giudice, G., Lattanzi, M., Valiante, N. M., Praestgaard, J., Huang, B., . . . Klickstein, L. B. (2014). mTOR inhibition improves immune function in the elderly. *Science Translational Medicine, 6*(268), 268ra179.

Marrkowitz, E. (2012). Immortality: the next great investment boom. *Inc.com.* Retrieved from https://www.inc.com/eric-markowitz/immortality-the-next-great-investment-boom.html

Maxmen, A. (2017, Jan. 13). Questionable "young blood" transfusions offered in US as an anti-aging remedy. *MIT Technology Review.* Retrieved from https://www.technologyreview.com/s/603242/questionable-young-blood-transfusions-offered-in-us-as-anti-aging-remedy/

Mercken, E. M., Mitchell, S. J., Martin-Montalvo, A., Minor, R. K., Almeida, M., Gomes, A. P., . . . de Cabo, R. (2014). SRT2104 extends survival of male mice on a standard diet and preserves bone and muscle mass. *Aging Cell, 13*(5), 787–796.

Methuselah Foundation. (2018). Retrieved from https://www.mfoundation.org

MetroBiotech International. (2018). Retrieved from http://www.massbiomed.org

Miller, R. A., Harrison, D. E., Astle, C. M., Baur, J. A., Boyd, A. R., & de Cabo, R. (2011). Rapamycin, but not resveratrol or simvastatin, extends life span of genetically heterogeneous mice. *Journals of Gerontology Series A: Biological Sciences and Medical Sciences, 66*(2), 191–201.

Mills, K. F., Yoshida, S., Stein, L. R., Grozio, A., Kubota, S., Sasaki, Y., . . . Imai, S.-I. (2016). Long-term administration of nicotinamide mononucleotide mitigates age-associated physiological decline in mice. *Cell Metabolism, 24*(6), 795–806.

Mitobridge. (2018). Retrieved from http://www.mitobridge.com

Moreno, M., Moreno-Navarrete, J. M., Serrano, M., Ortega, F., Delgado, E., Sanchez-Ragnarsson, C., . . . Fernández-Real, J. M. (2015). Circulating irisin levels are positively associated with metabolic risk factors in sedentary subjects. *PLoS ONE,* *10*(4), e0124100.

Mount Tam Biotechnologies. (2018). Retrieved from http://mounttambiotech.com/news.aspx

Mullin, E. (2015, Aug. 17). This serious scientist is working on an anti-aging pill—and taking it himself. *Health & Science, Washington Post.*

Narkar, V. A., Downes, M., Yu, R. T., Embler, E., Wang, Y.-W., Banayo, E., . . . Evans, R. M. (2008). AMPK and PPARdelta agonists are exercise mimetics. *Cell, 134*(3), 405–415.

Navarro, S., Reddy, R., Lee, J., Warburton, D., & Driscoll, B. (2017). Inhaled resveratrol treatments slow ageing-related degenerative changes in mouse lung. *Thorax, 72*(5), 451–459.

Neff, F., Flores-Dominguez, D., Ryan, D. P., Horsch, M., Schroeder, S., Adler, T., . . . Ehninger, D. (2013). Rapamycin extends murine lifespan but has limited effects on aging. *Journal of Clinical Investigation 123*(8), 3272–3291.

Palo Alto Longevity Prize. (2018). Retrieved from http://paloaltoprize.com

Park, S.-J, Ahmad, F., Philp, A., Baar, K., Williams, T., & Luo, T. (2012). Resveratrol ameliorates aging-related metabolic phenotypes by inhibiting cAMP phosphodiesterases. *Cell, 148*(3), 421–433.

PureTech Health. (n.d.). Building the biopharma company of the future. Retrieved from http://puretechhealth.com

Qiao, X., Nie, Y., Ma, Y., Chen, Y., Cheng, R., Yin, W., . . . Xu, L. (2016). Corrigendum: irisin promotes osteoblast proliferation and differentiation via activating the MAP kinase signaling pathways. *Scientific Reports, 6,* 21053.

Ramsey, L. (2017, July 7). A diabetes medication that costs 6 cents a pill could be a key to living longer. *Business Insider.* Retrieved from http://www.businessinsider.com/generic-metformin-anti-aging-drug-2017-7

Rangwala, S. M., Wang, X., Calvo, J. A., Lindsley, L., Zhang, Y., Deyneko, G., . . . Markovits, J. (2010). Estrogen-related receptor gamma is a key regulator of muscle mitochondrial activity and oxidative capacity. *Journal of Biological Chemistry, 285,* 22619–22629.

Rao, R. R., Long, J. Z., White, J. P., Svensson, K. J., Lou, J., Lokurkar, I., . . . Spiegelman, B. M. (2014). Meteorin-like is a hormone that regulates immune-adipose interactions to increase beige fat thermogenesis. *Cell, 157*(6), 1279–1291.

Regalado, A. (2017, Mar. 28). Is this the anti-aging pill we've all been waiting for? *MIT Technology Review.* Retrieved from https://www.technologyreview.com/s/603997/is this-the-anti-aging-pill-weve-all-been-waiting-for/

resTORbio, Inc. (2018). *resTORbio.com.* Retrieved from https://www.restorbio.com

Reynolds, G. (2013, July 17). Exercise in a pill? The search continues. *New York Times.* Retrieved from https://well.blogs.nytimes.com/2013/07/17/exercise-in-a-pill-the-search-continues/

Reynolds, G. (2016, Oct. 12). How exercise may turn white fat into brown. *New York Times.* Retrieved from https://www.nytimes.com/2016/10/12/well/move/how-exercise-may-fight-obesity-by-turning-white-fat-into-brown.html

Richardson, A. (2013). Rapamycin, anti-aging and avoiding the fate of Tithonus. *Journal of Clinical Investigation, 123*(8), 3204–3206.

Roberts, L. D., Bostrom, P., O'Sullivan, J. F., Schinzel, R. T., Lewis, G. D., & Dejam, A. (2014). B-aminoisobutyric acid induces browning of white fat and hepatic B-oxidation and is inversely correlated with cardiometabolic risk factors. *Cell Metabolism, 19*(1), 96–108.

Roy, A. (2016, Apr. 21). First gene therapy successful against human aging, American woman gets biologically younger after gene therapies. *BioViva*. Retrieved from https://bioviva-science.com/blog/2017/3/2/first-gene-therapy-successful-against-human-aging

Salk Institute. (2011, Jan. 6). When less is more: how mitochondrial signals extend lifespan. [Press release]. Retrieved from https://www.salk.edu/news-release/when-less-is-more-how-mitochondrial-signals-extend-lifespan/

Salk Institute. (2017) "Exercise in a pill" boosts athletic endurance by 70 percent. [Press release]. Retrieved from https://www.salk.edu/news-release/exercise-pill-boosts-athletic-endurance-70-percent/

Satoh, A., Imai, S., & Guarente, L. (2017). The brain, sirtuins, and ageing. *Nature Reviews Neuroscience, 18*(6), 362–374.

Schnyder, S., & Handschin, C. (2015). Skeletal muscle as an endocrine organ: PGC-1α, myokines and exercise. *Bone, 80*, 115–125.

Sierra Sciences. (2017). Retrieved from https://www.sierrasci.com/about_us

Sinclair, David, Ph.D. (2018). *Paul F. Glenn Center for the Biological Methods of Aging*. Retrieved from http://medapps.med.harvard.edu/agingresearch/index.php/about/staff/sinclair

Sirtris Pharmaceuticals. (2017). *Wikipedia*. Retrieved from https://en.wikipedia.org/wiki/Sirtris_Pharmaceuticals

Skinner, J. (2015, Oct. 26). Research on "exercise pill" raises many questions. *The Hill*. Retrieved from http://thehill.com/blogs/congress-blog/healthcare/257930-research-on-exercise-pill-raises-many-questions

Soliman, G. A., Steenson, S. M., & Etekpo, A. H. (2016). Effects of metyformin and a mammalian target of rapamycin (mTOR) ATP-competitive inhibitor on targeted metabolomics in pancreatic cancer cell line. *Metabolomics, 6*(3), 183.

Solt, L. A., Wang, Y., Banerjee, S., Hughes, T., Kojetin, D. J., Lundasen, T., . . . Burris, T. P. (2012). Regulation of circadian behavior and metabolism by synthetic REV-ERB agonists. *Nature, 485*, 62–68.

Sonntag, W. E., Csiszar, A., de Cabo, R., Ferrucci, L., & Ungvari, Z. (2012). Diverse roles of growth hormone and insulin-like growth factor-1 in mammalian aging: progress and controversies. *Journals of Gerontology Series A: Biological Sciences and Medical Sciences, 67A*(6), 587–598.

Sprecher, D. L., Massien, C., Pearce, G., Billin, A. N., Perlstein, I., & Willson, T. M. (2017). Triglyceride: high-density lipoprotein cholesterol effects in healthy subjects administered a peroxisome proliferator activated receptor delta agonist, *Arteriosclerosis, Thrombosis, and Vascular Biology, 27*, 359–365.

Strait, J. E. (2016, Oct. 27). Natural compound reduces signs of aging in healthy mice. *Washington University School of Medicine in St. Louis*. Retrieved from https://medicine.wustl.edu/news/natural-compound-nmn-reduces-signs-aging-healthy-mice/

Swaminathan, N. (2008, July 31). Could a pill replace exercise? Retrieved from https://www.scientificamerican.com/article/could-a-pill-replace-exercise/

T. A. Sciences. (n.d.). TA-65MD nutritional supplements. Retrieved from https://www.tasciences.com/what-is-ta-65/

Telegraph Reporters. (2017, Apr. 25). Miracle "exercise pill" could be used to mimic the effect of going to the gym. *The Telegraph*. Retrieved from https://www.telegraph.co.uk/news/2017/04/25/miracle-exercise-pill-could-used-mimic-effect-going-gym/

Twilley, N. (2017, Nov. 6). The exercise pill (Annals of Science). *New Yorker*.

Ulgherait, M. Rana, A., Rera, M., Graniel, J., & Walker, D. W. (2014). AMPK modulates tissue and organismal aging in a non-cell-autonomous manner. *Cell Reports, 8,* 1767–1780.

Ungvari, Z., Sonntage, W. E., de Cabo, R., Baur, J. A., & Csiszar, A. (2011). Mitochondrial protection by resveratrol. *Excercise and Sports Science Review, 39*(3), 128–132.

Unity Biotechnology. (2017). Retrieved from https://unitybiotechnology.com

University of New South Wales. (2017, Mar. 23). Scientists unveil a giant leap for anti-aging. *ScienceDaily.* Retrieved from www.sciencedaily.com/releases/2017/03/170323141340.htm

U.S. National Library of Medicine. (2017). Efficacy and safety of bimagrumab/BYM338 at 52 weeks on physical function, muscle strength, mobility in sIBM patients (RESILIENT). Retrieved from https://clinicaltrials.gov/ct2/show/NCT01925209

Verdin, E. (2015). NAD+ in aging, metabolism, and neurodegeneration. *Science, 350*(6265), 1208–1213.

Vina, J., Sanchis-Gomar, F., Martinez-Bello, V., & Gomez-Cabrera, M. C. (2012). Exercise acts as a drug: the pharmacological benefits of exercise. *British Journal of Pharmacology, 167*(1), 1–12.

Wade, N. (2011, Jan. 10). Doubt on anti-aging molecule as drug trial stops. *New York Times.* Retrieved from https://www.nytimes.com/2011/01/11/science/11aging.html

Watson, K., & Baar, K. (2014). mTOR and the health benefits of exercise. *Seminars in Cell and Developmental Biology, 36,* 130–139.

Wellness Fx. (2014). The IGF-1 trade-off: performance vs. longevity. Retrieved from http://blog.wellnessfx.com/2013/09/04/igf-1-trade-performance-vs-longevity/

Wein, H. (2012). Scientists find target for resveratrol, NIH Research Matters. *National Institutes of Health.* Retrieved from https://www.nih.gov/news-events/nih-research-matters/scientists-find-target-resveratrol

Weintraub, K. (2017, Jan. 6). Critics blast star-studded advisory board of anti-aging company. *MIT Technology Review.* Retrieved from https://www.technologyreview.com/s/603199/critics-blast-star-studded-advisory-board-of-anti-aging-company/

Woldt, E., Sebti, Y., Solt, L.A., Duhem, C., Lancel, S., & Eeckhoute, J. (2013). Reverb-alpha modulates skeletal muscle oxidative capacity by regulating mitochondrial biogenesis and autophagy. *Nature Medicine, 19,* 1039–1046.

World Anti-Doping Agency. (2018). What is prohibited: 2018 list of prohibited substances and method. Retrieved from https://www.wada-ama.org/en/content/what-is-prohibited/prohibited-at-all-times/hormone-and-metabolic-modulators

Zhang, H., Ryu, D., Wu, Y., Gariani, K., Wang, X., Luan, P., . . . Auwerx, J. (2016). NAD⁺ repletion improves mitochondrial and stem cell function and enhances life span in mice. *Science, 352*(6292), 1436–1443.

Zhu, Y., Tchkonia, T., Pirtskhalava, T., Gower, A.C., Ding, H., Giorgadze, N., . . . Kirkland, J. L. (2015). The Achilles' heel of senescent cells: from transcriptome to senolytic drugs. *Aging Cell, 14*(4), 644–658.

Wall Street Pit. (2017). A potential anti-aging pill promises to extend life for 5 cents a pop. Retrieved from http://wallstreetpit.com/114063-first-anti-aging-pill-promises-extend-life-5-cents-pop/

CHAPTER 15

American College of Obstetricians and Gynecologists. (2015). Exercise after pregnancy. Retrieved from https://www.acog.org/Patients/FAQs/Exercise-After-Pregnancy

American College of Obstetricians and Gynecologists. (2017). Exercise during pregnancy. Retrieved from https://www.acog.org/Search?Keyword=exercise+during+pregnancy

American Heart Association. (2017, Aug. 22). How do beta blocker drugs affect exercise? Retrieved from http://www.heart.org/HEARTORG/Conditions/More/MyHeartandStrokeNews/How-do-beta-blocker-drugs-affect-exercise_UCM_450771_Article.jsp#.WbGW8tOGMWo

Anaerobic Threshold. (1997, Dec.). *SportsMed Web*. Retrieved from http://www.rice.edu/~jenky/sports/anaerobic.threshold.html

Arem, H., Moore, S. C., Patel, A., Hartge, P., de Gonzalez, A. B., Visvanathan, K., & Matthews, C. E. (2015). Leisure time physical activity and mortality—a detailed pooled analysis of the dose-response relationship. *JAMA Internal Medicine, 175*(6), 959–967.

Atherton, P. J., Babraj, J., Smith, K., Singh, J., Rennie, M. J., & Wackerhage, H. (2005). Selective activation of AMPK-PGC-1alpha or PKB-TSC2-mTOR signaling can explain specific adaptive responses to endurance or resistance training-like electrical muscle stimulation. *FASEB Journal, 19*(7), 786–788.

Attwooll, J. (2008, Aug. 15), Michael Phelps—the extraordinary 12,000 calories diet that fuels greatest ever Olympian. *The Telegraph*. Retrieved from http://www.telegraph.co.uk/sport/olympics/2563451/Michael-Phelps-the-extraordinary-12000-calorie-diet-that-fuels-greatest-ever-Olympian-Beijing-Olympics-2008.html

Bailey, T. G., Cable, N. T., Aziz, N., Dobson, R., Sprung, V. S., Low, D. A., & Jones, H. (2016). Exercise training reduces the frequency of menopausal hot flushes by improving thermoregulatory control. *Menopause, 23*(7), 708–718.

Ballantyne, C. (2009, Jan. 2). Does exercise really make you healthier? *Scientific American*. Retrieved from https://www.scientificamerican.com/article/does-exercise-really-make/

Baron, K. G., Reid, K. J., & Zee, P.C. (2013). Exercise to improve sleep in insomnia: exploration of the bidirectional effects. *Journal of Clinical Sleep Medicine, 9*(8), 819–824.

Beaudouin, E., Renaudin, J. M., Morisset, M., Codreanu, F., Kanny, G., & Moneret-Vautrin, D. A. (2006). Food-dependent exercise-induced anaphylaxis: update and current data. *European Annals of Allergy and Clinical Immunology, 38*(2), 45–51.

Berardi, J. (2015, June 30). How to avoid jet lag: lifestyle tricks that work. *Huffington Post*. Retrieved from http://www.huffingtonpost.com/john-berardi-phd/jet-lag-tips_b_7571586.html

Berkeley Wellness. (2014, Sept. 10). The exercise detraining effect. *Berkeley Wellness, University of California*. Retrieved from http://www.berkeleywellness.com/fitness/exercise/article/exercise-detraining-effect

Bickel, C. S., Cross, J. M., & Bamman, M. B. (2011). Exercise dosing to retain resistance training adaptations in young and older athletes. *Medicine and Science in Sports and Exercise, 43*(7), 1177–1187.

Boseley, S. (2017, May 17). No such thing as "fat but fit," major study finds. *The Guardian*. Retrieved from https://www.theguardian.com/society/2017/may/17/obesity-health-no-such-thing-as-fat-but-fit-major-study

Bostrom, P., Wu, J., Jedrychowski, M. P., Korde, A., Ye, L., Lo, J., . . . Spiegelman, B. M. (2012). A PGC1-alpha-dependent myokine that drives brown-fat-like development of white fat and thermogenesis. *Nature, 4481*(7382), 463–468.

Boutcher, S. H. (2011). High-intensity intermittent exercise and fat loss. *Journal of Obesity, 2011*, 868305. Retrieved from http://doi.org/10.1155/2011/868305

Bower, B. (1987, Dec. 5). Hamster jet lag: running it off. *The Free Library*. Retrieved from https://www.thefreelibrary.com/Hamster+jet+lag%3A+running+it+off.-a06213751

Broom, D. R., Batterham, R. L., King, J. A., & Stensel, D. J. (2009). Influence of resistance and aerobic exercise on hunger, circulating levels of acylated ghrelin and peptide YY in healthy males. *American Journal of Physiology: Regulatory, Integrative and Comparative Physiology, 296*(1), R29–35.

Broom, D. R., Miyashita, M., Wasse, L. K., Pulsford, R., King, J. A., Thackray, A. E., & Stensel, D. J. (2017). Acute effect of exercise intensity and duration on acylated ghrelin and hunger in men. *Journal of Endocrinology, 232*(3), 411–422.

Bruno, N. E., Kelly, K. A., Hawkins, R., Bramah-Lawani, M., Amelio, A. I., & Nwachukwu, J. C. (2014). Creb coactivators direct anabolic responses and enhance performance of skeletal muscle. *EMBO Journal, 33*, 1027–1043.

Bryant, C. X. (2011, Feb. 8). Why is it important to vary my workout routines? *American Council of Fitness (ACE)*. Retrieved from https://www.acefitness.org/acefit/healthy-living-article/60/1210/why-is-it-important-to-vary-my-workout/

Caleyachetty, R., Thomas, G. N, Toulis, K. A., Mohammed, N., Gokhale, K. M., Balachandran, K., & Nirantharakumar, K. (2017). Metabolically healthy obese and incident cardiovascular disease events among 3.5 million men and women. *Journal of the American College of Cardiology, 70*(12), 1429–1437.

Carey, E. (2017, July 17). What exercises are safe in the first trimester? *HealthLine*. Retrieved from https://www.healthline.com/health/pregnancy/first-trimester-exercise-fitness#overview1

Carroll, A. E. (2015, June 15). To lose weight, eating less is far more important than exercising more. *New York Times*. Retrieved from https://www.nytimes.com/2015/06/16/upshot/to-lose-weight-eating-less-is-far-more-important-than-exercising-more.html

Centers for Disease Control and Prevention. (2016, Nov. 29). Current physical activity guidelines. Retrieved from https://www.cdc.gov/cancer/dcpc/prevention/policies_practices/physical_activity/guidelines.htm

Cheung, K., Hume, P., & Maxwell, L. (2003). Delayed onset muscle soreness: treatment strategies and performance factors. *Sports Medicine, 33*(2), 145–164.

Chtourou, H., & Souissi, N. (2012). The effect of training at a specific time of day: a review. *Journal of Strength and Conditioning Research, 26*(7), 1984–2005.

Circadian rhythms. (2017, Aug.). *National Institute of General Medical Science*. Retrieved from https://www.nigms.nih.gov/education/pages/Factsheet_CircadianRhythms.aspx

Coffey, V. G., Zhong, Z., Shield, A., Canny, B. J., Chibalin, A. V., Zierath, J. R., & Hawley, J. A. (2006). Early signaling responses to divergent exercise stimuli in skeletal muscle from well-trained humans. *FASEB Journal, 20*(1), 190–192.

Coren, S. (1996). Daylight savings time and traffic accidents. *New England Journal of Medicine, 334*, 924–925.

Coyle, E. F., Martin, W. H. 3rd, Sinacore, D. R., Joyner, M. J., Hagberg, J. M., & Holloszy, J. O. (1984). Time course of loss of adaptations after stopping prolonged intense endurance training. *Journal of Applied Physiology: Respiratory, Environmental, and Exercise Physiology, 57*(6), 1857–1864.

Crane, J. D., MacNeil, L. G., Lally, J. S., Ford, R. J., Bujak, A. D., & Brar, I. K. (2015). Exercise-stimulated interleukin-15 is controlled by AMPK and regulates skin metabolism and aging. *Aging Cell, 14*(4), 615–634.

Davis, J. (2017). How long does it take to lose your running fitness? *Runners Connect*. Retrieved from https://runnersconnect.net/how-long-does-it-take-to-lose-your-running-fitness/

Davis, R. J. (2017, Jun. 17). What is the best time of the day to exercise? It's not when you think. *Washington Post*. Retrieved from https://www.washingtonpost.com/national/health-science/what-is-the-best-time-of-day-to-exercise-its-not-when-you-think/2017/06/16/2020c3ba-51cf-11e7-be25-3a519335381c_story.html?utm_term=.bcf8239cd2ed

Di Mascio, D., Magro-Malosso, E. R., Saccone, G., Markhefka, G. D., & Berghella, V. (2016). Exercise during pregnancy in normal-weight women and risk of preterm birth: a systematic review and meta-analysis of randomized controlled trials. *American Journal of Obstetrics and Gynecology, 215*(5), 561–571.

Doheny, K. (n.d.). The truth about fat. *WebMD*. Retrieved from https://www.webmd.com/diet/features/the-truth-about-fat#1

Dusheck, J. (2017, May 24). Fitness trackers accurately measure heart rate but not calories burned. *Stanford Medicine News Center*. Retrieved from https://med.stanford.edu/news/all-news/2017/05/fitness-trackers-accurately-measure-heart-rate-but-not-calories-burned.html

Dwyer-Lindgren, L., Freedman, G., Engell, R. E., Fleming, T. D., Lim, S. S., Murray, C. J. L., & Mokdad, A. H. (2013). Prevalence of physical activity and obesity in US counties, 2001–2011: a road map for action. *Population Health Metrics, 11*, 7.

Eijsvogels, T. M. H., Molossi, S., Lee, D.-C., Emery, M. S., & Thompson, P. D. (2016). Exercise at the extremes. *Journal of the American College of Cardiology, 67*(3), 316–329.

Entis, L. (2017). Can you be fit and fat? The answer is complicated (and contentious). *Fortune*. Retrieved from http://fortune.com/2017/08/23/fit-fat-weight-health-heart-disease/

Exercise Addiction 101. (n.d.). Retrieved from https://www.addiction.com/addiction-a-to-z/exercise-addiction/exercise-addiction-101/

Ferguson, T., Rowlands, A. V., Olds, T., & Maher, C. (2015). The validity of consumer-level, activity monitors in healthy adults worn in free-living conditions: a cross-sectional study. *International Journal of Behavioral Nutrition and Physical Activity, 12*, 42.

Fitness Calculator. (2017). *Cardiac Exercise Research Group, NTNU*. Retrieved from https://www.ntnu.edu/cerg/vo2max

Foreman, J. (2008). Does exercise increase or decrease your appetite? *Boston Globe*. Retrieved from http://archive.boston.com/news/health/articles/2008/11/10/does_exercise_increase_or_decrease_your_appetite/

Foreman, J. (2008, Apr. 14). Women athletes win equal time on injury list. *Boston Globe*. Retrieved from http://judyforeman.com/columns/women-athletes-win-equal-time-injury-list/

Freimuth, M., Moniz, S., & Kim, S. R. (2011). Clarifying exercise addiction: differential diagnosis, co-occurring disorders, and phases of addiction. *International Journal of Environmental Research and Public Health, 8*(10), 4069–4081.

Frese, C., Frese, F., Kuhlmann, S., Saure, D., Reljic, D., Staehlel, H. J., & Wolff, D. (2015). Effect of endurance training on dental erosion, caries and saliva. *Scandinavian Journal of Medicine and Science in Sports, 25*(3), e319–326.

Fulco, C. S., Rock, P. B., Muza, S. R., Lammi, E., Cymerman, A., Butterfield, G., . . . Lewis, S. F. (1999). Slower fatigue and faster recovery of the adductor pollicis muscle in women matched for strength with men. *Acta Physiologica Scandinavica, 167*(3), 233–239.

Gans, R. (2016, Jun. 23). Did you know exercise is good for your eyes—and your vision? *Cleveland Clinic Health Essentials.* Retrieved from https://health.clevelandclinic.org/2016/06/know-exercise-good-eyes-vision/

Gibala, M. J., Little, J. P., MacDonald, M. J., & Hawley, J. A. (2012). Physiological adaptations to low-volume, high-intensity interval training in health and disease. *Journal of Physiology, 590*(5), 1077–1084.

Gillen, J. B., Martin, B. J., MacInnis, M. J., Skelly, L. E., Tarnopolsky, M. A., & Gibala, M. J. (2016). Twelve weeks of sprint interval training improves indices of cardiometabolic health similar to traditional endurance training despite a five-fold lower exercise volume and time commitment. *PLoS ONE, 11*(4), e0154075.

Gomez Escribano, L., Galvez Cases, A., Escriba Fernandez-Marcote, A. R., Tarraga Lopez, P., & Tarrago Marcos, L. (2017). Review and analysis of physical exercise at hormonal and brain level, and its influence on appetite. *Clinica e Investigacion en Arteriosclerosis, 29*(6), 265–274.

Graham, T. E. (2001). Caffeine and exercise: metabolism, endurance and performance. *Sports Medicine, 31*(11), 785–807.

Gu, C., Coomans, C. P., Hu, K., Scheer, F. A., Stanley, H. E., & Meijer, J. H. (2015). Lack of exercise leads to significant and reversible loss of scale invariance in both aged and young mice. *Proceedings of the National Academy of Sciences of the United States of America, 112*(8), 2320–2324.

Hakkinen, K., Alen, M., Kallinen, M., Newton, R. U., & Kraemer, W. J. (2000). Neuromuscular adaptation during prolonged strength training, detraining and re-strength training in middle-aged and elderly people. *European Journal of Applied Physiology, 83*(1), 51–62.

Hawley, J. A., Hargreaves, M., Joyner, M. J., & Zierath, J. R. (2014). Integrative biology of exercise. *Cell, 159*(4), 745.

Henselmans, M. (2015). 9 reasons why women should not train like men. *Bayesian Bodybuilding.* Retrieved from https://bayesianbodybuilding.com/why-women-should-not-train-like-men/

Hewings-Martin, Y. (2017, Dec. 19), Why do my muscles feel sore after exercise? *Medical News Today.* Retrieved from https://www.medicalnewstoday.com/articles/320415.php

Heyward, V. H. (1998) Normative data for VO2max. In *The physical fitness specialist certification manual, The Cooper Institute for Aerobics Research, advanced fitness assessment & exercise prescription,* 3rd ed. Retrieved from http://www.machars.net/v02max.htm

Hickson, R. C. (1980). Interference of strength development by simultaneously training for strength and endurance. *European Journal of Applied Physiology and Occupational Physiology, 45*(2–3), 255–263.

Hosey, R., Carek, P. J., & Goo, A. (2001). Excercise-induced anaphylaxis and urticaria. *American Family Physician, 64*(8), 1367.

Hu, F. B., Willett, W. C., Stampfer, M. J., Colditz, G. A., & Manson, J. E. (2004). Adiposity as compared with physical activity in predicting mortality among women. *New England Journal of Medicine, 351*(26), 2694–2703.

Hu, K., Van Someren, E. J. W., Shea, S. A., & Scheer, F. A. J. L. (2009). Reduction of scale invariance of activity fluctuations with aging and Alzheimer's disease: involvement of the circadian pacemaker. *Proceedings of the National Academy of Sciences of the United States of America, 106*(8), 2490–2494.

Hutchinson, A. (2011). *Which comes first, cardio or weights?* New York, NY: William Morrow.

Hutchinson, A. (2017, July 7). What really determines your VO2max? *Runner's World.* Retrieved from https://www.runnersworld.com/sweat-science/what-really-determines-your-vo2-max

Internicola, D. (2013, Feb. 11). Exercise with a cold: is it safe to work out while sick? *Huffington Post, Healthy Living.* Retrieved from https://www.huffingtonpost.com/2013/02/11/exercise-with-a-cold-work-out-while-sick-flu_n_2660465.html

Jaret, P. (2011, Apr. 15). Exercise for healthy skin. *WebMD.* Retrieved from http://www.webmd.com/skin-problems-and-treatments/acne/features/exercise#1

Johns, D. J., Hartmann-Boyce, J., Jebb, S. A., & Aveyard, P. (2014). Diet or exercise interventions vs. combined behavioral weight management programs: a systematic review and meta-analysis of direct comparisons. *Journal of the Academy of Nutrition and Dietetics, 114*(10), 1557–1568.

Katzmarzyk, P. T., Gagnon, J., Leon, A. S., Sinner, J. S., Wilmore, J. H., Rao, D. C., & Bouchard, C. (2001). Fitness, fatness, and estimated coronary heart disease risk: the HERITAGE Family Study. *Medicine and Science in Sports and Exercise, 33*(4), 585–590.

Kim, J. H., Malhotra, R., Chiampas, G., d'Hemecourt, P., Troyanos, C., Cianca, J., Race, & Associated Cardiac Arrest Event Registry (RACER) Study Group. (2012). Cardiac arrest during long-distance running races. *New England Journal of Medicine, 366*(2), 130–140.

Klok, M. D., Jakobsdottir, S., & Drent, M. L. (2007), The role of leptin and ghrelin in the regulation of food intake and body weight in humans: a review. *Obesity Reviews, 8*(1), 21–34.

Kokkinos, P., Myers, J. (2010). Exercise and physical activity. *Circulation, 122,* 1637–1648.

Kravitz, L. (2014). High-intensity interval training. *American College of Sports Medicine.* Retrieved from https://www.acsm.org/docs/brochures/high-intensity-interval-training.pdf

Laddu, D. R., Rana, J. S., Munilo, R., Sorel, M. E., Quesenberry, C. P., & Allen, N. B. (2017). 25-year physical activity trajectories and development of subclinical coronary artery disease as measured by coronary artery calcium: the Coronary Artery Risk Development in Young Adults (CARDIA) study. *Mayo Clinical Proceedings, 92*(11), 1660–1670.

Larson-Myer, D. E., Palm, S., Bansal, A., Austin, K. J., Hart, A. M., & Alexander, B. M. (2012). Influence of running and walking on hormonal regulators of appetite in women. *Journal of Obesity, 2012,* 730409.

Laskowski, E. D. (2017, Feb. 9). Is it ok to exercise if I have a cold? *Mayo Clinic.* Retrieved from http://www.mayoclinic.org/healthy-lifestyle/fitness/expert-answers/exercise/faq-20058494

Lassale, C., Tzoulaki, I., Moons, K. G. M., Sweeting, M., Boer, J., Johnson, L., ... Butterworth, A. S. (2017). Separate and combined associations of obesity and metabolic health with coronary artery disease: a pan-European case-cohort analysis. *European Heart Journal, 39*(5), 397–406.

Lavelle, J. (2015, Oct. 8). New brain effects behind "runner's high." *Scientific American.* Retrieved from https://www.scientificamerican.com/article/new-brain-effects-behind-runner-s-high/

Lawson, E. C., Han, M. K., Sellers, J. T., Chrenek, M. A., Hanif, A., Gogniat, M. A., ... Pardue, M. T. (2014). Aerobic exercise protects retinal function and structure from light-induced retinal degradation. *Journal of Neuroscience, 34*(7), 2406–2412.

Lee, D.-C., Brellenthin, A. G., Thompson, P. D., Sui, X., Lee, I.-M., & Lavie, C. J. (2017). Running as a key lifestyle medicine for longevity. *Progress in Cardiovascular Diseases, 60*(1), 45–55.

Lee, I.-M., & Shiroma, E. J. (2014). Using accelerometers to measure physical activity in large-scale epidemiological studies: issues and challenges. *British Journal of Sports Medicine, 448*, 197–201.

Lee, J.-K., Luchian, T., & Park, Y. (2015). Effect of regular exercise on inflammation induced by drug-resistant *Staphylococcus aureus* 3089 in ICR mice. *Scientific Reports, 5*, 16364.

Lee, R. (2015, Jan.). Ask the doctor: does a beta blocker interfere with exercise? *Harvard Health Publications, Harvard Medical School.* Retrieved from https://www.health.harvard.edu/drugs-and-medications/does-a-beta-blocker-interfere-with-exercise

Lucas, R. (2016). Is exercise an effective therapy for menopause and hot flashes? *Menopause, 23*(7), 701–703.

Lynch, W. K. J., Piehl, K. B., Acosta, G., Peterson, A. B., & Hemby, S. E. (2010). Aerobic exercise attenuates reinstatement of cocaine-seeking behavior and associated neu-roadaptions in the prefrontal cortex. *Biological Psychiatry, 68*(8), 774–777.

Maldonado-Martin, S., Camara, J., James, D. V. B., Fernandez-Lopez, J. R., & Artetxe-Gezuraga, X. (2017). Effects of long-term training cessation in young top-level road cyclists. *Journal of Sports Sciences, 35*(14), 1396–1401.

Maron, D. F. (2015, Aug. 11). Can you lose weight with exercise alone? *Scientific American.* Retrieved from https://www.scientificamerican.com/article/can-you-lose-weight-with-exercise-alone1/

Mayo Clinic Staff. (2016, Jun. 9). Pregnancy and exercise: baby, let's move! *Mayo Clinic.* Retrieved from http://www.mayoclinic.org/healthy-lifestyle/pregnancy-week-by-week/in-depth/art-20046896?pg=1

Mayo Clinic Staff. (2017, Mar. 14). How fit are you? See how you measure up. *Mayo Clinic.* Retrieved from http://www.mayoclinic.org/healthy-lifestyle/fitness/in-depth/fitness/art-20046433

Mayo Clinic Staff. (2017, May 19). Exercise intensity: how to measure it. *Mayo Clinic.* Retrieved from https://www.mayoclinic.org/healthy-lifestyle/fitness/in-depth/exercise-intensity/art-20046887?pg=1

Mayo Clinic Staff. (2017, Aug. 8). Muscle cramps: symptoms and causes. *Mayo Clinic.* Retrieved from http://www.mayoclinic.org/diseases-conditions/muscle-cramp/symptoms-causes/dxc-20186052

McMaster, D. T., Gill, N., Cronin, J., & McGuigan, M. (2013). The development, reten-tion and decay rates of strength and power in elite rugby union, rugby league and American football: a systematic review. *Sports Medicine, 43*(5), 367–384.

McPhate, Mike. (2016, May 25). Just how accurate are Fitbits? The jury is out. *New York Times.* Retrieved from https://www.nytimes.com/2016/05/26/technology/per-sonaltech/fitbit-accuracy.html

Meeusen, R., Roelands, B., & Spriet, L. L. (2013). Caffeine, exercise and the brain. *Nestle Nutrition Institute Workshop Series, 76*, 1–12. Retrieved from https://doi.org/10.1159/000350223

Mekary, R. A., Grontved, A., Despres, J. P., De Moura, L. P., Asgarzadeh, M., & Willett, W. C. (2015). Weight training, aerobic physical activities, and long-term waist cir-cumference change in men. *Obesity (Silver Spring), 23*(2), 461–467.

Miller, A. M. (2017, July 7), Does exercise make you hungry or suppress your appetite? *US News.*

Mora-Rodriguez, R., Ortega, J. F., Hamouti, N., Fernandez-Elias, V. E., Garcia-Prieto, J. C., & Guadalupe-Grau, A. (2014). Time-course effects of aerobic interval training and detraining in patients with metabolic syndrome. *Nutrition, Metabolism and Cardiovascular Disease, 24*(7), 792–798.

Mujika, I., & Padilla, S. (2000), Detraining: loss of training-induced physiological and performance adaptations, part I. *Sports Medicine, 30*(2), 79–87.

Mujika, I., & Padilla, S. (2001). Cardiorespiratory and metabolic characteristics of detraining in humans. *Medicine and Science in Sports and Exercise, 33*(3), 413–421.

Myllymäki, T., Kyröläinen, H., Savolainen, K., Hokka, L., Jakonen, R., Juuti, T., . . . Rusko, H. (2011). Effects of vigorous late-night exercise on sleep quality and cardiac autonomic activity. *Journal of Sleep Research, 20*(1 Pt 2), 146–153.

National Sleep Foundation. (2017). How does exercise help those with chronic insomnia? Retrieved from https://sleepfoundation.org/ask-the-expert/how-does-exercise-help-those-chronic-insomnia

Needleman, I., Ashley, P., Petrie, A., Fortune, F., Turner, W., & Jones, J. (2013). Oral health and impact on performance of athletes participating in the London 2012 Olympic Games: a cross sectional study. *British Journal of Sports Medicine, 47*(16), 1054–1058.

Neighmond, P. (2010, July 5). Can you be fat and fit? More health experts say yes. *NPR, Morning Edition.* Retrieved from https://www.npr.org/templates/story/story.php?storyId=128267723

Nelson, M. B., Kaminsky, L. A., Dickin, D. C., & Montove, A. H. (2016). Validity of consumer-based physical activity monitors for specific activity types. *Medicine and Science in Sports and Exercise, 48*(8), 1619–1628.

Nichols, A. W. (1992), Exercise-induced anaphylaxis and urticarial. *Clinics in Sports Medicine, 11*(2), 303–312.

Nordqvist, C. (2017, Dec. 1). Causes and treatment for leg cramps. *Medical News Today.* Retrieved from https://www.medicalnewstoday.com/articles/180160.php

North American Menopause Society. (2013, July 31). Exercise is good for you, but it won't cut hot flashes. [Press release]. *Eureka Alert.* Retrieved from https://www.eurekalert.org/pub_releases/2013-07/tnam-eig073013.php

O'Connor, P. J., Poudevigne, M. S., Cress, M. E., Motl, R. W., & Clapp, J. F. III (2011). Safety and efficacy of supervised strength training adopted in pregnancy. *Journal of Physical Activity and Health, 8*(3), 309–320.

O'Hagan, F. T., Sale, D. G., MacDougall, J. D., & Garner, S. H. (1995), Response to resistance training in young women and men. *International Journal of Sports Medicine, 16*(5), 314–321.

O'Hare, R. (2017, Aug. 15). "Fat but fit" are at increased risk of heart disease. *Imperial College London, Science Daily.* Retrieved from https://www.sciencedaily.com/releases/2017/08/170815095202.htm

O'Keefe, J. H., Patil, H. R., Lavie, C. J., Magalski, A., Vogel, R. A., & McCullough, P. A. (2012). Potential adverse cardiovascular effects from excessive endurance exercise. *Mayo Clinic Proceedings, 87*(6), 587–595.

Ogasawara, R., Yasuda, T., Naokata, I., & Abe, T. (2013). Comparison of muscle hypertrophy following 6 months of continuous and periodic strength training. *European Journal of Applied Physiology, 113*(4), 975–985.

Ogasawara, R., Yasuda, T., Sakamaki, M., Ozaki, H., & Abe, T. (2011). Effects of periodic and continued resistance training on muscle CSA and strength in previously untrained men. *Clinical Physiology and Functional Imaging, 31*(5), 399–404.

Olson, D., Sikka, R. S., Hayman, J., Novak, M., & Stavig, C. (2009). Exercise in pregnancy. *Current Sports Medicine Reports, 8*(3), 147–153.

Paffenbarger, R. S. Jr., Hyde, R. T., Wing, A. L., & Hsieh, C. C. (1986). Physical activity, all-cause mortality, and longevity of college alumni. *New England Journal of Medicine, 314*(10), 605–613.

Paulsen, G., Hamarsland, H., Cumming, K. T., Johansen, R. E., Hulmi, J. J., Borsheim, E., ... Raastad, T. (2014). Vitamin C and E supplementation alters protein signaling after a strength training session, but not muscle growth during 10 weeks of training. *Journal of Physiology, 592*(24), 5391–5408.

Pedersen, B. K., & Saltin, B. (2006). Evidence for prescribing exercise as therapy in chronic disease. *Scandinavian Journal of Medicine & Science in Sports, 16*(Suppl 1), 3–63.

Perrault, K., Bauman, A., Johnson, N., Britton, A., Rangul, V., & Stamatakis, E. (2017). Does physical activity moderate the association between alcohol drinking and all-cause, cancer and cardiovascular mortality? A pooled analysis of eight British population cohorts. *British Journal of Sports Medicine, 51*(8), 651–657.

Perry, E. (2011, Apr. 3). Target fat loss: myth or reality? *Yale Scientific.* Retrieved from http://www.yalescientific.org/2011/04/targeted-fat-loss-myth-or-reality/

Peter Magnusson, S., Hansen, M., Langberg, H., Miller, B., Haraldsson, B., Kjoeller Westh, E., ... Kjær, M. (2007). The adaptability of tendon to loading differs in men and women. *International Journal of Experimental Pathology, 88*(4), 237–240.

Place, N., Ivarsson, N., Venckunas, T., Neyroud, D., Brazaitis, M., Cheng, A. J., ... Westerblad, H. (2015). Ryanodine receptor fragmentation and sarcoplasmic reticulum Ca2+ leak after one session of high-intensity interval exercise. *Proceedings of the National Academy of Sciences of the United States of America, 112*(50), 15492–15497.

Predel, H.-G. (2014). Marathon run: cardiovascular adaptation and cardiovascular risk. *European Heart Journal, 35*(44), 3091–3098.

Rabin, R. C. (2017, Oct. 26). "Fat but fit?" The controversy continues. *New York Times.* Retrieved from https://www.nytimes.com/2017/10/26/well/eat/fat-but-fit-the-controversy-continues.html

Ramirez-Campillo, R., Andrade, D. C., Campos-Jara, C., Henriques-Olguin, C., & Izquierdo, M. (2013). Regional fat changes induced by localized muscle endurance resistance training. *Journal of Strength and Conditioning Research, 27*(8), 2219–2224.

Ready, A. E., & Quinney, H. A. (1982). Alterations in anaerobic threshold as the result of endurance training and detraining. *Medicine and Science in Sports and Exercise, 14*(4), 292–296.

Reference Health. (n.d.). How many steps burn 1000 calories? Retrieved from https://www.reference.com/health/many-steps-burn-1000-calories-cb780cf847073dbd#

Reid, K. J., Baron, K. G., Lu, B., Naylor, E., Wolfe, L., & Zee, P. C. (2010). Aerobic exercise improves self-reported sleep and quality of life in older adults with insomnia. *Sleep Medicine Research, 11*(9), 934–940.

Reilly, T. (1990). Human circadian rhythms and exercise. *Critical Reviews in Biomedical Engineering 18*(3), 165–180.

Reynolds, G. (2012, Dec. 12). Why afternoon may be the best time to exercise. *New York Times.* Retrieved from https://well.blogs.nytimes.com/2012/12/12/why-afternoon-may-be-the-best-time-to-exercise/

Reynolds, G. (2013). How exercise can help us eat less. Retrieved from https://well.blogs.nytimes.com/2013/09/11/how-exercise-can-help-us-eat-less/

Reynolds, G. (2013, Aug. 21). How exercise can help us sleep better. *Phys Ed, New York Times.* Retrieved from https://well.blogs.nytimes.com/2013/08/21/how-exercise-can-help-us-sleep-better/

Reynolds, G. (2014, Mar. 26). Exercising for healthier eyes. *Well, New York Times*. Retrieved from https://well.blogs.nytimes.com/2014/03/26/exercising-for-eye-health

Reynolds, G. (2014, Apr. 16). Younger skin through exercise. *Well, New York Times*. Retrieved from https://well.blogs.nytimes.com/2014/04/16/younger-skin-through-exercise/

Reynolds, G. (2014, June 25). For fitness, push yourself. *Well, New York Times*. Retrieved from https://well.blogs.nytimes.com/2014/06/25/for-fitness-push-yourself/

Reynolds, G. (2014, Sept. 24). Is exercise bad for your teeth? *Well, New York Times*. Retrieved from https://well.blogs.nytimes.com/2014/09/24/is-exercise-bad-for-your-teeth/

Reynolds, G. (2014, Oct. 15). What's your fitness age? *Well, New York Times*. Retrieved from https://well.blogs.nytimes.com/2014/10/15/whats-your-fitness-age/

Reynolds, G. (2014, Nov. 26). Why antioxidants don't belong in your workout. *Well, New York Times*. Retrieved from https://well.blogs.nytimes.com/2014/11/26/why-antioxidants-dont-belong-in-your-workout/

Reynolds, G. (2015, Apr. 8). Mothers' exercise may lower heart risks in newborns. *Phys Ed, New York Times*. Retrieved from https://well.blogs.nytimes.com/2015/04/08/exercise-may-lower-heart-risks-in-newborns-study-suggests/

Reynolds, G. (2015, May 20). Lack of exercise can disrupt the body's rhythms. *Phys Ed, New York Times*.

Reynolds, G. (2015, Dec. 16). How exercise may help us fight off colds. *Well, New York Times*. Retrieved from https://well.blogs.nytimes.com/2015/12/16/how-exercise-may-help-us-fight-off-colds/

Reynolds, G. (2016, Apr. 27). 1 minute of all out exercise may equal 45 minutes of moderate exertion. *Well, New York Times*. Retrieved from https://well.blogs.nytimes.com/2016/04/27/1-minute-of-all-out-exercise-may-equal-45-minutes-of-moderate-exertion

Reynolds, G. (2016, Aug. 3). Exercise may ease hot flashes, provided it's vigorous. *Well, New York Times*. Retrieved from https://well.blogs.nytimes.com/2016/08/03/exercise-may-ease-hot-flashes-provided-its-vigorous/

Reynolds, G. (2016, Oct. 12). How exercise may turn white fat into brown. *New York Times*. Retrieved from https://www.nytimes.com/2016/10/12/well/move/how-exercise-may-fight-obesity-by-turning-white-fat-into-brown.html

Reynolds, G. (2017, Apr. 12). An hour of running may add 7 hours to your life. *New York Times*. Retrieved from https://www.nytimes.com/2017/04/12/well/move/an-hour-of-running-may-add-seven-hours-to-your-life.html

Reynolds, G. (2017, Aug. 9). Exercise as a weight loss strategy. *Well, New York Times*. Retrieved from https://www.nytimes.com/2017/08/09/well/eat/exercise-as-a-weight-loss-strategy.html?rref=health

Reynolds, G. (2017, Dec. 6). How exercise can make for healthier fat. *New York Times*. Retrieved from https://www.google.com/search?source=hp&ei=BmXPXIezGZGc_Qag97iwBA&q=How+exercise+can+make+for+healthier+fat&btnK=Google+Search&oq=How+exercise+can+make+for+healthier+fat&gs_l=psy-ab.3..0i22i30l2.3300.3300..6128...1.0..0.92.173.2......0....2j1..gws-wiz.....6..35i39._utw3Y4oi9U

Rim, T. H., Kim, H. K., Kim, J. W., Lee, J. S., Kim, D. W., & Kim, S. S. (2018). A nationwide cohort study on the association between past physical activity and neovascular age-related macular degeneration in an East Asian population. *JAMA Ophthalmology, 136*(2), 132–139.

Ristow, M., Zarse, K., Oberbach, A., Klöting, N., Birringer, M., Kiehntopf, M., . . . Blüher, M. (2009). Antioxidants prevent health-promoting effects of physical exercise in humans. *Proceedings of the National Academy of Sciences of the United States of America, 106*(21), 8665–8670.

Ross, R., Blair, S. N., Arena, R., Church, T. S., Després, J.-P., Franklin, B. A., ... Stroke Council. (2016). Importance of assessing cardiorespiratory fitness in clinical practice: a case for fitness as a clinical vital sign: a scientific statement from the American Heart Association. *Circulation, 134*(24), e653–e699.

Safdar, A., Bourgeois, J. M., Ogborn, D. I., Little, J. P., Hettinga, B. P., Akhtar, M., ... Tarnopolsky, M. A. (2011). Endurance exercise rescues progeroid aging and induces systemic mitochondrial rejuvenation in mtDNA mutator mice. *Proceedings of the National Academy of Sciences of the United States of America, 108*(10), 4135–4140.

Scherbina, A., Mattsson, C. M., Waggott, D., Salisbury, H., Christle, J. W., Hastie, T., ... Ashley, E. A. (2017). Accuracy in wrist-worn, sensor-based measurements of heart rate and energy expenditure in a diverse cohort. *Journal of Personalized Medicine, 7*(2).

Schroeder, A. M., Truong, D., Loh, D. H., Jordan, M. C., Roos, K. P., & Colwell, C. S. (2012). Voluntary scheduled exercise alters diurnal rhythms of behaviour, physiology and gene expression in wild-type and vasoactive intestinal peptide-deficient mice. *Journal of Physiology, 590*(Pt 23), 6213–6226.

Schulkey, C. E., Regmi, S. D., Magnan, R. A., Danzo, M. T., Luther, H., Hutchinson, A. K., ... Jay, P. Y. (2015). The maternal-age-associated risk of congenital heart disease is modifiable [letter]. *Nature, 520,* 230–233.

Schwingshackl, L., Dias, S., & Hoffman, G. (2014). Impact of long-term lifestyle programmes on weight loss and cardiovascular risk factors in overweight/obese participants: a systematic review and meta-analysis. *Systematic Reviews, 3,* 130.

Scientific American. (n.d.) Food matters. Antioxidant supplements: too much of a kinda good thing. Retrieved from https://blogs.scientificamerican.com/food-matters/antioxidant-supplements-too-much-of-a-kinda-good-thing/

Selin, Z., Orsini, N., Ejdervik Lindblad, B., & Wolk, A. (2015). Long-term physical activity and risk of age-related cataract: a population-based prospective study of male and female cohorts. *Ophthalmalogy, 122*(2), 274–280.

Shiota, M., Sudou, M., & Ohshima, M. (1996). Using outdoor exercise to decrease jet lag in airline crewmembers. *Aviation, Space, and Environmental Medicine, 67*(12), 1155–1160.

Should you exercise when you are sick? (2017, Jan. 26). *Scripps Health.* Retrieved from https://www.scripps.org/news_items/4360-should-you-exercise-when-you-re-sick

Sim, A. Y., Wallman, K. E., Fairchild, T. J., & Guelfi, K. J. (2014), High-intensity intermittent exercise attenuates ad-libitum energy intake. *International Journal of Obesity (London), 38*(3), 417–422.

Skarmulis, L. (n.d.). What's the best time to exercise? *WebMD.* Retrieved from https://www.webmd.com/fitness-exercise/features/whats-the-best-time-to-exercise#1

Spriet, L. L. (2014). Exercise and sport performance with low doses of caffeine. *Sports Medicine, 44*(Suppl 2), 175–184.

Storrs, C. (2016, Jan. 27). Exercise during menopause could reduce hot flashes, study says. *CNN Health.* Retrieved from http://www.cnn.com/2016/01/27/health/menopause-hot-flashes-exercise/index.html

Sui, X., LaMonte, M. J., & Laditka, J. N. (2007). Cardiorespiratory fitness and adiposity as mortality predictors in older adults. *Journal of the American Medical Association, 298*(21), 2507–2516.

Sussman, S., Lisha, N., & Griffiths, M. (2011). Prevalence of the addictions: a problem of the majority or the minority. *Evaluation and the Health Professions, 34,* 3–56.

Thivel, D., Isacco, L., Montaurier, C., Boirie, Y., Duche, P., & Morio, B. (2012), The 24-h energy intake of obese adolescents is spontaneously reduced after intensive exercise: a randomized controlled trial in calorimetric chambers. *PLoS ONE, 7*(1), e29840.

Thomas, D. M., Bouchard, C., Church, T., Slentz, C., Kraus, W. E., Redman, L. M., . . . Heymsfield, S. B. (2012). Why do individuals not lose more weight from an exercise intervention at a defined dose? An energy balance analysis. *Obesity Reviews, 13*(10), 835–847.

Tobias, D. K., Zhang, C., van Dam, R. M., Bowers, K., & Hu, F.B. (2011). Physical activity before and during pregnancy and risk of gestational diabetes mellitus: a meta-analysis. *Diabetes Care, 34*(1), l223–1229.

Troiano, R. P., McClain, J. J., Brychta, R. J., & Chen, K. Y. (2014). Evolution of accelerometer methods for physical activity research. *British Journal of Sports Medicine, 48,* 1019–1023.

Tzur, A. (2017, Apr. 13). The science of detraining: how long you can take a break from the gym before you lose muscle mass, strength, and endurance. *Sci-Fit: The Science of Fitness.* Retrieved from http://sci-fit.net/2017/detraining-retraining/

Van Pelt, D. W., Guth, L. M., & Horowitz, J. F. (1985). Aerobic exercise elevates markers of angiogenesis and macrophage IL-6 gene expression in the subcutaneous adipose tissue of overweight-to-obese adults. *Journal of Applied Physiology, 123*(5), 1150–1159.

Villaneuva, C., & Kross, R. D. (2012), Antioxidant-induced stress. *International Journal of Molecular Science, 13*(2), 2091–2109.

Villareal, D. T., Chode, S., Parimi, N., Sinacore, D. R., Hilton, T., Armamento-Villarreal, R., . . . Shah, K. (2011). Weight loss, exercise, or both and physical function in obese older adults. *New England Journal of Medicine, 364*(13), 1218–1229.

Vina, J., Sanchis-Gomar, F., Martinez-Bello, V., & Gomez-Cabrera, M. (2012). Exercise acts as a drug; the pharmacological benefits of exercise. *British Journal of Pharmacology, 167*(1), 1–12.

Walts, C. T., Hanson, E. D., Delmonico, M. J., Yao, L., Wang, M. Q., & Hurley, B. F. (2008). Do sex or race differences influence strength training effects on muscle or fat? *Medicine and Science in Sports and Exercise, 40*(4), 669–676.

Wasserman, K. (1986), The anaerobic threshold: definition, physiological significance and identification. *Advances in Cardiology, 35,* 1–23.

Wessel, L. (2016, Aug. 18). Is there such a thing that as "fat and fit"? *Scientific American, STAT.* Retrieved from https://www.scientificamerican.com/article/is-there-such-a-thing-as-fat-but-fit/

What causes leg cramps? (2002, May 28). *Scientific American.* Retrieved from https://www.scientificamerican.com/article/what-causes-leg-cramps/

White, C. (2017, May 31). Should men and women train differently? *ABC Health and Well Being, Australia.* Retrieved from http://www.abc.net.au/news/health/2017-06-01/should-men-and-women-train-differently/8568396

Wilhelm, M. (2014). Atrial fibrillation in endurance athletes. *European Journal of Preventive Cardiology, 21*(8), 1040–1048.

Wilkerson, Rick. (2017, June). Muscle cramps. *OrthoInfo, American Academy of Orthopaedic Surgeons.* Retrieved from http://orthoinfo.aaos.org/topic.cfm?topic=a00200

Williams, P. T. (2009). Prospective study of incident age-related macular degeneration in relation to vigorous physical activity during a 7-year follow up. *Investigative Ophthalmology and Visual Science, 50*(1), 101–106.

Williams, P. T. (2013). Walking and running are associated with similar reductions in cataract risk. *Medicine and Science in Sports and Exercise, 45*(6), 1089–1096.

Wolff, G., & Esser, K. A. (2012). Scheduled exercise phase shifts the circadian clock in skeletal muscle. *Medicine and Science in Sports and Exercise, 44*(9), 1663–1670.

World Fitness Level. (n.d.). How fit are you, really? Retrieved from https://www.worldfitnesslevel.org/#/

Zhang, Y., Xie, C., Wang, H., Foss, R. M., Clare, M., George, E. V., . . . Yang, L. J. (2016). Irisin exerts dual effects on browning and adipogenesis of human white adipocytes. *American Journal of Physiology, Endocrinology and Metabolism, 311*(2), E530–535.

CHAPTER 16

Arias, E. (2015). United States life table. *National Vital Statistics Reports, 64*(11). Retrieved from http://www.cdc.gov/nchs/products/nvsr.html

Centers for Disease Control and Prevention. (2010). *10 leading causes of death and injury, United States* [data set]. Retrieved from http://www.cdc.gov/injury/wisqars/leadingcauses.html

Fraser, G. E. (2003). *Diet, life expectancy, and chronic disease: studies of Seventh-Day Adventists and other vegetarians.* Oxford, UK; New York, NY: Oxford University Press.

Heron, M. (2016). Deaths: leading causes for 2013. *National Vital Statistics Reports, 65*(2), 1. Retrieved from http://www.cdc.gov/nchs/data/nvsr/nvsr65/nvsr65_02.pdf

Kincel, B. (2014). The centenarian population: 2007–2011. *American Community Survey Briefs.* Retrieved from https://www.census.gov/prod/2014pubs/acsbr12-18.pdf.

Kochanek, K. D., Murphy, S. L., Xu, J. Q., & Arias, E. (2017) *Mortality in the United States,* NCHS Data Brief No. 293. Hyattsville, MD: National Center for Health Statistics.

National Institute of Aging. (2011). *Global health and aging.* Retrieved from https://www.nia.nih.gov/research/publication/global-health-and-aging/living-longer

Sun, F., Sebastiani, P., Schupf, N., Bae, H., Andersen, S. L., McIntosh, A., . . . Perls, T. T. (2015). Extended maternal age at birth of last child and women's longevity in the Long Life Family Study. *Menopause, 22*(1), 26–31.

Xu, J., Murphy, L. S., Kochanek, K. D., & Bastian B. A. (2016). Deaths: final data for 2013. *National Vital Statistics Reports, 65.*

INDEX